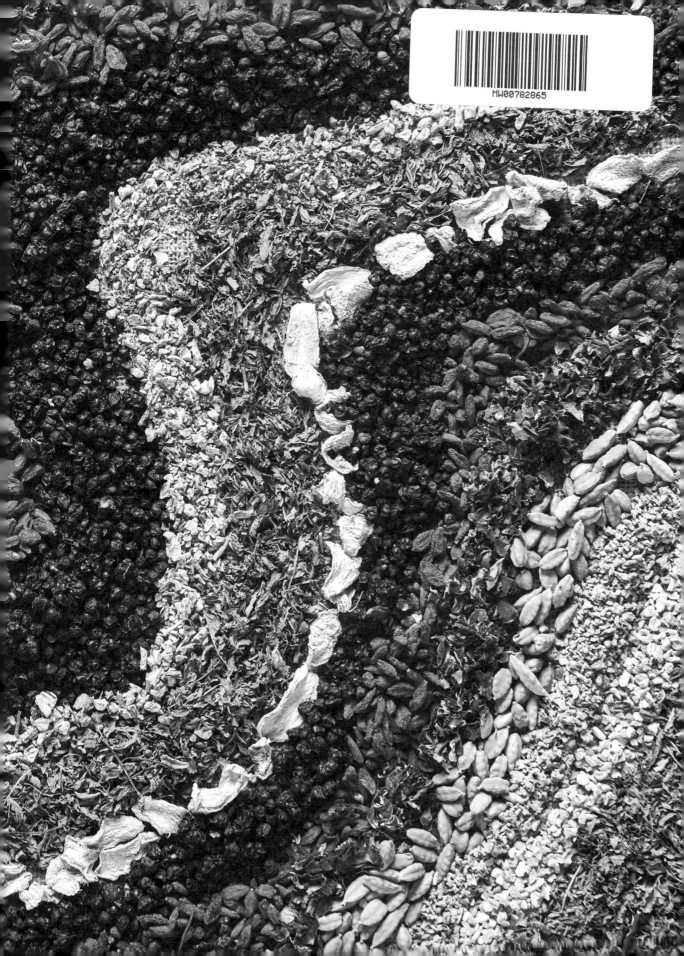

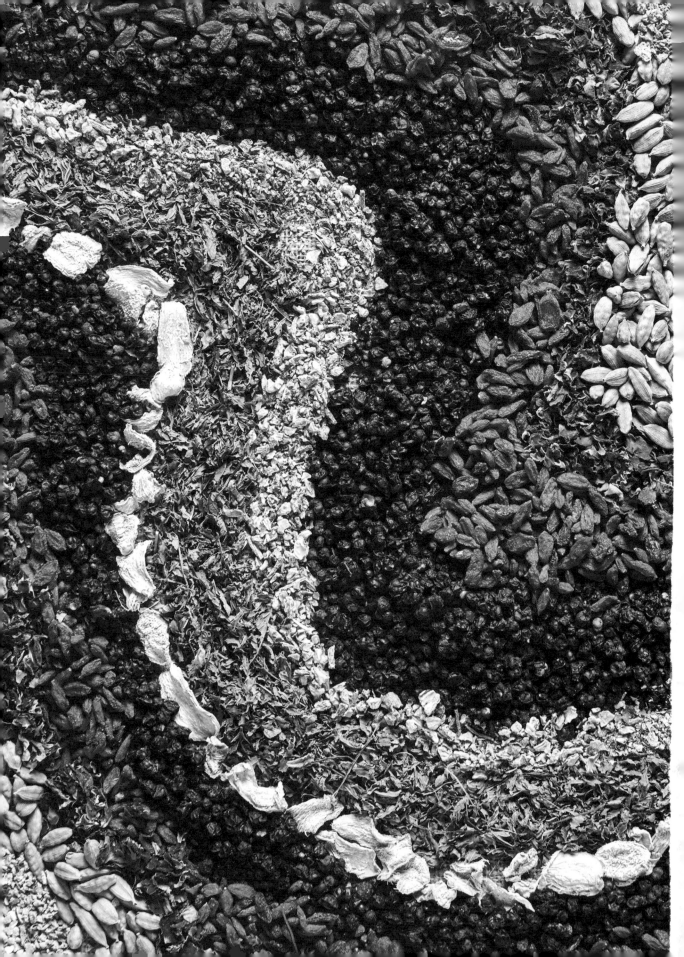

The
PLANT
MEDICINE
PROTOCOL

The
PLANT
MEDICINE
PROTOCOL

Unlocking the Power of
Plants for Optimal Health
and Longevity

WILLIAM SIFF, LAc

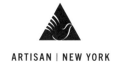

ARTISAN | NEW YORK

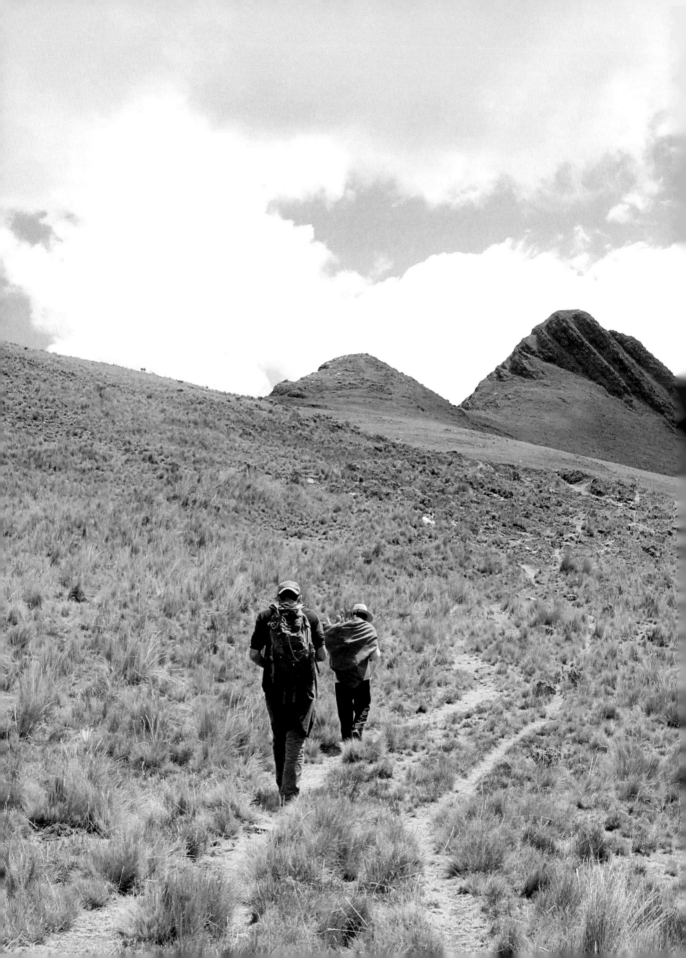

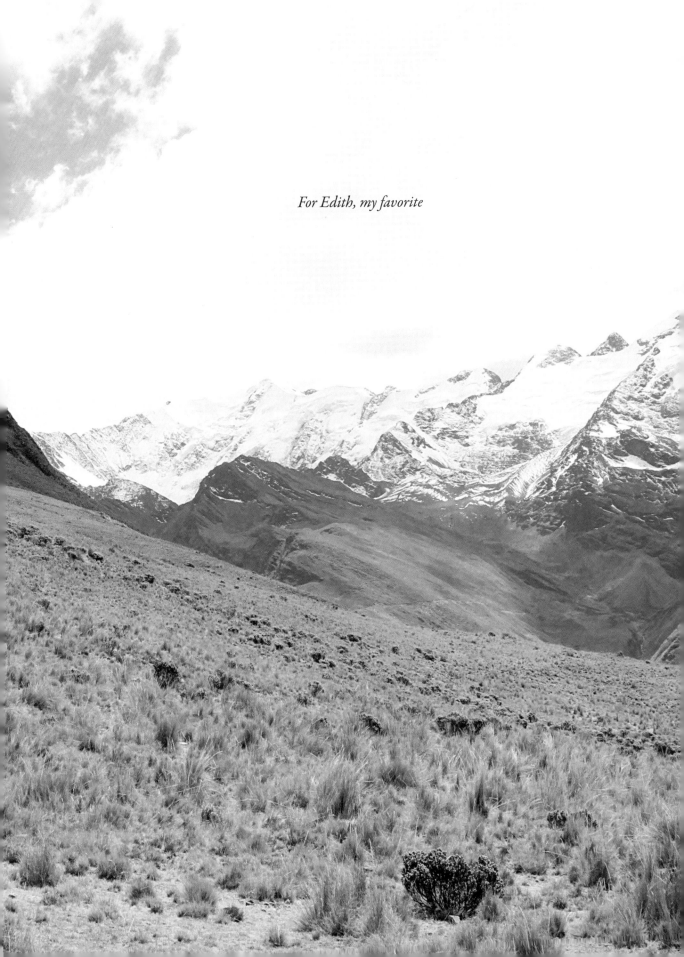

For Edith, my favorite

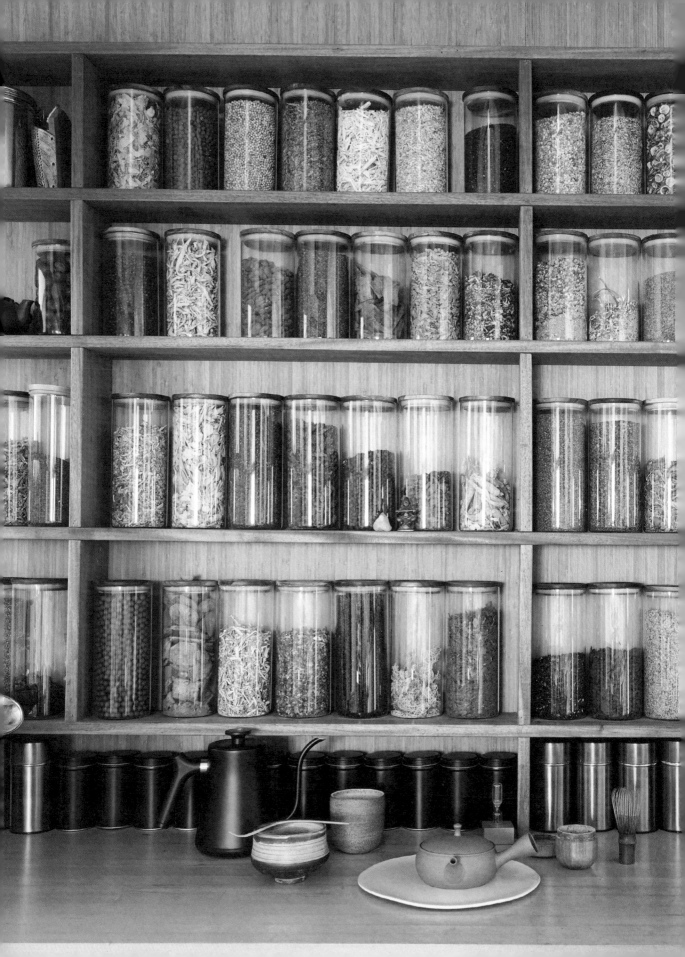

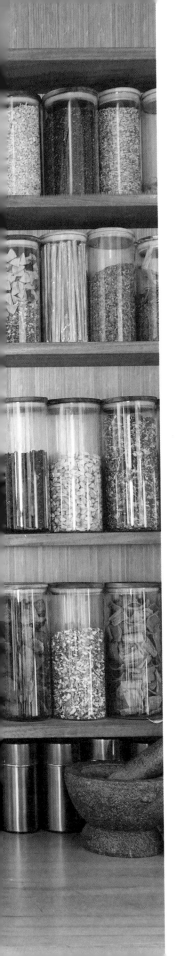

Contents

Preface   8

Introduction   16

PART I: NATURAL MEDICINE FUNDAMENTALS   24

Principles of Natural Medicine   27

Our Essential Body Systems   37

Medicinal Plant Categories   59

PART II: THE PLANT MEDICINE PROTOCOL   86

Getting Started   88

STEP 1: Culinary Herbs, Spices & Bitters   101

Japanese Green Tea: Mindfulness & Mastery   136

STEP 2: Nutritives   145

Cacao: Food of the Gods   168

STEP 3: Demulcents   175

STEP 4: Nervines   197

Kava: Get Happy   226

STEP 5: Adaptogens   235

Protocol FAQs   257

Beginning Your New Plant-Powered Life   260

PART III: THE PLANT-POWERED HOME   266

Your Home on Plants   269

Home Apothecary   287

A Word on Kids & Medicinal Plants   296

PART IV: PLANT PROFILES   300

Resources   352

Further Reading   356

Acknowledgments   357

Notes   360

Index   374

Photography Credits   383

PREFACE

TO UNDERSTAND THE POWER OF MEDICINAL PLANTS, look no further than the black pepper that's probably sitting next to the salt on your and everyone else's dinner table right now. Anywhere there are people on this planet, you'll most likely find black pepper within arm's reach. In fact, the International Space Station probably has some pepper on hand. No other spice has been so widely used over such a long time span by so many.

Once known as black gold, black pepper comes from the Malabar Coast of southern India. A climbing vine with clusters of small green seeds, the black pepper plant (*Piper nigrum*) grows in the dappled sunlight within the understory of India's tropical forests. Just a few hundred years ago, vast fleets regularly made the perilous journey across the ocean seeking these tiny, pungent seeds. The spice was considered so essential it was equal in value to precious metals and accepted as a form of currency. Sure, pepper has an amazing flavor and aroma, but the risks people were willing to take to obtain it were also motivated by a fundamental quest for health and longevity. Their empirical understanding of black pepper's benefits has now been validated by modern science and medicine. One of its primary and most well-researched compounds, piperine, is a powerful antioxidant that enhances nutrient absorption, increases circulation to the digestive tract, quells inflammation, improves cognitive health, boosts metabolism, neutralizes pathogens, stabilizes blood sugar, boosts immunity, and increases energy levels. All of this good stuff is available to us in every little sprinkle of pepper. The shaker on your table is a superhero hiding in plain sight.

"My approach to practicing natural medicine is to make it as easy as possible to access the power of these medicinal plants in our everyday lives for optimal health."

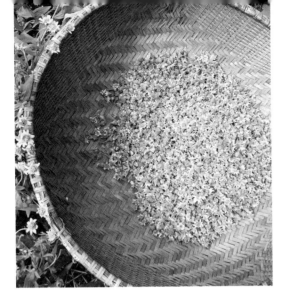
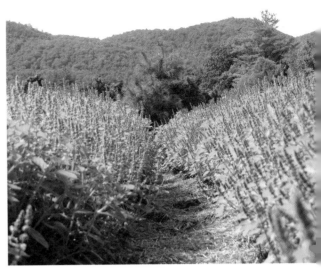
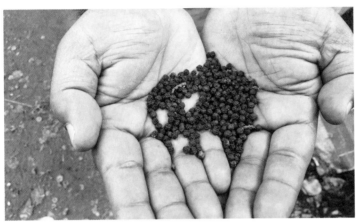

Top: Arnica flower harvest (left) and rows of tulsi plants (right) at the Goldthread farm in Massachusetts

Bottom: Harvesting black pepper in the cardamom forests of Kerala, India

As an acupuncturist and clinical herbalist, much of my work centers on commonplace medicinal plants like black pepper that have maintained their essential role in cultures throughout the world for thousands of years. My approach to practicing natural medicine is to make it as easy as possible to access the power of these medicinal plants in our everyday lives for optimal health.

I opened my first clinical practice in natural medicine with a few other acupuncturists in a town on the coast of Maine. To build the practice, I gave presentations about acupuncture, Traditional Chinese Medicine, and Ayurvedic medicine, my areas of expertise, for garden clubs and small groups at places like the local Elks lodge and the American Legion—essentially anywhere I could find an audience. This community was mostly made up of builders, lobstermen, office workers, parents, teachers, administrators—everyday people going about their lives. They weren't particularly fascinated by the philosophy or esoteric aspects of natural medicine. They just wanted to know if it works. I'd often treat people who weren't able to find the relief or results

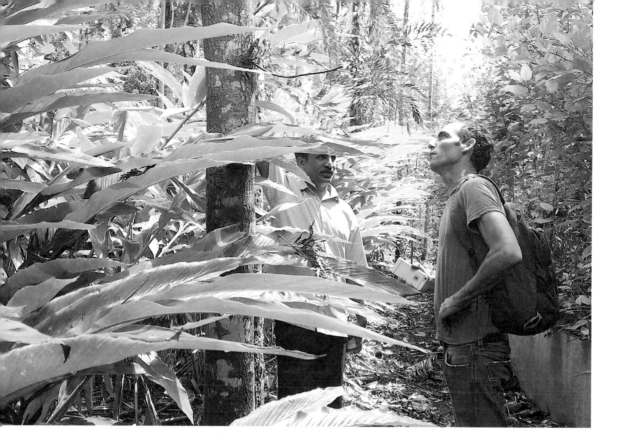

they were looking for through standard Western medicine and were giving acupuncture and herbs a shot as a last resort. My practice grew gradually through word of mouth because I was able to get results. This was an important lesson to learn at the beginning of my career: Above all else, natural medicine had to be practical and effective.

I moved to a progressive city in Massachusetts a few years later and set up a new practice inspired by the Asian models I'd encountered, where natural medicine is thoroughly integrated into everyday life and medicinal plants play a central role. The result was a combination clinical practice and herbal apothecary called Goldthread, and plants were the stars of the show. The apothecary was an aesthetically pleasing and inviting space, with eye-catching displays of medical plants and preparations. This curated collection came from around the world and included bottles of all shapes and sizes filled with roots, barks, leaves, flowers, and berries. I had tinctures, elixirs, tonics, essential oils, pastes, powders, tablets, and capsules—essentially every conceivable preparation one could think of or need. Customers and patients were naturally attracted to the medicinal plants presented this way and could easily envision them becoming part of their lives.

Goldthread offered people a place to walk in and get medicinal plants along with credible professional advice about how to use them: the preparations that would work best for them, the appropriate dosage, when to take them during the day, how long to use them, potential contraindications or considerations to keep in mind, and any dietary and lifestyle adjustments that could make the medicinal plants more effective. Sometimes I would recommend a preparation off the shelf; other times I would formulate something custom for them on the spot. If their issues were complex and multifaceted enough to require a more in-depth diagnosis and treatment plan, I would see them as a patient. Working this way gave me the unique opportunity to see thousands of people in a setting normally not available in private practice, and to focus largely on dispensing medicinal plants to help people achieve an optimal level of health.

> "The direct experience of consuming medicinal plants conveys their power and efficacy directly to the body in a way that words don't."

My goal in the clinic was to make sure each person's encounter with natural medicine extended beyond their appointment with me into their everyday life. I recommended medicinal plants and preparations that reinforced what I was doing in the clinic and that accelerated progress between visits. I formulated hundreds of preparations to facilitate this process (many of which are included in this protocol). People began to recognize the power of medicinal plants as invaluable tools not simply to treat illness but to optimize their health and developed the confidence and familiarity to use them daily. Many went on to become students in programs that I taught in the apothecary (and later at the farm), to deepen their understanding and extend the benefits of medicinal plants to their families and communities.

Around this time, I started a 5-acre (2 ha) farm in the hills outside of town with the intention to supply the apothecary and clinic with local medicinal plants. We began growing over a hundred species, distilling essential oils commercially and creating an educational program, called Farm to Pharmacy, that ran throughout the season. Students were taught the fundamentals of cultivating, harvesting, and processing medicinal plants through hands-on work, combined with the principles of Traditional Chinese Medicine and Ayurveda, and they ultimately learned how to administer the plant medicines they were growing to people in the apothecary. It was a one-of-a-kind immersive program that attracted students from around the country and the world, leading to the addition of several weeklong intensive programs to accommodate those traveling from a distance.

The Farm to Pharmacy program gave students the knowledge and skills necessary to reinvigorate a form of grassroots, plant-centered health care. The program was based on experiential learning: Being immersed in the elements, working with the medicinal plants on the farm, and consuming substantial amounts of them every day were the catalysts for a new way of living. All of the students would leave the program far healthier than when they arrived.

More than two decades of working in clinical practice, running the apothecary and farm, teaching hundreds of students, and formulating products, all while living a plant-saturated life myself, has convinced me that medicinal plants are an essential aspect of both individual and societal health. I was determined to transform Goldthread into something that could reach even more people and create widespread empowerment and proficiency in the use of medicinal plants. So I formulated a line of functional beverages, made with medicinal plants sourced through a global network of generational farmers, that would be a tangible expression of the power of medicinal plants, adapted for people living busy modern lives.

In our society, change often comes through the marketplace, and certain products create awareness and inspire curiosity in a way that can be transformative and beneficial. Things that people may not have recognized as having value suddenly become indispensable. Goldthread tonics are a way to bring the power of plants to places and people that I could never reach as just one person. The direct experience of consuming medicinal plants conveys their power and efficacy directly to the body in a way that words don't.

The mission behind my clinical practice, the Goldthread apothecary, farm, educational programs, and tonic line continues with *The Plant Medicine Protocol*. The highest goal of medicine according to Ayurveda is for individuals to achieve optimal health so that we can actualize our potential and make a positive impact on society. When you make your life better, you make the world around you better. This book represents the synthesis of a decades-long pursuit of the most practical and effective way to create a medicinal plant–powered lifestyle for everyone who wants one, and to restore plants to the foundation of health care where they belong.

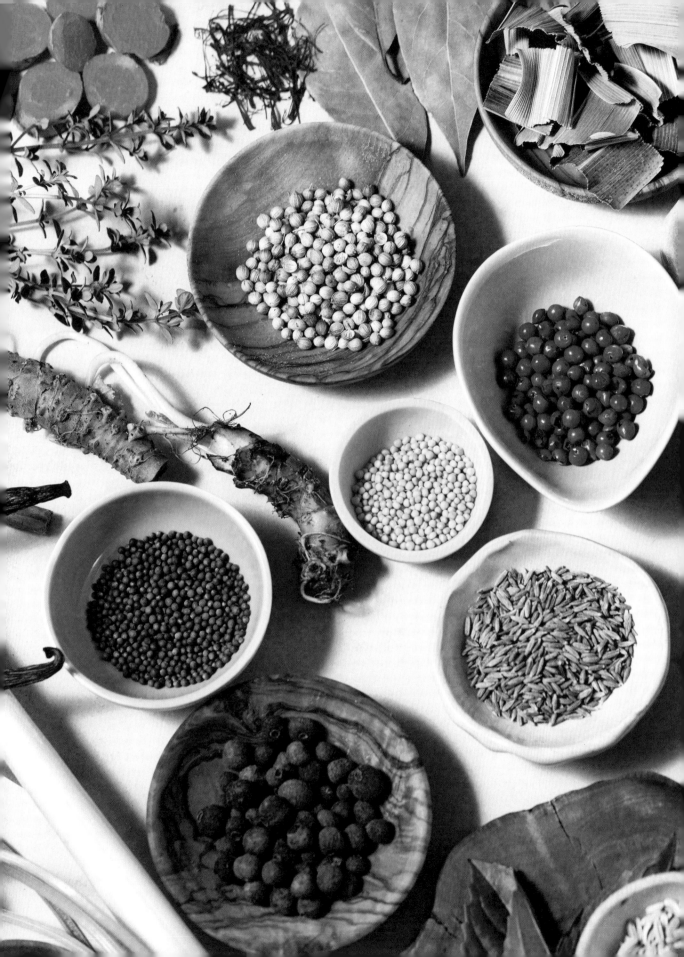

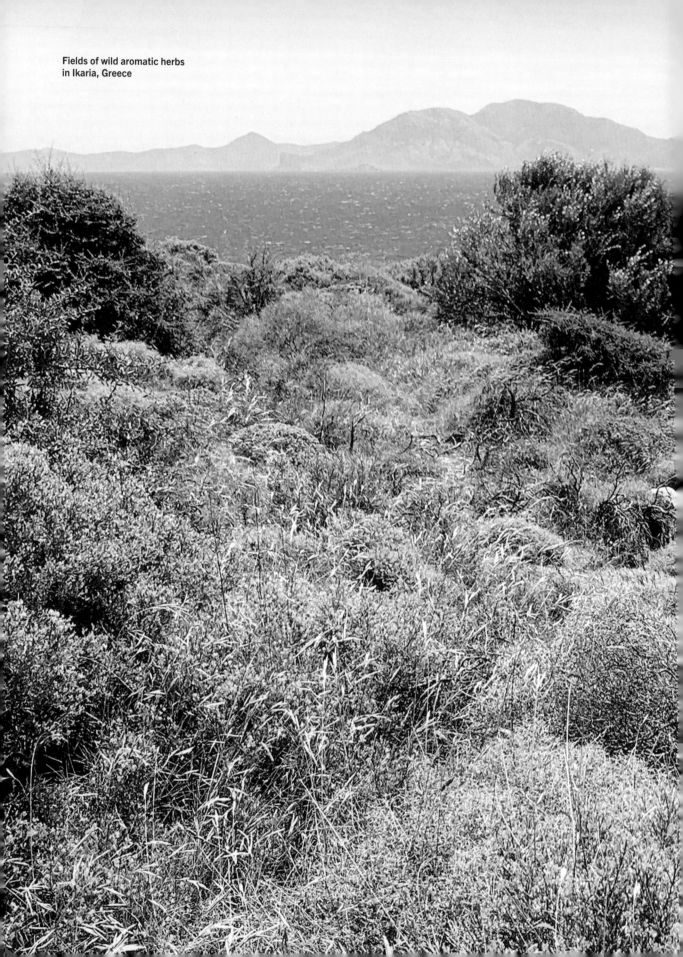

Fields of wild aromatic herbs
in Ikaria, Greece

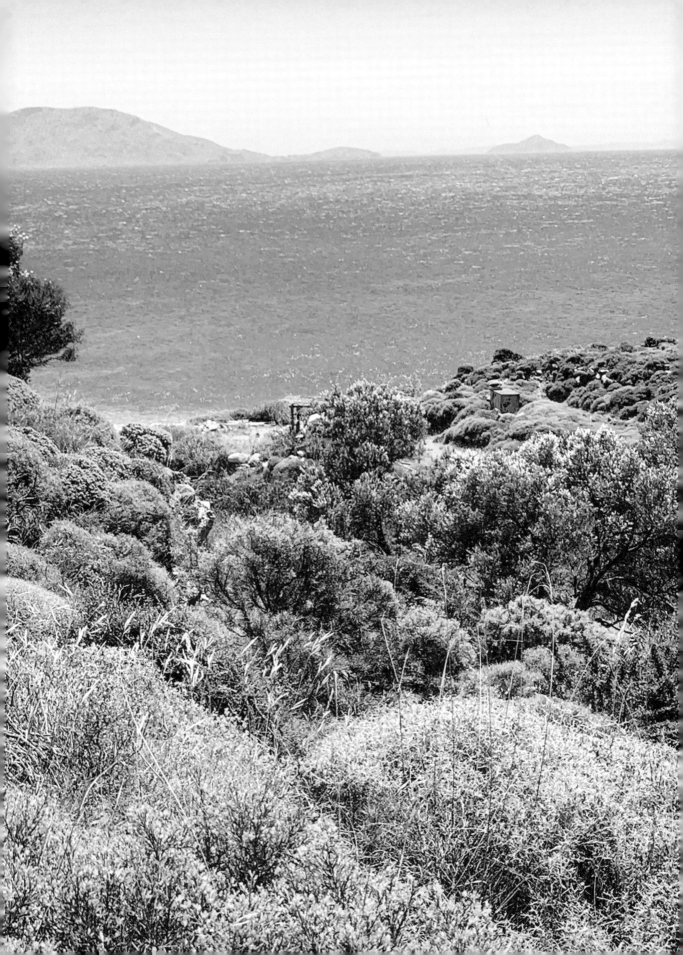

INTRODUCTION

I WOKE UP THIS MORNING AND DRANK A GLASS OF water with a fresh slice of aloe vera gel, some basil seeds, and a splash of lemon juice mixed in, to rehydrate after a long night of sleep. After changing out of my pajamas, I made a Cacao-Reishi-Cordyceps Latte (page 249), with some vanilla and a dash of cinnamon powder: a delicious elixir to kick off the day with sustainable energy and immune enhancement. I diffused a little rosemary oil into the air to bring focus and clarity to the morning and had a Ginger-Turmeric Shot (page 124) to kindle my appetite and digestive energy. For breakfast, I soaked chia seeds in cashew milk and topped them with granola, walnuts, hemp seeds and flaxseeds, and a handful of blueberries and goji berries. Afterward, I took a small swig of aromatic bitters as both a digestif and liver tonic. As I switched into work mode, I made a strong infusion of peppermint tea to relax the gut and encourage a state of flow in the nervous system. Lastly, I took a few deep inhalations of frankincense essential oil to clear the mind. By 9:00 a.m., I was well on my way to being fully saturated with powerful compounds and phytochemicals found only in medicinal plants.

My plant-powered routine continues throughout the day, incorporating a variety of other medicinal plants for improving many more essential functions—right up to the evening's calming dose of sleep-enhancing herbs. Then I wake up and start all over again. These rituals and habits are part of the natural flow of my life and are easy to maintain. I may miss one or two of these plant encounters on a given day, but by virtue of the number of opportunities I create to ingest them, I'm guaranteed to get the powerful phytonutrients I need to keep each key system of the body functioning at its best. This is what it looks like to live a medicinal plant–powered lifestyle, and this book offers a step-by-step guide for creating a personalized version in your own life.

If all of this seems overly complicated, time-consuming, expensive, or extravagant, trust me: It isn't. Over the years,

I've gotten thousands of patients, students, friends, and family members to embark on their own versions of the plant-powered lifestyle. Why? These plants represent one of the most effective, enjoyable, affordable, self-empowering, and environmentally sustainable ways to optimize health.

The Power of Medicinal Plants

We've all heard about traditional cultures around the globe where people routinely live long, healthy lives well into their eighties, nineties, and beyond with remarkably low incidence of chronic disease. Researchers studying these cultures often cite diet, regular exercise, deep social bonds, meaningful work, and living close to nature as clear factors in their longevity. There's something else they all have in common: the plentiful consumption of wild and medicinal plants. In these cultures, culinary spices and medicinal herbs are both a foundational aspect of diet and lifestyle and a means for enhancing health.

My work has brought me to visit dozens of these remarkably healthy cultures around the world, and I'm always struck by the uncommon level of vibrancy, energy, and contentment among the people who live in these places. Many of the medicinal plants and recipes presented in this book are directly attributable to the inspiring people and places I have been lucky enough to visit and the ethnobotanical wisdom they shared with me along the way.

When spending time in Greece, for example, I regularly consumed pots of mountain tea alongside meals that included wild dandelion greens; fragrant salads adorned with fresh oregano, thyme, and basil; and of course plenty of olive oil. Greek mountain tea, a daily tonic that improves digestion and immunity, is part of what keeps the eighty-year-old farmers spry enough to hike the steep mountains each day with ease and enjoyment. In India, meals overflowed with savory tropical spices, like cardamom, cinnamon, turmeric, cumin, and ginger; prized for their flavors and ability to enhance digestive power, they also provide an abundance of antioxidants that keep inflammation at bay. In Kyoto, a modern metropolis steeped in ancient culture, I sipped matcha at a teahouse that had been in continuous operation for more

> "These plants represent one of the most effective, enjoyable, affordable, self-empowering, and environmentally sustainable ways to optimize health."

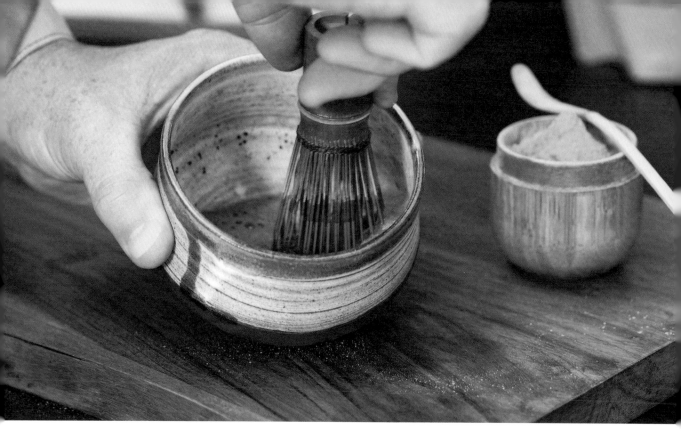

Whisking a bowl of Japanese matcha
(see page 143)

than four hundred years—one among dozens around the city treasured as places to enjoy a moment of presence and tranquility courtesy of this Japanese "elixir of longevity." While on a sourcing trip to Fiji, I participated in traditional kava ceremonies where friends gathered at night to celebrate around big wooden bowls full of this earthy root tonic, famous for promoting a sense of physical and mental ease and relaxation.

In these and many other cultures, there is little distinction between food and medicine. Ingesting medicinal plant compounds in moderate amounts every day adds up, contributing to a natural resilience and vitality that fortifies them for a long, healthy life.

Today, as people strive for more self-empowered ways to be healthy, there is a renewed interest in medicinal plants—and for good reason. Don't be put off by the word *medicinal*, either. In some ways kale and chamomile, peppermint and carrots are not so different—all provide health benefits to the body. The distinctions between them are how, when, and for what purpose you're using them. The kinds of medicinal plants I'm talking about in this book occupy their own lane as a fundamental tool for well-being. They are not technically food, but they do contain essential nutrients and often appear as delicious elements of the diet. They aren't medicine per se, defined as something used exclusively to remedy a disease, though they're full of beneficial effects that improve functionality in all our vital organs and systems. Think of them as extensions of the plants you already consume to keep you healthy and make you healthier.

We ask a lot of our bodies. Vital organs and systems accumulate wear and tear over time, requiring upkeep to extend their warranty. Medicinal plants contain a host of vital nutrients and unique phytochemicals that accelerate healing and repair while encouraging essential body systems and cellular mechanisms to function better. Enhancing digestion, calming the nervous system, increasing energy, improving sleep, promoting resilience to stress, reducing inflammation, elevating mood and cognition, increasing libido and fertility, boosting immunity, supporting detoxification, nourishing the microbiome, and rehydrating the system are among the many benefits. These are necessary prerequisites for both feeling good now and generating health in the long term.

A Plant-Powered Protocol

As a practitioner of natural medicine, I often treat advanced issues and chronic health conditions in the clinic using medicinal plants as a primary modality. I use custom-formulated herbal preparations and supplements to correct and reverse serious and intractable disease processes and bring my patients' systems back into balance. I get the best results when I also use plant protocols to address the roots of imbalance and strengthen the terrain of the body. This involves incorporating additional medicinal plants, like the ones presented in this book, into the diet and lifestyle as various tonics, elixirs, teas, powders, fresh herbs, and culinary spices. Unlike stronger prescriptive preparations, which can be discontinued once the immediate problem is alleviated, there is no graduating from these plants—these good habits are meant to be maintained for life. The plants you'll encounter here have universal applicability and appeal.

The big-picture goal of the Plant Medicine Protocol is to help you strategically incorporate a wide variety of medicinal plants into your routine, in moderate amounts, allowing the benefits to steadily accumulate and ultimately elevate the health of all of your essential body systems. The simple formula: Variety + Consistency + Time = Elevated Health. Though the effects of each individual plant can be subtle, once you begin infusing your days with them, you'll experience an unmistakable improvement in your health and resilience.

If you picked up this book hoping to address a specific health issue, the protocol will lead to improvement in your symptoms. If you're already feeling pretty good about your health and aspire to ever higher levels of wellness, this book will fulfill that purpose, too. I encourage you to think of your health as something you can achieve, unlock, and expand. There's no top end. A lifestyle rich in medicinal plants works on multiple levels, the most important of which is optimization. Unlike approaching your health from the mode of prevention, or holding back something that is inevitable for as long as possible, setting your sights on optimization means focusing on enjoying better and better health and letting prevention take care of itself along the way. It's a subtle shift, but an important one.

How to Use This Book

This book is the ultimate guide to a plant-powered lifestyle: Part I offers an overview of the foundations of natural medicine, the core systems of the body, and the categories of herbs that keep these systems humming. This essential context will ensure that you'll get the most out of the protocol. In Part II, we get down to brass tacks. The design of the Plant Medicine Protocol closely mirrors the methodology I use as a clinician to help individuals establish a medicinal plant–powered lifestyle. This simple, step-by-step process will help you find your own best ways to incorporate medicinal plants into your daily routine, and it includes the recipes and preparations I use myself. Throughout Part II, I'll also share plantventures that explore the amazing places these medicinal plants come from and the people who live closest to them. Pour yourself an herbal tonic or inhale your favorite essential oil and experience the plants coming to life in stories and settings that you'll want to go and see for yourself. Part III focuses on the home and creating living spaces that actualize your new plant-powered lifestyle. It includes tips on setting up a home pharmacy and a functional approach to using medicinal plants for some of the common ailments we all experience from time to time. Part IV is a deep dive into the most essential medicinal plants, covering their traditional uses, functional benefits, and how to use them. Finally, the

PLANTS + ADVENTURE = PLANTVENTURE

One of the best parts of my work is traveling around the world, sourcing medicinal plants and learning directly from the people with a long tradition of growing and using them. These trips are a unique way to experience cultures through the lens of the medicinal plants that they hold dear. This is how the word *plantventure* came to me. What I ultimately realized, though, is that whenever I'm sharing medicinal plants with someone, when plants and people come together to unlock an adventure of aliveness, we're in the midst of a plantventure. The real plantventure happens inside of us—through the novel sensations and experience of heightened vitality that only medicinal plants create.

Resources section at the back of the book contains recommended sources for herbs and products from companies that are doing a great job.

It should be said that many important factors when it comes to optimizing our health fall into the realm of diet, exercise, and lifestyle considerations that are outside the scope of this book. Medicinal plants are not a replacement for a healthy diet, good sleep, proper exercise, time spent in nature, meaningful work, nurturing relationships, and so on. Medicinal plants enhance our ability to implement and actualize all of these and other necessary fundamentals of healthy living. I say it often, and I live it: Medicinal plants separate health from super health. This is no empty promise, fad, or silver bullet—using them daily and often represents a practical, effective, achievable approach to optimizing health that has stood the test of time.

> "Adopting a medicinal plant–powered lifestyle is one of the best ways to stay connected to the natural world on a daily basis."

One way or another, nature is the source of our health. Adopting a medicinal plant–powered lifestyle is one of the best ways to stay connected to the natural world on a daily basis. Medicinal plants are saturated with the positive, life-enhancing force of nature, and it's my mission to get more and more of them into more and more people. Healthy individuals create a healthy society, and healthy societies in turn support healthy individuals. Medicinal plants have been nature's universal health-care plan for tens of thousands of years. Why stop now?

The Health-Care Pyramid

The health-care pyramid shown below represents a practical, effective, economically sound, and sustainable health-care system for individuals, society, and the planet. The more we rely on the base tiers of the pyramid, the less we need to engage with the ones on top, which by and large are more invasive, are designed to suppress symptoms, often create side effects, and can be overtly detrimental to long-term health.

The base of the pyramid is essential for both maintaining and regenerating health. Barring accidents and injuries, we need fewer drugs and surgeries when we take care of ourselves with medicinal plants and natural techniques, along with the cutting-edge insights emerging from the science of wellness—taking advantage of Western medicine where it makes sense, but within a broader holistic framework. These methods address the roots of imbalance, making us less susceptible to the epidemic of chronic disease that Western medicine finds increasingly difficult to treat. And when we do require the upper tiers, medicinal plants and natural medicine are equally essential for their ability to support the body's vitality, dramatically accelerate healing, and encourage the complete resolution or reversal of the issues at hand.

tier **4**
tier **3**
tier **2**
tier **1**

Tier 1
Natural Medicine Fundamentals

These simple, natural methods and techniques create and sustain optimal health, prevent illness, and treat relatively common and uncomplicated conditions that don't require a higher level of medical intervention. Specifically, we're talking about the use of medicinal plants (including culinary herbs, adaptogenic tonics, medicinal mushrooms, essential oils, teas, tinctures, elixirs, vitamins, supplements, and a range of other preparations); a nutritious, whole-foods diet; proper exercise; good sleep; and vitality-enhancing practices like hydrotherapy, saunas, cold plunges, fasts and seasonal cleanses, yoga, meditation, tai chi, time in nature, massage, and breathing techniques, among others. Ideally, everyone learns these fundamentals of self-care and prevention from a young age.

Tier 2
Natural and Functional Medicine Professionals

Acupuncturists, naturopaths, chiropractors, professional herbalists, Ayurvedic practitioners, and integrative and functional medicine doctors diagnose and treat more-complex and challenging conditions. These professionals use tools, techniques, and tenets from Tier 1—including medicinal plants and supplements in more concentrated forms, and therapeutic and prescriptive methods—as well as general health screenings, bloodwork, and diagnostics interpreted in a holistic framework.

Tier 3
Western Medicine

This tier comprises the majority of standard modern medicine techniques, including advanced diagnostic tests, imaging, over-the-counter and prescription pharmaceuticals, and specialized disciplines. The emphasis is on managing the symptoms of chronic diseases and performing surgical interventions.

Tier 4
Emergency Medicine

This tier includes the aspects of Western medicine related to advanced technological, surgical, and pharmaceutical techniques as well as lifesaving interventions for acute trauma, rescue operations, and stabilization.

In most modern societies, the pyramid is often inverted: The strongest, potentially most harmful (and expensive) techniques are commonly used first to address many health issues rooted in lifestyle. The tendency is to turn to natural methods, such as the use of medicinal plants, only when all else fails—and to engage with them so sparingly as to often be ineffectual.

Conversely, relying on medicinal plants when Western medicine is the appropriate choice can also be problematic. Each tier of the pyramid is necessary for an intact functional approach to health care, and all have their strengths and limitations. Understanding how to use them in the proper proportions and at the appropriate times is key to empowering individuals to take greater responsibility for their own health and well-being. This model shows us how to put the information in this book to best use, and where medicinal plants fit among the range of health and wellness options.

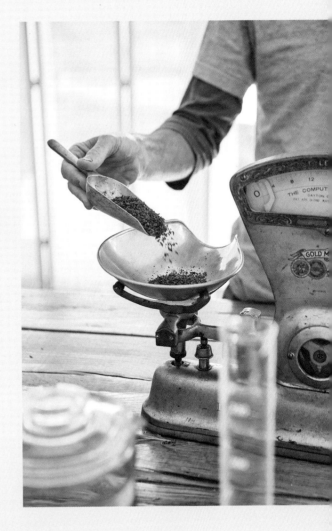

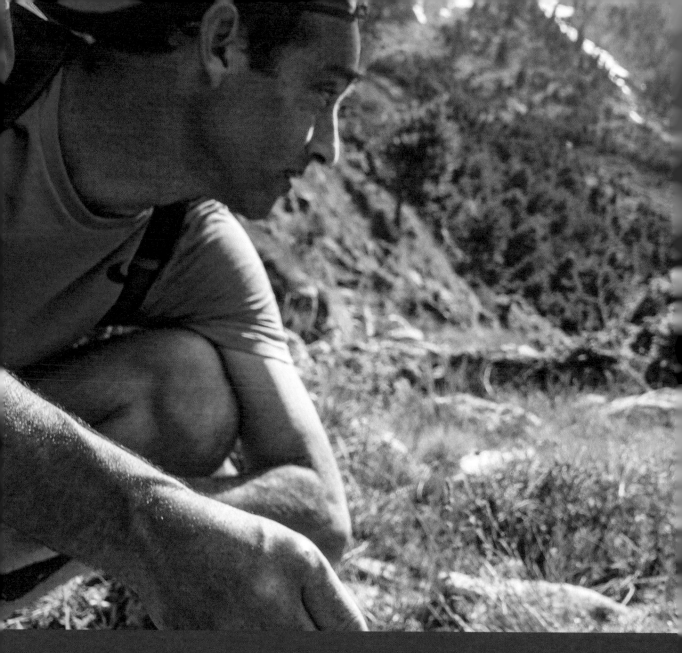

Part I

NATURAL MEDICINE FUNDAMENTALS

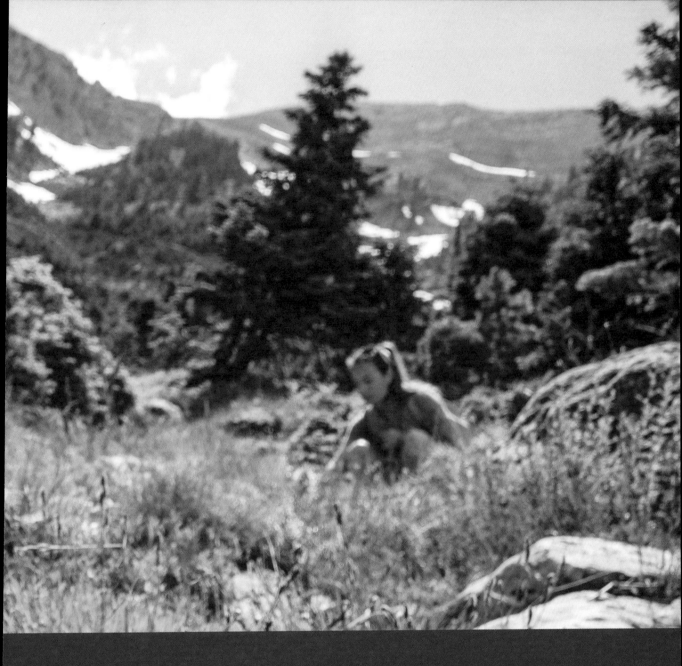

Part I explores the principles of natural medicine, the essential body systems, and the categories of medicinal plants you'll be using every day. All traditional health and healing modalities are based on a set of simple, practical principles that anyone can apply. Here I'll introduce you to the core tenets that are foundational to all natural medicine systems, including my specialties: Traditional Chinese Medicine (TCM) and Ayurveda. The focus of these systems is on nourishing, strengthening, and vitalizing the body to reinforce the roots of wellness. The most direct way to accomplish this is through supporting the major physiological mechanisms that govern digestion, detoxification, hydration, and the nervous, endocrine, and immune systems. These systems are the foundation upon which health is created and sustained. Optimal health inevitably results when our essential body systems are functioning at their best. Part I sets the stage for the protocol in Part II, where you'll learn to put the power of plants to work in your daily life to optimize each of these systems.

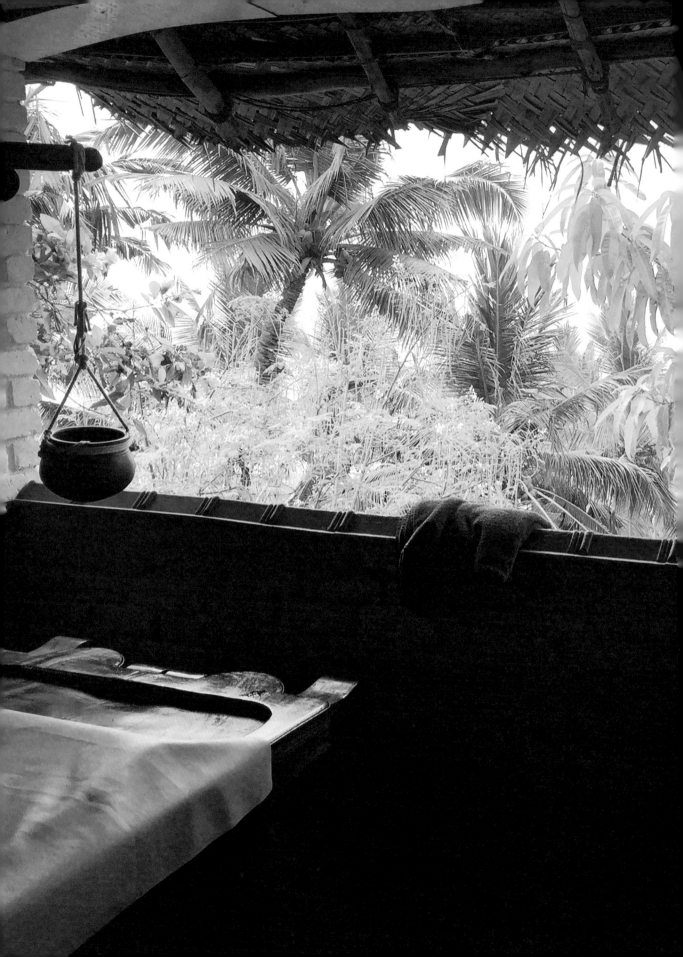

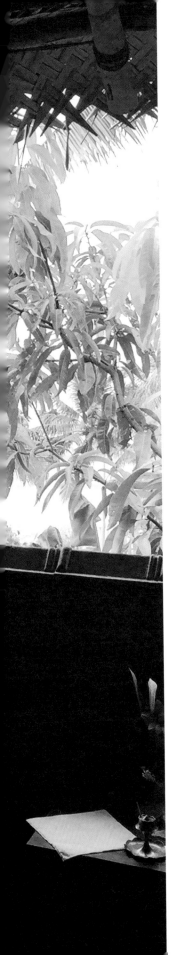

Principles of Natural Medicine

ACCORDING TO THE WORLD HEALTH ORGANIZATION, natural medicine is "the sum total of the knowledge, skill, and practices based on the theories, beliefs, and experiences indigenous to different cultures, whether explicable or not, used in the maintenance of health as well as in the prevention, diagnosis, improvement, or treatment of physical and mental illness."

Natural medicine developed out of necessity, as a commonsense, practical way to maintain health by cultures contending with the challenges of living intimately within nature. Over time, the knowledge and practices coalesced into systems that were passed down, continuously evolving over centuries of use into the world's great natural medicine traditions. Traditional Chinese Medicine and Ayurveda are perhaps the two most familiar and widely practiced in the world today, and are foundational to the design of the protocol.

The Body in Balance

Through careful observation of the way nature works—the movement of weather; the rhythms of the seasons; patterns of light and dark, cold and heat; and the cycles of the sun and moon over long periods of time—ancient peoples recognized that the body is a microcosm of the outside world. The underlying principles, energies, and forces within nature are the same mechanisms that animate and sustain the workings of our mind and body. We are a reflection of nature, thoroughly intertwined, interdependent, and inseparable from it. The water inside our body literally originated as clouds and rain, the heat that powers our metabolism was generated by the sun 93 million miles (150 million km) away, the minerals and trace elements that form our bodily structure come from the soil, the oxygen we breathe is produced by plants to form the atmosphere we are immersed in—and all of these elements are in a continuously circulating cycle in the space both within and outside our bodies.

This realization is beautifully expressed in the Ayurvedic theory that sees everything in the universe, including our bodies, as being made up of five universal elements: earth, water, fire, air, and space. Understanding the qualitative characteristics of these elements and observing how they function in nature gives us a sense of how they operate inside our bodies. Each of the five universal elements is composed of specific qualities that we

experience subjectively with our own senses: the feeling of heat or coolness, dampness or dryness, stillness or movement, heaviness or lightness, and many others.

As shown in the chart opposite, each element and its corresponding qualities play a vital role in our physiology, and health results from maintaining a balance among them. The familiar black-and-white yin-yang symbol in ancient Chinese philosophy similarly illustrates this same essential point: Life is a balancing act between opposing qualities continuously acting on each other in dynamic tension. Becoming aware of these qualities and their impact on us informs our choices and helps us live in a way that supports optimal health.

The protocol will show you how to use medicinal plants to harmonize the ratios and manifestations of the five elements within the body. Using our senses to give us the necessary data in real time about how we are feeling qualitatively guides us toward medicinal plants with either opposing or similar qualities to create balance. If we are feeling cold, for example, we may use pungent herbs like ginger or cinnamon to make tea that warms us. If we are experiencing dryness in our skin or throat, we may use demulcent plants like aloe vera or marshmallow to moisten and rehydrate. Conversely, if we are already feeling hot and we consume herbs with heating qualities (like cayenne pepper), we may create an imbalance.

THE FIVE ELEMENTS OF AYURVEDA

Fire

The principle of transformation

Qualities: Sharp, hot, bright, spreading, penetrating

Bodily systems: Digestion, metabolism, chemical reactions, cognition, eyesight, anything involved with combustion and transformation

Medicinal plants: Ginger, cayenne pepper, cinnamon, wasabi, spices of all kinds

Air

The principle of movement

Qualities: Subtle, light, mobile, changeable

Bodily systems: Nerve current, blood circulation, heartbeat, respiration, circadian rhythms, any movement in the body

Medicinal plants: Chamomile, nervines, mint, eucalyptus, green tea, yerba maté

Water

The principle of cohesion

Qualities: Cool, moist, heavy, dense, fluid

Bodily systems: Blood, saliva, lymph, sweat, and all other liquids

Medicinal plants: Aloe vera, chia seed, marshmallow root, Irish moss, all demulcents

Space

The principle of emptiness

Qualities: Cold, light, subtle, expansive

Bodily systems: Mind, consciousness, the space between everything, hollow organs

Medicinal plants: Bitters, frankincense, palo santo, sage

Earth

The principle of stability

Qualities: Heavy, stable, cool, hard, dense

Bodily systems: Bones, teeth, muscles, all aspects of our structure

Medicinal plants: Adaptogens, roots, nettles, alfalfa, sea vegetables, mushrooms, goji berries, maca root

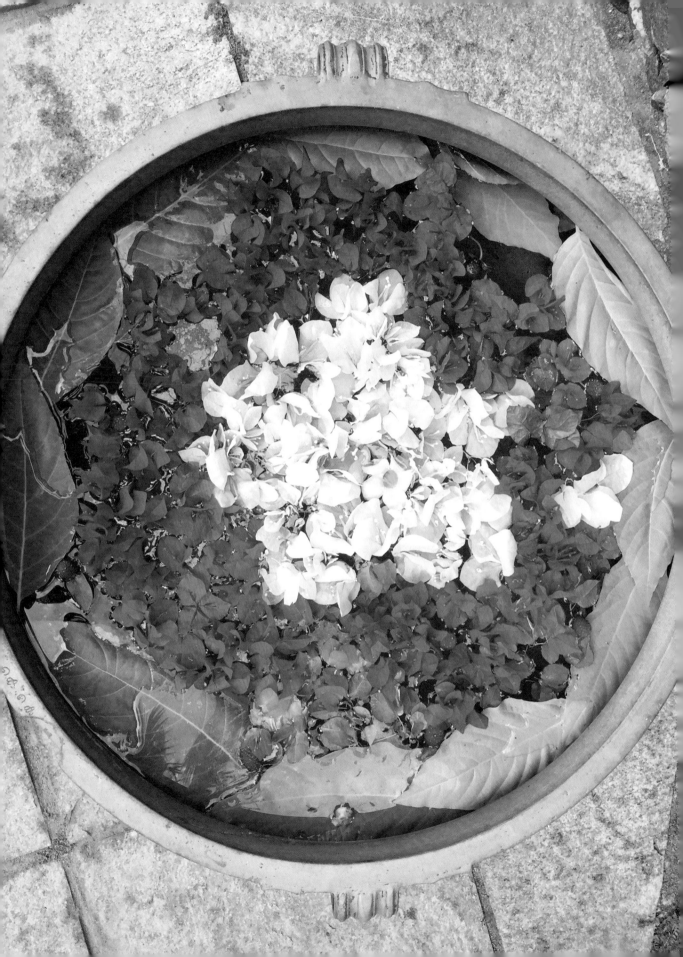

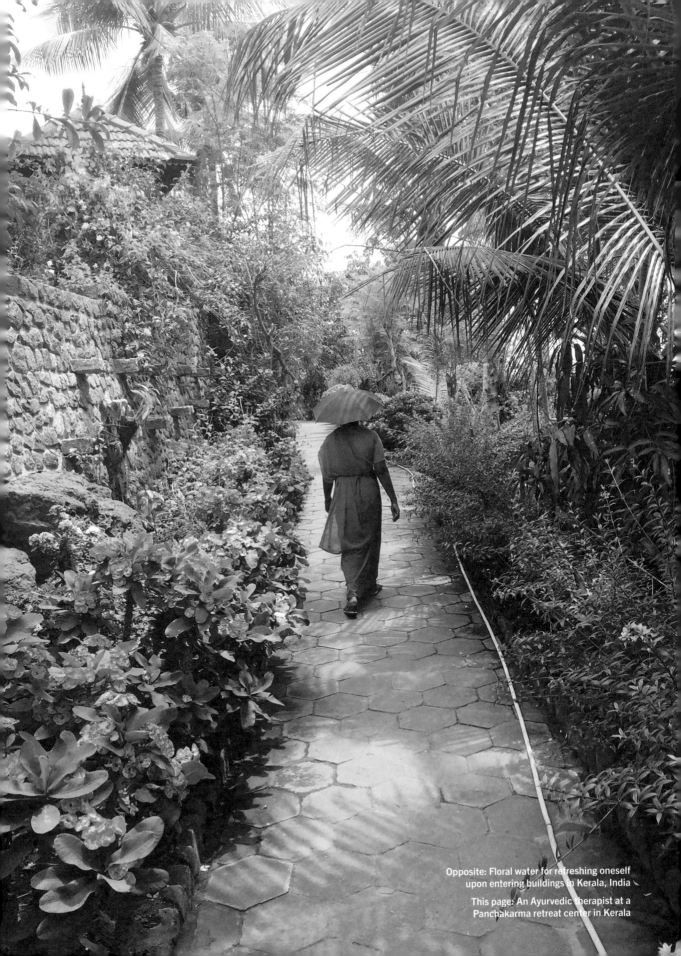

Opposite: Floral water for refreshing oneself
upon entering buildings in Kerala, India

This page: An Ayurvedic therapist at a
Panchakarma retreat center in Kerala

The Tenets of Natural Medicine

What follows are a set of universal principles essential to all systems of natural medicine.

01
Nature's Healing Power

Natural medicine recognizes the existence of an intelligent, self-healing vital energy that is perpetually sustaining the health of our body. Known as *qi* in TCM and *prana* in Ayurveda, this energy flows through us and every part of nature. All physiological functions are coordinated and maintained by this vital life force.

Right now your heart is beating, blood is circulating, hormones are being manufactured, injuries are healing, food is being digested, eyes are seeing. Something like one hundred billion distinct operations are happening in the brain alone every second, without a conscious thought. Ask yourself, for example, are you involved in the myriad detoxification processes your liver is performing right now? Did you consciously manufacture the specific enzymes needed to digest your breakfast? Are you controlling the delicate balance of blood gases needed to oxygenate the body? Extrapolate this out to every other physiological system, down to the cellular level, and we find there is very little that we are directly responsible for within our physiology, and yet here we are, alive.

When this vital force is blocked or weakened in the body, the result is impaired functioning and illness. The tools and techniques of natural medicine are designed to strengthen and liberate its flow.

02
Cause and Effect

The Ayurvedic concept of prajnaparadha, meaning "crimes against wisdom," describes the small ways we create imbalances in our health by willfully or unknowingly transgressing the wisdom of the body. As Hippocrates said, "Illnesses do not come upon us out of the blue. They are developed from small daily sins against Nature. When enough sins have accumulated, illnesses will suddenly appear." It is the ongoing small, sometimes subtle—other times blatant—choices that subvert the wisdom of the body that eventually lead to illness. Overeating, skipping meals, burning the candle at both ends, not getting enough sleep, and being sedentary, among many other examples, are the kinds of choices that compound to the point that the body is pushed out of alignment, eventually resulting in more serious imbalances. The more attuned we become to listening to our bodies, the better our chances of acting while imbalances are slight and easily corrected.

03
Prevent and Optimize

The tools and techniques of natural medicine are intended to be used daily to enhance health and resilience. By proactively optimizing how the body functions every day, we preempt issues from developing or address them when they're still minor and manageable.

Natural medicine views health as more verb than noun, a moving target that's dynamic and never static. The goal of natural medicine is to actualize the highest expression of health possible for each individual moment to moment.

04
Know Thyself

There is no one-size-fits-all when it comes to health. Everyone is born with a unique constitution that has its inherent strengths, weaknesses, and tendencies. Our constitutions are impacted by age, genetics, lifestyle habits, dietary choices, socioeconomic factors, and the physical environments around us. Understanding and honoring our own unique constitution informs the choices we make to ensure a lifetime of good health.

05
Mind-Body Connection

Natural medicine sees no separation between the mind and body; they exist as a mutually interdependent whole. How we feel mentally, emotionally, and spiritually has a direct influence on the physical body, for good or ill. Likewise, our physical state will impact our mind, emotions, and spirit. Integration of body and mind is how we stay connected to the present moment, allowing us to feel what is actually occurring and make informed choices that promote health. Therefore, developing a stable and present mind that is relaxed and at ease—even in the midst of stimulation and activity—is an essential consideration when it comes to optimal health.

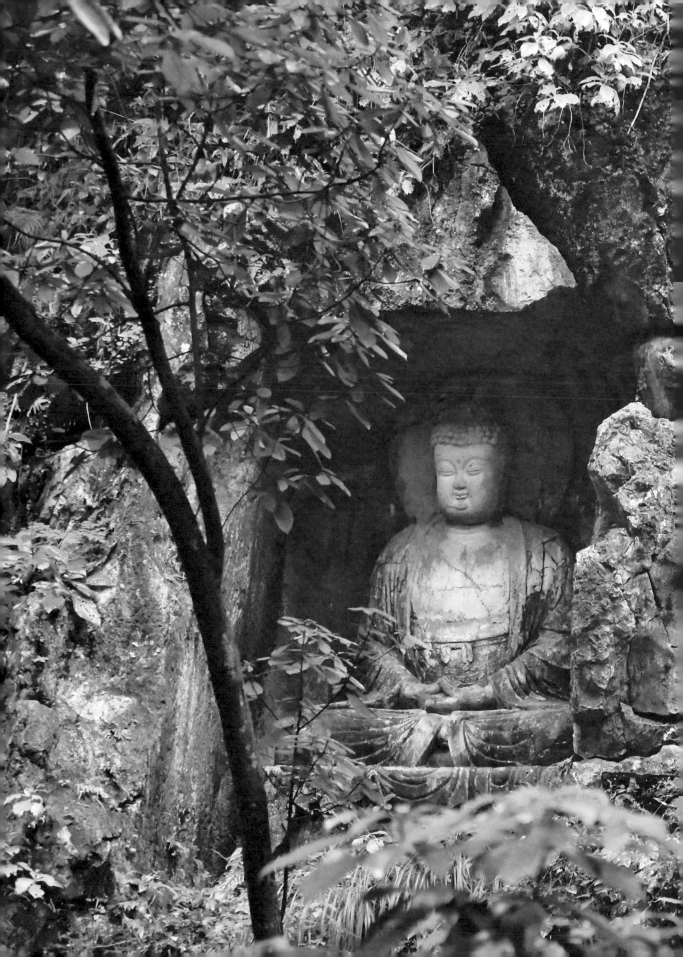

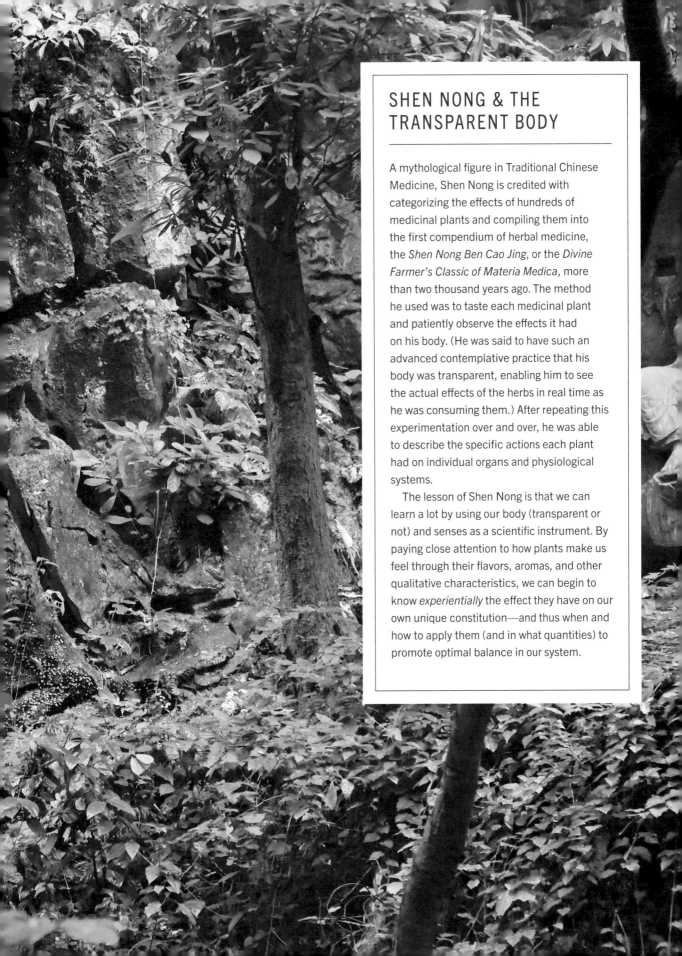

SHEN NONG & THE TRANSPARENT BODY

A mythological figure in Traditional Chinese Medicine, Shen Nong is credited with categorizing the effects of hundreds of medicinal plants and compiling them into the first compendium of herbal medicine, the *Shen Nong Ben Cao Jing*, or the *Divine Farmer's Classic of Materia Medica*, more than two thousand years ago. The method he used was to taste each medicinal plant and patiently observe the effects it had on his body. (He was said to have such an advanced contemplative practice that his body was transparent, enabling him to see the actual effects of the herbs in real time as he was consuming them.) After repeating this experimentation over and over, he was able to describe the specific actions each plant had on individual organs and physiological systems.

The lesson of Shen Nong is that we can learn a lot by using our body (transparent or not) and senses as a scientific instrument. By paying close attention to how plants make us feel through their flavors, aromas, and other qualitative characteristics, we can begin to know *experientially* the effect they have on our own unique constitution—and thus when and how to apply them (and in what quantities) to promote optimal balance in our system.

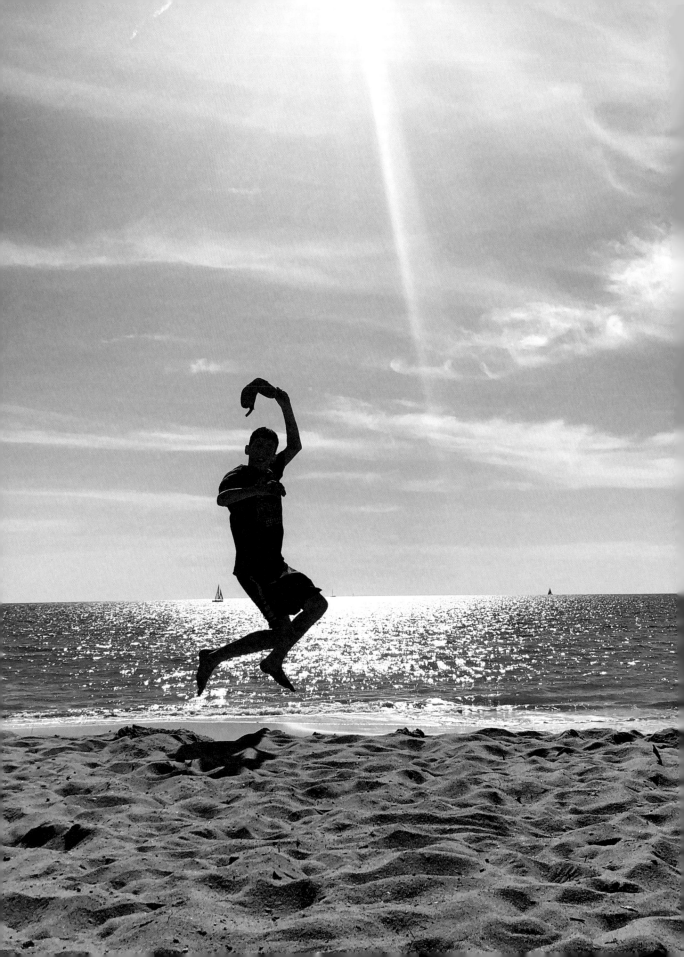

Our Essential Body Systems

THE BODY HAS A NUMBER OF ESSENTIAL FUNCTIONS THAT are a nonnegotiable foundation for achieving optimal health. The Plant Medicine Protocol focuses on five of these, chosen for their large impact on the body as a whole: digestion, detoxification, hydration, the nervous system, and core energy. These systems are interrelated and interdependent. Like gears on a clock, each one affects the functioning of the rest.

Understanding and appreciating the importance of these critical systems starts with regaining a feel for how they are supposed to function when working optimally. We often don't notice the beginning stages of declining health, or we dismiss or normalize them. Before a problem becomes diagnosable, it manifests in these signs and symptoms that we choose to ignore. Slight deviations from optimal functioning build on each other over time until they turn into chronic diseases.

The plant-powered approach works synergistically, strengthening all of the body's core systems to create the foundation of optimal health. In the pages that follow, I'll give you the diagnostic framework that will build your confidence and capacity to enhance each system using medicinal plants.

The Digestive System
Metabolize & Nourish

"If you have a good diet, you don't need doctors and drugs;
if you don't have a good diet, you don't need doctors and drugs."
—AYURVEDIC SAYING

All systems of traditional medicine recognize good digestion as the most essential requirement for health. The primary function of digestion is to break down the components of what we eat into smaller molecules that are absorbed by our cells for energy, growth, and repair. All aspects of physiology depend on the nutrients made available through digestion. The vast majority of chronic health problems originate with poor digestive functioning, and their resolution depends on correcting it.

Many people haven't experienced good—let alone optimal—digestion for so long that they forget what it feels like. Of the thousands of patients I have seen over the years, the vast majority experience some type of digestive disharmony, sometimes without even knowing it. It's easy to ignore poor digestion in its early stages and adjust to it as somehow "normal," but anything less than optimal digestion invariably has a cumulative negative effect on the rest of our health. In other words, having a digestive system that's working at 75 percent efficiency means that the other 25 percent is creating problems down the road.

Restoring digestive function if it isn't working well (and improving it if it is) begins with familiarizing and sensitizing ourselves to the workings of our digestive system. This means paying attention to how we feel before, during, and after every meal. Are you satisfied or feeling overly full? Are you bloated and gassy, or feeling fiery and acidic? Are you often tired and lethargic after you've eaten or light and energized? How about your thinking: Is it clear or muddled?

The body is a finely tuned instrument, always sending us signals that let us know when something is off. Experiencing occasional symptoms of poor digestion is one thing; if they occur with frequency over a long period of time, that's another. Listening to our body's early-warning signs is key: It's a lot easier to restore balance to digestion when issues are minor and manageable. And improving digestion is the quickest and most direct way to experience positive benefits in *all* aspects of health.

The digestive system takes up a lot of real estate in our body, and the process of digestion requires a considerable amount of energy. We want an efficient, clean-burning system that uses the least amount of energy to extract the maximum amount of nutrients while producing the smallest amount of residual waste. The functions of our gut act like a furnace. The glowing warmth of metabolism liberates energy from our food to fuel our cells. It should operate like a factory running on clean, renewable energy, not a smoggy smokestack.

The gastrointestinal (GI) tract starts in the mouth and moves down into the esophagus, stomach, and small and large intestines; it also includes the workings of the liver, gallbladder, and pancreas. Food mixes with saliva, then

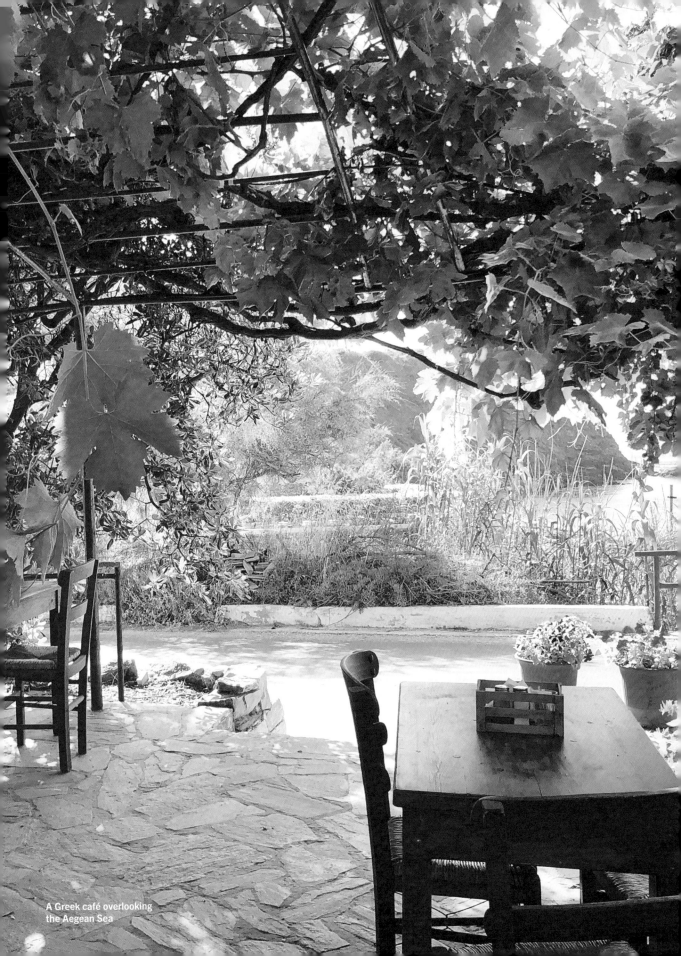

A Greek café overlooking
the Aegean Sea

travels down the GI tract at just the right pace, combining with cascades of digestive enzymes, acids, bile, and hormones along the way. These fluids break food down to its constituent parts, making it easily assimilable by the millions of tiny villi lining the small intestine. This nutrient essence is absorbed into the bloodstream and filtered through the liver, where any remaining toxins are disposed of before it moves on to feed hungry cells. Farther down the GI tract, primarily in the large intestine, our beneficial bacteria continue breaking down proteins, complex carbohydrates, and fiber, while synthesizing key vitamins and short-chain fatty acids. When the microbiome is finished assimilating all remaining nutrients, the waste left over is removed from the body.

In Ayurvedic medicine, the transformative power of metabolism is called *agni*, meaning "fire" in Sanskrit. While agni functions throughout the body, the gut and digestive system are the core reactor, where it's most concentrated. The stronger our agni, the more efficient our digestive system is at breaking down food and liberating the nutrients it contains, resulting in greater nourishment and fewer residual wastes. "Weak agni" describes a gut that is essentially undercooking the food we ingest, due in part to lowered amounts of digestive acids and enzymes. This prevents us from becoming properly nourished and leaves behind an accumulation of wastes and toxins that is the basis for inflammation. It's like a fireplace that doesn't burn logs efficiently, leaving behind soot and black smoke that clogs everything. The old axiom "You are what you eat" should be more like "You are what you digest."

The gut is also the most concentrated area of immune activity in our bodies. The lymph glands lining our GI tract, known as the gut-associated lymphoid tissue (GALT), contain 60 to 70 percent of the body's total immune cells. GALT filters out toxins and harmful pathogens so they aren't absorbed into the bloodstream. Gut immunity is designed to screen for and burn up the inevitable toxins and microbes that ride in on the food we eat. Incompletely broken-down proteins in our diet can trigger the immune system, making even healthy diets a potential source of inflammation when not digested properly. Not to mention the artificial and processed ingredients, refined sugars, hydrogenated oils, and other weird things we call food these days that are indigestible even in the best of circumstances.

If this pattern becomes chronic, inflammation builds up, irritating the gut lining and making it more permeable, which allows more incompletely digested proteins to slip through. Eventually the inflammatory process in the gut lining can no longer be contained and spreads like a brush fire, negatively impacting the entire body. This hyperactive immune response and subsequent breakdown of the gut lining caused by weakened agni is what is called "leaky gut" syndrome.

This pattern of gut dysfunction and its resulting systemic inflammation impacts virtually all body systems and has implications for most every chronic disease and condition, from joint pain and skin issues to low energy, anxiety, insomnia, migraines, cardiovascular and autoimmune issues, cognitive decline, obesity, and diabetes. If the pattern smolders for years, inflammation begins impacting fundamental metabolic processes and the health of our organs. In medical science, it's now well established that most of the debilitating conditions affecting us at epidemic levels today are built on a foundation of chronic inflammation, and the gut is the primary site where it all begins.

One of the most effective ways to strengthen and support the digestive fire is through the regular use of digestive-supporting medicinal plants. Getting antioxidant-rich culinary herbs and spices (page 102) into our diet on a consistent basis is a valuable and time-honored means of improving and maintaining good digestion. Aromatic oils and other constituents in culinary spices enhance the production of the acids and enzymes needed to break down and assimilate what we eat. Consuming culinary spices with our meals is like preheating the digestive system to ensure food is cooked (digested) properly.

Bitter herbs (page 105) are another essential plant category that contributes to optimal digestion. Bitters enhance the liver's capacity to break down fats and proteins while promoting the elimination of wastes and toxins.

Moisture-rich demulcents (page 175) act as a soothing balm, neutralizing excess gastric acids, hydrating, lubricating, and restoring the protective mucous membranes lining the GI tract.

Finally, fragrant relaxants (page 198) calm the nerves in the gut, easing tension and creating the space necessary for our food to mix and churn and allow for complete assimilation.

elimination is another sign of poor digestion—whether a tendency toward loose, sometimes urgent or frequent bowel movements or the opposite, constipation.

In general, there is always a reason for not digesting well. Before you can resolve the issue, you may need to become a digestion detective of sorts. Ask yourself: *What were the circumstances when I was eating—did I feel rushed, was I eating fast, or not chewing enough? Was I feeling stressed or paying attention to other things?* Most important, *What food might I have eaten that didn't agree with my system?* It may take a few experiences to narrow down and remove the cause. Improving eating habits along with consuming medicinal plants that improve agni is a highly effective combination for optimal digestive health.

When Your Digestion Is Out of Balance

Poor digestion exists on a continuum, usually starting with minor, intermittent signs of imbalance that sometimes go unnoticed. Depending on the individual, some signs and symptoms of poor digestion include frequent belching and feeling bloated, gassy, nauseous, or hyperacidic after meals. If digestive agni is low, one may have a diminished appetite or feel excessively full or fatigued after eating. Poor digestion can also lead to foggy, muddled thinking; headaches; and cravings for sweets and sugar.

When our bodies don't digest well, we may experience congestion often soon after eating. We may become puffy, gain weight, or experience borborygmus (the sound of water rumbling around in the gut). Irregular

8 SIGNS YOUR DIGESTION IS OUT OF BALANCE

1) Inconsistent appetite

2) Bloating and fullness after meals

3) Acidity and reflux issues

4) Brain fog and significant fatigue after eating

5) Excessive sweets cravings

6) Unexpected weight gain

7) General discomfort in your gut

8) Intestinal disorders, like irregular bowel movements or constipation

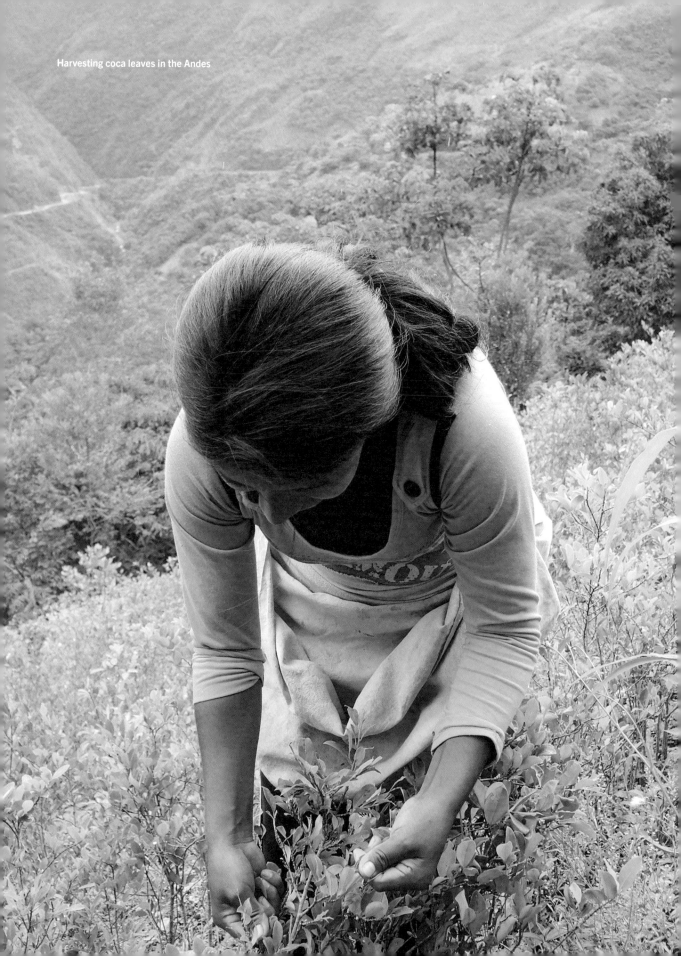

Harvesting coca leaves in the Andes

Detoxification
Cleanse & Renew

"Illnesses do not come out of the blue. They are developed from small daily sins against Nature."
—HIPPOCRATES

The desire to detoxify makes intuitive sense. All of the body's metabolic processes naturally create residual waste. The idea that cleansing ourselves of this toxic junk will make us feel better isn't all that different from the impulse to keep our house clean and take out the trash on a regular basis. Everyone feels better living in a neat, uncluttered home compared to one where the garbage needs emptying, dishes fill the sink, and laundry has piled up. Similarly, we feel better when our bodies aren't burdened with excess metabolic toxins and wastes clogging our systems. Thankfully, the body has developed specialized mechanisms to transform waste into inert substances and remove them through various pathways.

Detoxification happens every minute of every day inside our bodies through the collective action of the lungs, kidneys, colon, skin, lymphatic system, immune system, and liver, which work as a team to remove and transform wastes and toxins. The lungs filter out carbon dioxide and other impurities from the air we breathe. The kidneys are the body's internal water filter, charged with removing urea and nitrogenous wastes from the blood. The dirty work of removing solid waste falls, of course, to the colon. The skin provides the largest avenue for the removal of toxins via sweat, and the lymphatic vessels are a vast network of drainpipes for transforming and eliminating cellular wastes. The LeBron James of detoxification is the liver, which uses enzymes and bile to disassemble harmful chemicals, ammonia, fat-soluble toxins, and cholesterol. On top of all of that, the body's innate immune system is constantly clearing out old or damaged cells to make room for new, healthy ones.

If the organs and mechanisms charged with detoxifying become overwhelmed and fall behind in their tasks, common metabolic wastes can accumulate and turn toxic. The detoxification process is like the regularly scheduled trash pickup in your neighborhood: It happens as part of the ordinary course of living, and you usually don't think much about it. Now imagine that your neighborhood just hosted Mardi Gras. After days of thousands of people parading through the streets, piling up empty beer cups and strands of beads, there are now heaps more trash to deal with. That's fine for one week of the year. The sanitation department puts in for overtime, and it's all good. If our bodies are dealing with the aftermath of Mardi Gras *every single day*, however, the usual mechanisms of waste removal, as excellent as they are, invariably fall behind, and impurities pile up.

Detoxification is interconnected with all of the other essential systems that maintain our health, especially digestion, which is often the largest source of metabolic wastes. Subpar functioning in one or more of these systems burdens the organs of detoxification, and compromised detoxification in turn weakens other systems. The following are simple examples of how detoxification and the essential body systems affect one another.

Endocrine system. All hormones are chemicals that must be broken down and removed like other waste products. It's the liver's role to deactivate and detoxify these endocrine messengers once they have served their function. If the liver falls behind in its detoxification duties, hormones like cortisol and adrenaline will continue to circulate, prolonging the stress response and disrupting vital systems. The sluggish breakdown of hormones like estrogen and progesterone can disrupt ovulation, leading to irregular menstruation, PMS, and fertility issues.

Sleep. During sleep, the body redirects its energy inward toward detoxification, regeneration, and renewal. The organs of detoxification do most of their work during our deepest sleep cycles. Blood returns to the liver to be filtered, lymphatic vessels drain toxins and inflammatory proteins from the brain, and deeper, slower breathing allows the lungs to discharge more carbon dioxide and other waste gases. If our sleep quality is poor or we aren't getting enough, the critical work of cleansing the system of impurities is compromised.

Hydration. Detoxification requires a well-hydrated system. Water is essential for diluting and dissolving toxins, flushing them through the liver, kidneys, and lymphatic system, keeping the intestines moist, and removing wastes from the body.

Nutrition. The enzyme systems and biological pathways that break down wastes and toxins at the cellular level depend on a variety of specific micronutrients to function properly. Deficiencies in our micronutrient reserves diminish the capacity of detoxification organs to do their job.

Digestive system. Poor digestion creates an excess accumulation of wastes and toxins in the GI tract. This congests the gut's lymphatic drainage, causing inflammation and an imbalanced microbiome, contributing to a range of systemic issues over time (see below).

Never before in human history have our systems of detoxification been under such constant strain as they are today. We are exposed to literally tens of thousands of novel human-manufactured toxins in the air we breathe, the food we eat, and the water we drink. Add to this alcohol, tobacco, pharmaceuticals, preservatives, and artificial ingredients in food, and what you have is a real mess. When our bodies are inundated with both normal metabolic wastes as well as these potent external toxins, our detoxification organs are being asked to go way above and beyond what they are designed to do.

Supporting these overburdened organs is essential. Using plants to help cleanse the body of wastes and toxins is a key strategy for prevention and healing in all traditional medicine systems. Bitter herbs (page 105) are especially helpful for enhancing the body's ability to break down and remove wastes and toxins.

When Our Detoxification System Is Out of Balance

Ayurveda considers the accumulation of toxins, called *ama* in Sanskrit, to be the basis for inflammation, immune dysfunction, and the underlying cause of chronic disease and metabolic disorders. Traditional Chinese Medicine has a similar concept, referring to excessive wastes and toxins as an accumulation of "dampness" in the body. As in the external environment, dampness weighs things down, making us feel heavy, lethargic, and fatigued. It's frequently associated with sluggish metabolism, weight gain, "brain fog," poor memory or concentration, and other cognitive issues.

Some telltale signs that you may be experiencing an overload of toxins include inflammatory reactions showing up in various parts of the body: random aches and pains in the muscles and joints; rashes or skin conditions like psoriasis or acne; constipation, gas, and other digestive imbalances. Microbiome imbalances can also develop over time due to excess toxins and are a major contributing factor in yeast infections, candidiasis, and inflammatory bowel issues, such as irritable bowel syndrome (IBS) and colitis. One of the liver's main jobs is to remove excess cholesterol and break down fats during digestion. If it's not working well, triglyceride and cholesterol levels rise, both risk factors in cardiovascular disease. When the immune system is continuously dealing with an excess of toxins, vulnerability to common pathogens increases as well as risk of developing more serious and entrenched illness.

12 SIGNS YOUR DETOXIFICATION IS OUT OF BALANCE

1) Low energy

2) Constipation, bloating, and other digestive issues

3) High blood sugar, cholesterol, or triglycerides

4) Weight gain

5) Acne, rashes, cysts

6) Mood issues, muddled thinking, fogginess

7) Dental cavities

8) Strong-smelling body odor, urine, bowel movements, or breath

9) Menstrual irregularities and PMS

10) Inflammatory joint issues

11) Chronic colds, coughs, headaches

12) Weakened immunity

The Nervous System
Ease & Flow

"Be formless, shapeless, like water."
—BRUCE LEE

Physiologically, our nervous systems are more or less the same today as they were fifty thousand years ago. Immersed in the sounds, sights, and smells of nature (and nothing else), they developed a tempo and rhythm that reflected those environments. Most of what occurs in nature is pretty chill. A butterfly floats around a flower, clouds drift across the sky, the sun rises and sets, ocean waves lap against the shore. Sure, there were hurricanes, tornadoes, forest fires, and the proverbial saber-toothed tiger to contend with, but those were intermittent interruptions in a world that was otherwise moving quite slowly. Fast-forward to now and the modern world around us is filled with car alarms, artificial lights, sirens, and smartphones. Our ancient nervous system is being forced to adapt, in an extremely short period of time (evolutionarily speaking), to a cacophonous backdrop of near-constant stimulation. Absorbing all of this sensory data creates chaotic vibrations in the nervous system, and assimilating it in real time is a big challenge.

Imagine one of those old telephone switchboard rooms, with rows of operators receiving and connecting calls in a complex system of plugs and wires. It may look like chaos from the outside, but somehow all the information gets sorted and calls are connected properly. In a similar way, our nervous system sends information as electrical impulses and chemical neurotransmitters through a vast network of nerve fibers, syncing our bodies with the outside world.

With 37 miles (60 km) of nerve fibers containing more than 7 trillion neurons, our nervous system is more 5G internet than a switchboard. The nervous system consists of the brain, spinal cord, all the nerves that branch out through the rest of the body, and all the associated neurotransmitters they generate. It has two basic modes that counterbalance each other: sympathetic and parasympathetic. The sympathetic, or "fight or flight," mode prepares the body for action and perceived threats. The parasympathetic, or "rest and digest," mode keeps things on an even keel and promotes relaxation and restoration. Optimal nervous system health occurs when the majority of our time is spent in a steady parasympathetic state, with the occasional bursts of sympathetic activity when needed.

The vagus nerve, an essential part of our parasympathetic nervous system, is a bidirectional pathway connecting the brain to the lungs, heart, and GI tract. When properly toned, it helps regulate stress, deepen breathing, relax muscles in the gut, lower blood pressure, and promote good digestion. The vagus nerve also communicates with the more than 100 million neurons lining our GI tract—often referred to as our "second brain." Enteric nerves in the gut produce 80 to 90 percent of the body's neurotransmitters (serotonin, dopamine, and gamma-aminobutyric acid, aka GABA) responsible for an alert, happy, and stable mood.

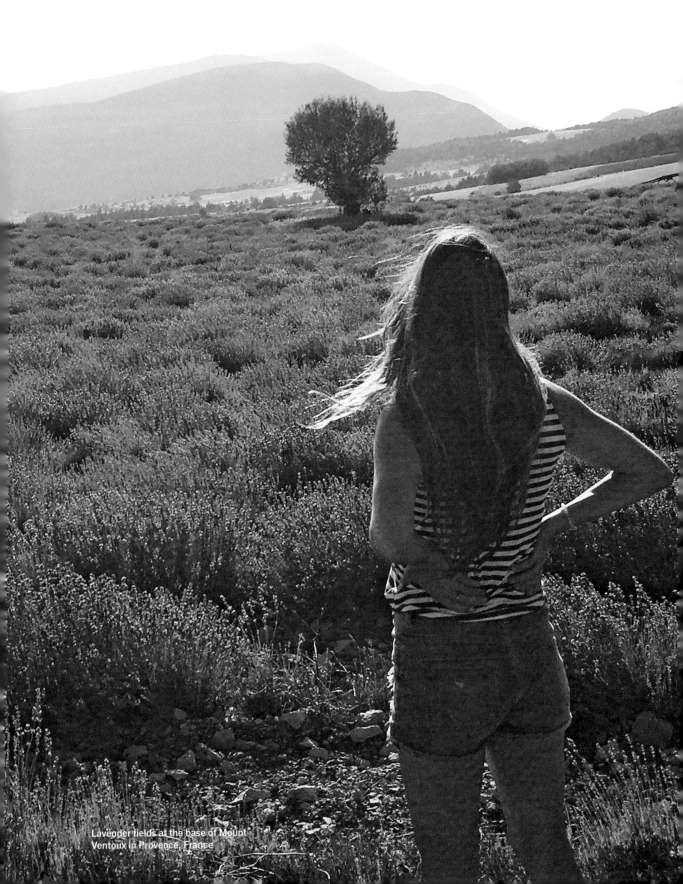

Lavender fields at the base of Mount Ventoux in Provence, France

By calming enteric nerves in the gut, both vagal nerve tone and heart-rate variability (HRV) are increased—two key metrics that indicate a balanced nervous system.

HRV is another good indicator of nervous system function and a way to measure tension, in an objective way. Heart-rate variability measures the variation in time between heartbeats, which is controlled by the autonomic nervous system. A higher HRV is associated with increased activation of the parasympathetic branch of the nervous system, which leads to deeper sleep, faster recovery from exercise, improved cardiovascular and immune functioning, better mental health, and enhanced resilience to stress. Studies show that people who have a high HRV have increased cardiovascular fitness and greater resilience to stress.

The term *brain wave* is a measurement of the way electrical impulses flow in the brain. Neuroscientists generally recognize five distinct types of brain waves ranging in frequency, from fastest to slowest: gamma, beta, alpha, theta, and delta. The higher the frequency, the more active the brain and therefore the nervous system. The lower frequencies occur when we are relaxed, sleeping, and experiencing states of flow. Good health requires access to all these different frequencies; each one has its purpose, and ideally we fluctuate seamlessly between them throughout the day.

The beta brain wave state is characterized by an alert, active logical-thinking and problem-solving mind. Spending too much time in the beta state can feel like there's a Tasmanian devil spinning around in our head. Modern life makes it hard to transition out of this state. If we are worried and anxious all the time, multitasking with devices in both hands, drinking way too much caffeine, and getting too little sleep, our hyperstimulated nervous system starts short-circuiting like a flickering lightbulb with faulty wiring. This leads to a chaotic and intermittent supply of nerve force flowing into our vital organ systems, like rolling blackouts, weakening and disrupting their functioning. This is a problem because, as we've said, the nervous system is the communications network that directs the flow of life energy.

The nervous system is the maestro conducting the orchestra of our physiology, and it must maintain a harmonious tempo for our bodies to function at their best. Nerve currents should

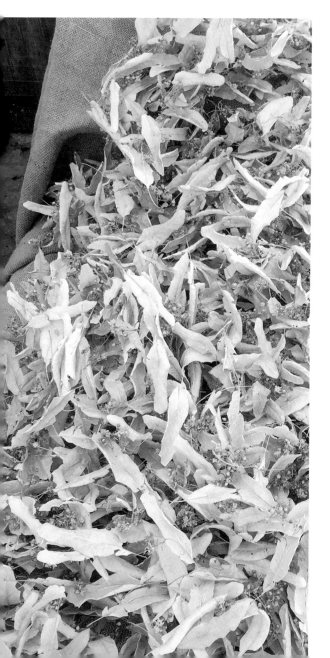

Linden flowers at the farmers' market in Buis-les-Baronnies, France

flow through the system unimpeded, in a slow, steady, rhythmic Bob Marley reggae beat, to balance circadian rhythms related to mood, cognition, sleep, digestion, energy levels, and reproduction, among many others. In Traditional Chinese Medicine, there is a strong emphasis on keeping qi, or life energy, flowing smoothly as a major determinant of health. Flowing qi closely corresponds to the way nerve impulses move throughout the nervous system. Occupying an internal stance of nonresistance allows qi energy to flow *through* the nervous system rather than accumulate inside as residual tension. In TCM, a healthy nervous system is akin to bamboo, a plant that bends and flexes in the wind, withstanding harsh elements without breaking.

Encouraging a balanced nervous system that promotes flow, ease, and mind-body integration, as well as the capacity for deep rest and renewal, is an essential aspect of achieving optimal health and happiness. Incorporating nervine herbs, fragrant relaxants, and euphoric floral essential oils into our lifestyle can enhance the body's ability to achieve this state of balance.

When Your Nervous System Is Out of Balance

We want to become aware of the subtle signs of nervous system imbalance before we end up like cartoon robots with steam coming out of our ears and sparks flying everywhere. Because our thoughts and emotions have such a strong influence on the state of our nervous system, chronic mood imbalances and/or cognitive issues are among the first indicators that something is awry. Having excessive, unproductive thoughts driving emotions like anxiety, chronic worry, anger, and depression can mean we are spending too much time in higher-frequency brain wave patterns and not accessing other states of being to balance them.

The disruption of normal physiological patterns like sleep is another early consequence of nervous system imbalance. Truly restorative sleep occurs only when we are fully relaxed and immersed in the most stable low-frequency brain wave patterns. Difficulty falling and/ or staying asleep, diminished REM or deep-sleep cycles, and restlessness all point to an imbalanced nervous system.

The overall level of tension in our bodies is also a clear indicator of nervous system stress. Nerve and muscle fibers are intertwined like a cable-knit sweater. A chronically overstimulated nervous system builds up more electrical charge than can be circulated. The muscles act like a reservoir, storing excess energy as tension. Tight neck and shoulders, the urge to crack our joints, intermittent dull headaches, and general stiffness often reflect an accumulation of potential energy getting stuck in our body.

---

8 SIGNS YOUR NERVOUS SYSTEM IS OUT OF BALANCE

---

1) Chronic muscle tension

2) Difficulty falling or staying asleep and/or waking up feeling unrested

3) Inability to breathe deeply and rhythmically

4) Gut tension leading to digestive symptoms including poor appetite, indigestion, frequent belching and hiccuping, bloating, hyperacidity, elimination issues

5) Frequent mood swings, anxiety, depression

6) Poor concentration

7) Irregular menstrual cycles

8) Fatigue

Hydration
Moisten & Replenish

"When the well's dry, we know the worth of water."
—BENJAMIN FRANKLIN

Traditional Chinese Medicine views health as the successful balancing of opposing forces continuously acting upon one another, as depicted by the yin-yang symbol. According to TCM, water is the cooling, moistening, lubricating yin counterpart to the hot, active, drying yang aspects of life. Water's cooling (yin) properties act to balance the body's heat-generating metabolic processes (yang). One of the main reasons dehydration is so prevalent (yin deficiency) is because our fast-paced modern lifestyle is so excessively yang. Like a car, the faster we rev, the hotter we run. Sympathetic ("fight or flight") dominant nervous system states, characterized by chronic stimulation and stress, dramatically increase our rate of water usage and cause our systems to become dried out.

Other causes of yin deficiency include: Overexertion. Spending too much time looking at digital devices. Using our brains for too much abstract beta-wave mental work. Insufficient sleep. Eating a denatured, heavily processed diet. Smoking or drinking too much alcohol, caffeine, or diuretic beverages. Taking pharmaceuticals. Spending too much time in dry indoor living environments or living in arid regions.

Water is the liquid superconductor that powers our physiology. Every cellular process occurs within an electrochemically charged membrane filled with water. Our energy levels and the quality of our health depend on our ability to store and transmit these electric impulses through well-hydrated cells. Think of the body as one big battery that relies on water to maintain the charge necessary to carry out all its vital functions.

Water is also the body's liquid highway and universal solvent, the major network through which everything moves. As the main component of blood, water transports vital nutrients and oxygen into our cells and maintains proper blood volume, which directly affects circulation and blood pressure. The body's detoxification systems require water to dilute, filter, and transport metabolic wastes through the kidneys, ultimately to be excreted as urine. Immune cells rely on water to transport them through the lymphatic vessels, gobbling up pathogens and removing cellular debris along the way. The action of sweating cools us down, maintaining the optimal temperature range required for vital physiological processes to occur.

A well-hydrated body has the flexibility, protection, and resilience needed to live in a tough and turbulent world. It's the shock absorber and lubricant that gives our joints and tendons the ability to stretch and flex. Water forms the barrier on our skin and mucous membranes that insulates the inside world from the outside. Everything we eat, drink, or breathe is separated from the inner workings of our blood and organs by this thin, water-rich border. These membranes need to be well hydrated to allow passage of oxygen,

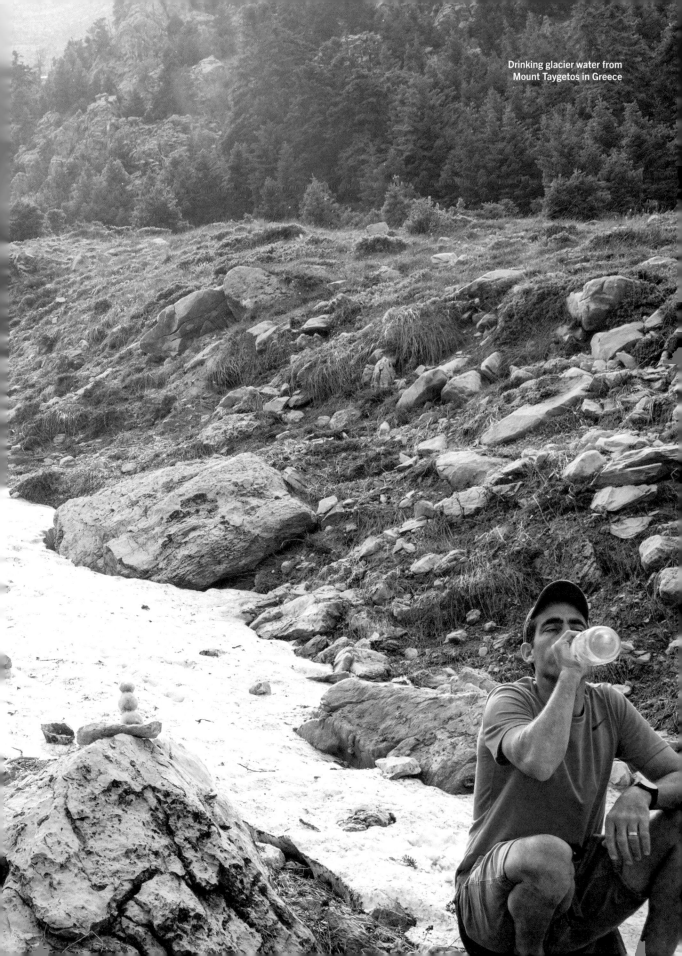

Drinking glacier water from
Mount Taygetos in Greece

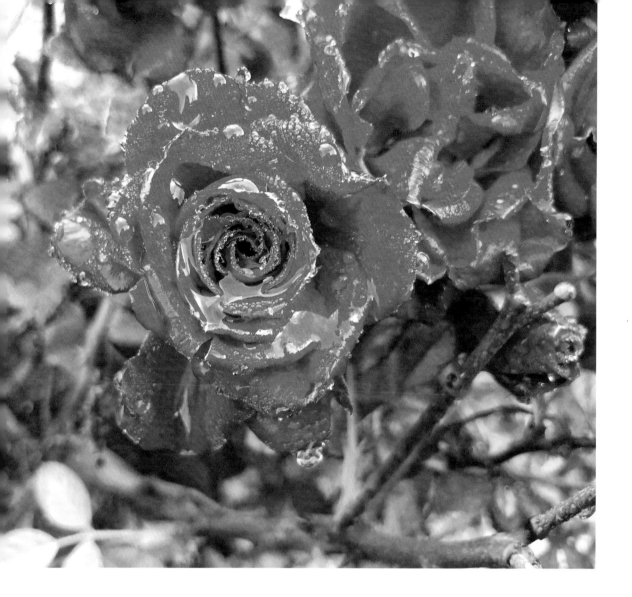

carbon dioxide, and other gases in and out of our respiratory system, ensure assimilation of nutrients through the GI tract, and provide protection from potential invasive pathogens.

The importance of proper hydration for health is drilled into us from an early age, and yet it is estimated that 70 percent of us—including children—are still chronically dehydrated. Recent literature suggests that all it takes is a 1 to 2 percent decrease in the body's water content to begin experiencing diminished functioning of essential body systems. To be properly hydrated, we need to think beyond the basic guidance of drinking eight glasses of water a day. Thankfully, there are plants that can help hydrate us much more effectively than water alone. Known as demulcents (page 175), these herbs have a gel-like, colloidal consistency that holds water like a sponge, releasing it slowly for optimal saturation.

When Our Hydration System Is Out of Balance

Thirst is not necessarily the first reliable signal that our body needs more water. By the time thirst arises, it's likely we're already in a state of mild dehydration—enough to experience a variety of detrimental effects.

When we run low on water, it's like a computer going into the power-save mode. The aspects of our physiology that require a lot of energy, like the brain, go a bit dim, leading to poor focus and concentration, muddled thinking, and vague feelings of anxiety or restlessness. We may become noticeably fatigued and prone to lightheadedness or low-grade headaches. It is easy to mistake these sensations for hunger, but often the real culprit is the need for water. If we feel low energy, it might be a message that we need to top off our fluids. This is particularly evident during heavy physical or mental exertion when the body is firing on all cylinders.

In the GI tract, a lack of water leads to weakened digestion—there just isn't enough juice to mix with and break down food. This, combined with dryness in the intestines, increases the time required for food to travel down the GI tract, which leads to constipation. The lack of moisture and lubrication contributes to inflammation in the gut lining, increased intestinal permeability, and hyperacidity. The thriving of our gut microbiome is also highly dependent on adequate hydration in the colon.

When we feel tightness and achiness in our muscles and joints, it's another sign we need to hydrate. Like the Tin Man in *The Wizard of Oz*, we get rusty and stiff without adequate lubrication. We become less flexible and suffer diminished physical endurance and capacity when we exercise. Our range of motion in muscles, tendons, ligaments, and joints is reduced, making us more susceptible to sprains and strains. Rebuilding muscles after exertion and/or recuperating from injuries also requires a lot of hydration.

11 SIGNS YOU MAY BE DEHYDRATED

1) Thirst

2) Dry mouth, eyes, lips

3) Dry skin and hair

4) Constipation

5) Foggy thinking

6) Dizziness or lightheadedness

7) Fatigue

8) Infrequent urination

9) Dark yellow urine

10) Headaches

11) Muscle cramps

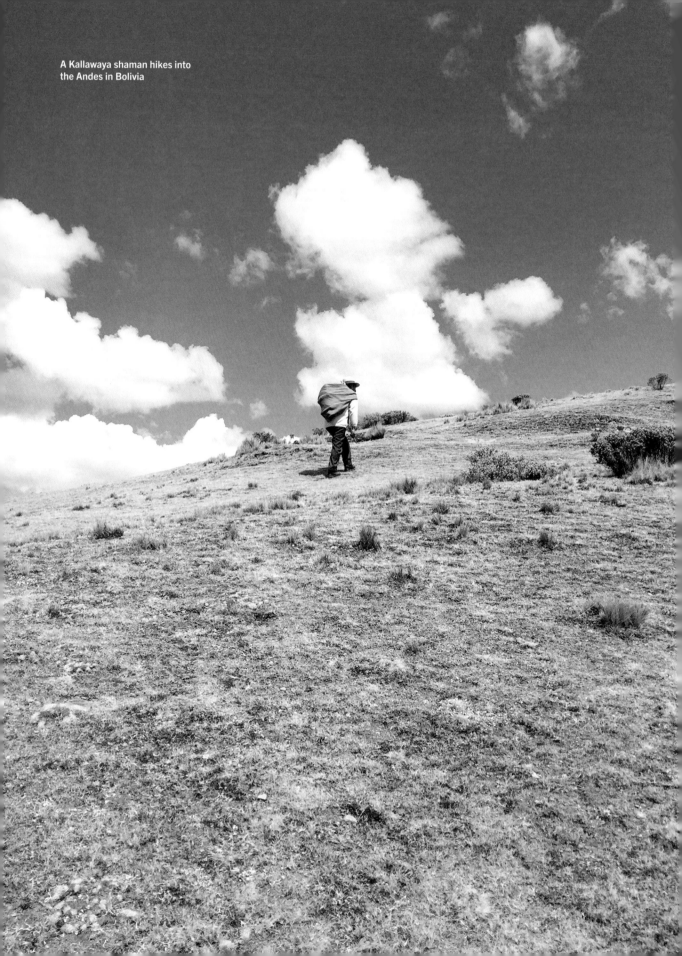
A Kallawaya shaman hikes into
the Andes in Bolivia

Core Energy
Adapt & Evolve

"It's not the strongest of the species that survives, nor the most intelligent that survives. It is the one that is most adaptable to change."
—CHARLES DARWIN

The pursuit of health is really part of a larger quest for a better quality of life, one in which we have abundant energy for all the things we want to do in the world. Our capacity to adjust to challenges and changes is a large part of what determines both the quality and quantity of energy we have access to. Life is a constant parade of demands that push us to reorient ourselves physically and mentally. The same physiological mechanisms of adaptation that enabled our ancestors to survive living in rugged conditions and harsh elements are still at work within us. The endocrine system continually adjusts our inner environment, adapting it to an outside world that is always in flux, balancing the intricate workings of the body with the frenzied rhythms of twenty-first-century life.

The amount of energy we have is a factor of both how much we can accumulate through food, water, oxygen, and other sources and how efficiently that energy is distributed throughout the body for core physiological functions such as metabolism, growth and development, mood and cognition, heart rate, sleep cycles, immunity, and reproductive capacity.

Both Traditional Chinese Medicine and Ayurveda have long recognized that wise management of our hormonal essence is the key to abundant energy. This concept—called *jing* in TCM and *ojas* in Ayurveda—represents the body's deepest reservoir of *potential* energy. Hormones are produced by the endocrine system to maintain the dynamic balance of our body systems and distribute energy for essential functions. They are precious resources that determine the rate at which we burn energy, like the flame in a lantern. The faster and brighter it burns, the quicker the oil is used up.

Continually trying to do more than we have the resources for is unsustainable and is one of the primary ways core energy gets depleted. Chronic and unproductive stress—our mind's anxious reaction to circumstances driving a physiological response—is another way energy reserves are exhausted.

The stress response to immediate threats, whether real or imagined, mobilizes resources and speeds up the rate at which energy is expended. Hormones like adrenaline, cortisol, and thyroid-stimulating hormone (TSH) accelerate heart and respiratory rates, raise glucose levels, and increase muscle tension, blood pressure, and the production of inflammatory chemistry. Once the threat has passed, the system dials everything back to ensure balance and recovery. Prolonged stress disrupts essential functions such as digestion, sleep, and immunity, setting the stage for deeper imbalances to manifest over time. Chronic stress is energy intensive: The more resources we spend sustaining stress physiology, the fewer are available to fuel other vital processes.

A balanced endocrine system has the flexibility to mount an efficient response to stress, spending only the energy needed to deal with the situation at hand and then quickly restoring physiology to a state of equilibrium. In other words, it has the ability to recognize unproductive stress and tone it down before it gets out of hand—thereby conserving energy for more important things. With a balanced endocrine system, our energy is steady and we're able to think with more clarity and focus. We have a sharper memory and a brighter mood. We become proactive rather than reactive in dealing with challenges and make better choices. We have a reliable, consistent libido, enhanced fertility, and deeper, more restorative sleep. We recover more quickly from physical and mental exertion. We are less likely to come down with opportunistic illnesses and become far less susceptible to developing chronic degenerative conditions like heart disease, diabetes, and autoimmune disorders.

The goal is having enough energy to get through our days feeling good and a surplus that lets us stretch beyond our perceived limits, so that we see change not as a stumbling block

Korean ginseng at a market in Seoul, South Korea

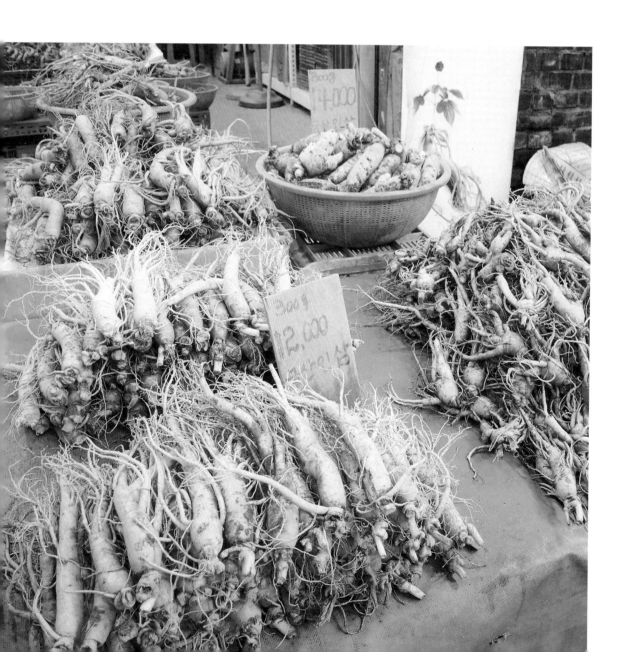

but as a catalyst for growth and opportunity to step out of our comfort zones. With this orientation, our relationship to many stressors can be developmental and transformational. Like athletic training, delivering a big presentation at work, or the feeling of nervous anticipation before a first date, challenges can lead to breakthroughs and higher levels of performance. Pushing boundaries and being an excited participant in life are indicators of a healthy, well-regulated endocrine system with powerful adaptive capabilities.

We can enhance our body's ability to adjust to life's changing demands using medicinal plants known as adaptogens (page 235). Adaptogens improve the way our endocrine system responds to stress and restore the body to a state of equilibrium.

handle even life's small changes and challenges is diminished. Fundamental rhythms underlying sleep, digestion, elimination, and menstruation, among others, become noticeably disrupted.

When our energy reserves become depleted, we're more susceptible to injuries and slow to recuperate. We catch colds and flus more often, and they linger longer than they should. Stress diverts energy we otherwise need for deep immunological functions and the maintenance and daily repair of our cells. Every major chronic health issue has stress-fueled depletion as some aspect of its origin.

When Our Core Energy Is Out of Balance

Overextending ourselves—forcing our body to exert physical and mental resources beyond its capacity—means an unsustainable reliance on stress chemistry as a default source of energy. This can be so hardwired in us that we don't even realize it's happening. Even the way we respond to positive life events can be driven by subtle anxieties and pressures that keep a low-level stress response simmering. That's why stress is known as the "silent killer"—it becomes the norm rather than the exception, sapping vitality needed to maintain essential systems along the way. The longer stress and tension go on, the greater the degree of imbalance and the more systems become impacted.

When we're under chronic stress, the recuperative response becomes inadequate and fails to really restore us. Just when we conclude one stress cycle, another starts right up. It's like riding a stress roller coaster, making us feel fatigued, tapped out, and lacking a zest for life. Our endurance wanes, and we become brittle, tense, and emotionally reactive. Our capacity to

12 SIGNS YOUR CORE ENERGY IS OUT OF BALANCE

1) Fatigue

2) Digestive issues

3) Chronic insomnia

4) Low libido

5) Irregular menstrual cycle, PMS, fertility issues

6) Achy joints, lower-back pain

7) Hair loss

8) High blood pressure

9) Weight loss or gain

10) Craving sugar/stimulants, addictions

11) Certain autoimmune conditions

12) Frequent colds or flus

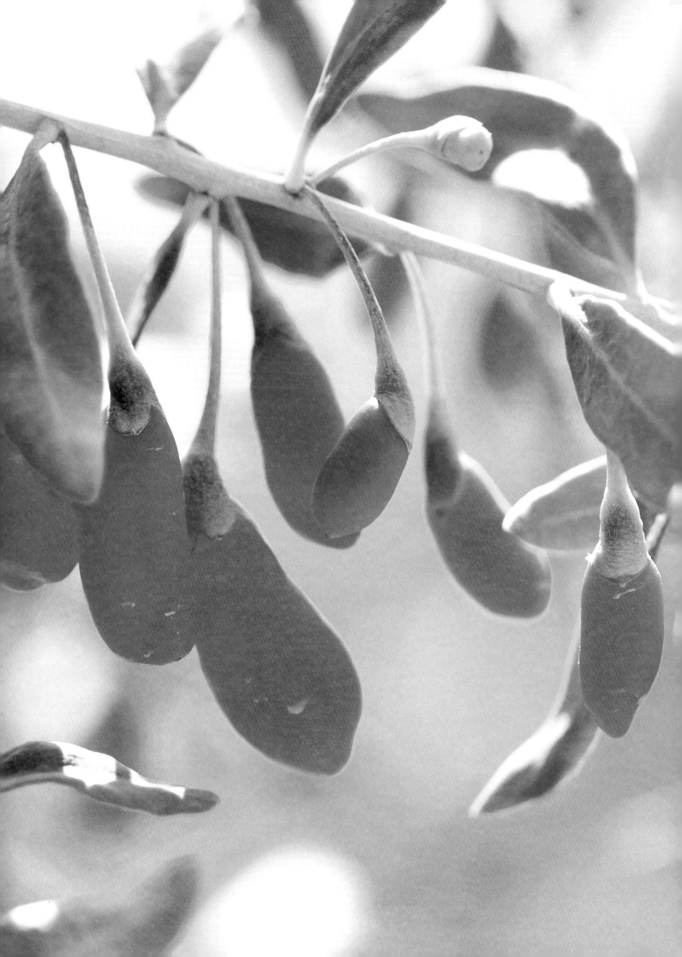

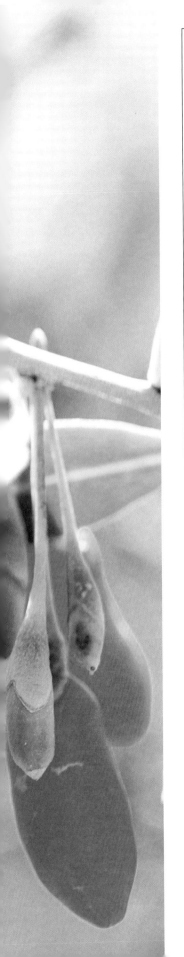

Medicinal Plant Categories

AS A SPECIES, WE EVOLVED EATING HIGHLY DIVERSE DIETS that included wild and medicinal plants abundant in health-enhancing phytochemicals. These days, the average diet includes fewer than twenty out of literally thousands of edible plants. As a result, most of us are experiencing a real phytochemical deficiency, with serious implications for our health.

Plants produce phytochemicals to defend against opportunistic insects and microbes, protect them from too much sun and harsh elements, retain moisture, signal neighboring plants, and attract pollinators—in addition to many other reasons we're just beginning to understand. Phytochemicals are what give plants their vibrant colors, flavors, and aromas. All plants produce phytochemicals, yet medicinal plants contain a wider variety and richer concentration than the cultivated crops that are the mainstay of our diet. This is because medicinal plants are closer to their wild origins, where they developed potent chemistry to help them adapt to their challenging environments.

Science has discovered more than twenty-five thousand distinct phytochemicals, many of which have established benefits for our health. Phytochemicals have been shown to reduce inflammation, boost immunity, protect against damage by free radicals (unstable atoms that harm healthy cells), increase metabolic flexibility, and activate cellular mechanisms to increase longevity. The more of these compounds we consume on a regular basis—and the wider the range and variety—the healthier we will be. There is no RDA minimum daily requirement for phytochemicals like there is for vitamins and minerals, yet given their proven benefits, we clearly cannot attain optimal health without phytochemical-rich medicinal plants.

Each of the categories of medicinal plants presented here complements and enhances the functioning of the specific body systems discussed on pages 37–57.

The Potency Spectrum

All of the plants that we consume for food and medicine occupy a spectrum. On one end are plants we commonly eat as part of a healthy diet: fruits, vegetables, nuts, seeds, grains, and legumes. On the other end are potent medicinal plants primarily used to treat acute illness under the guidance of a professional. As we move from the familiar side of the spectrum to the potent side, flavors and aromas become stronger and plants become more concentrated with micronutrients and phytochemistry, benefiting and enriching health in myriad ways. This book is focused on the plants that are staples in the everyday lives of most of the healthiest people around the world.

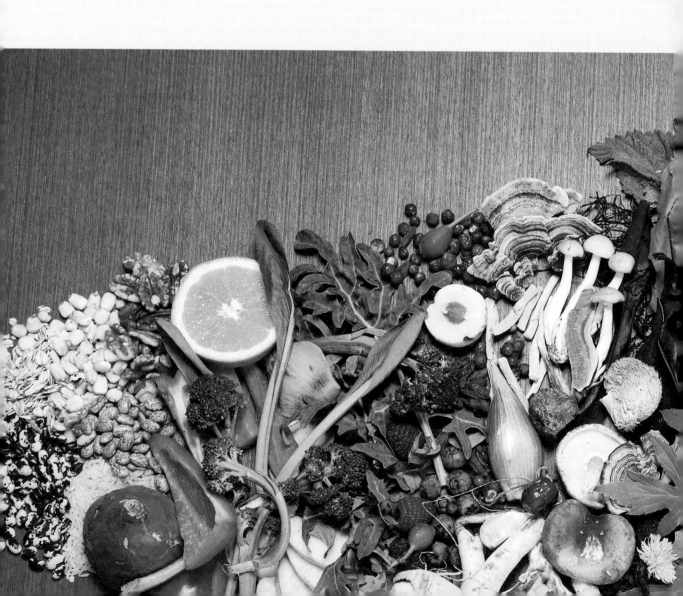

When do vegetables and food plants morph into medicinal plants? It happens somewhere around the dark leafy green zone. From there we arrive at wild greens like dandelions and nettles; super berries like acai, schisandra, and goji; tonic roots like ginseng, shatavari, and ashwagandha; and immune-boosting mushrooms such as reishi, maitake, and chaga. Further along are aromatic herbs like chamomile and peppermint, green tea, bitters, and culinary spices like turmeric, ginger, and rosemary that are rich in essential oils. All of these plants are abundant in beneficial healing compounds and vital nutrients.

The stronger the medicinal plant, the less we need to consume to get the beneficial effects. Plants for the home apothecary, like echinacea and andrographis, are used primarily as antimicrobial immune stimulators in cases of colds, flus, and minor infections. At the very far end of the spectrum are those powerful plants needed only occasionally and preferably administered under the guidance of a professional. These medicinal plants are still biocompatible relative to synthetic drugs, but their constituents are too potent for long-term use or inclusion in a daily diet.

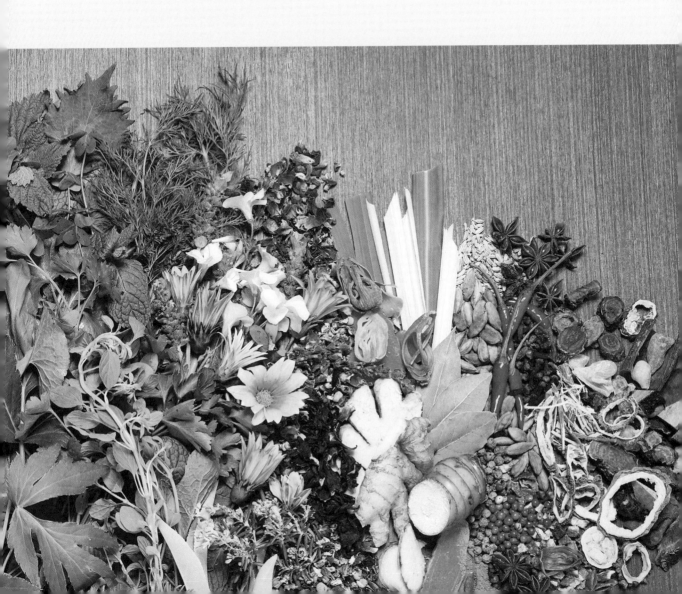

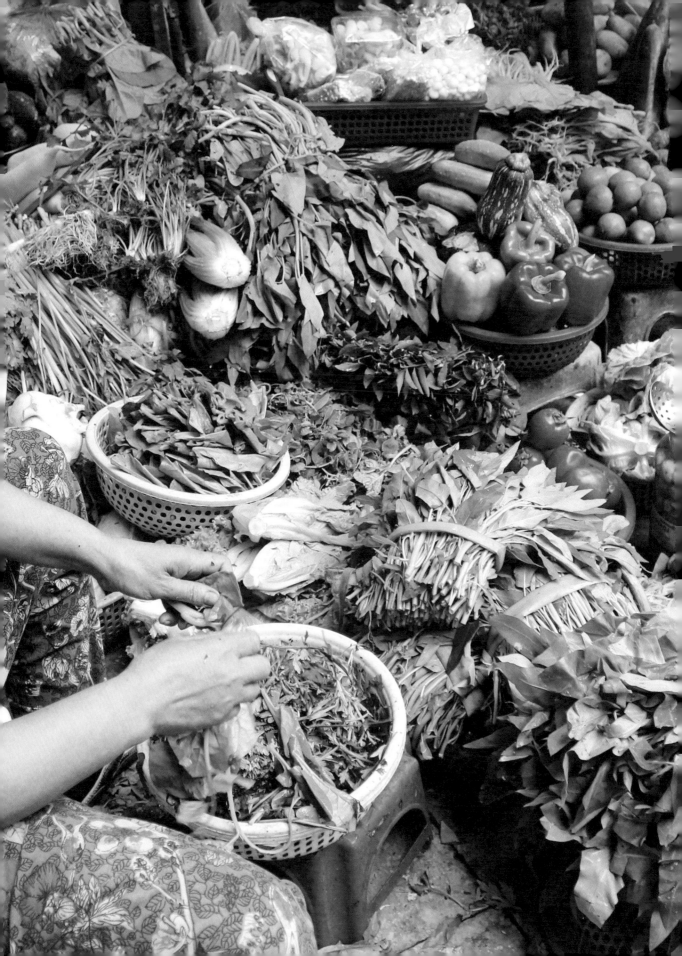

Culinary Herbs & Spices | FLAVORFUL & AROMATIC PLANTS THAT KINDLE THE METABOLISM

Culinary herbs and spices have always been the foundation of the world's healthiest cuisines. Traditional diets developed as both art and science, the centerpiece of enduring cultures. Beyond their tantalizing flavors and aromas, culinary herbs and spices are some of the most powerful and readily accessible medicinal plants available to us, with wide-ranging, health-enhancing effects.

Most spices originate in hot, sunny places—like the tropics and Mediterranean regions—where there is an abundance of solar energy. Plants soak up sunlight and transform it into pungent, aromatic compounds they store in their seeds, leaves, bark, and roots. When we consume these spices, that stored sunlight is transferred to us, igniting our metabolic fire and kindling agni (digestive fire). Aromatic oils within spices increase circulation to the digestive system, stimulating production of the hydrochloric acid and enzymes that break down our food, enhance nutrient absorption, increase energy, and prevent excess gas and bloating.

In addition to their digestive-enhancing benefits (and obvious sensory appeal), culinary herbs and spices have powerful antimicrobial effects. Countless invisible microbes hitching a ride on our food end up in our GI tract, where the harmful ones are filtered out by the immune system. Some herbs and spices are particularly potent at neutralizing pathogens, including wasabi (Japanese horseradish), oregano, thyme, and garlic. The antimicrobial constituents in these plants are also highly biocompatible, meaning they won't harm the friendly bacteria living in our gut. In fact, their abundance of beneficial phytochemicals provides a valuable source of nourishment to the microbiome.

Culinary herbs and spices are some of the most antioxidant-rich plants we can consume. Having daily doses of spices such as turmeric, ginger, cinnamon, and garlic in our food is an excellent way to reduce inflammation and prevent free radical damage to healthy cells. Compared with other plants like leafy greens or blueberries, they are far more concentrated in antioxidants—meaning you don't need to eat a bowl of turmeric or ginger for dinner. Consuming small servings of these powerful plants on a consistent basis will produce these and many other substantial benefits over time.

A vendor selling culinary herbs at a market in Hanoi, Vietnam

KEY CULINARY HERBS AND SPICES

Allspice	Cloves	Horseradish (wasabi)	Red pepper flakes
Basil	Coriander	Lemongrass	Rosemary
Bay leaf	Cumin	Mace	Saffron
Black pepper	Dill	Mustard seed	Sage
Cardamom	Fennel	Nutmeg	Star anise
Cayenne pepper	Fenugreek	Oregano	Thyme
Chile	Galangal	Pandan leaf	Turmeric
Chives	Garlic	Paprika	Vanilla
Cilantro	Ginger	Parsley	
Cinnamon	Green pepper	Red pepper	

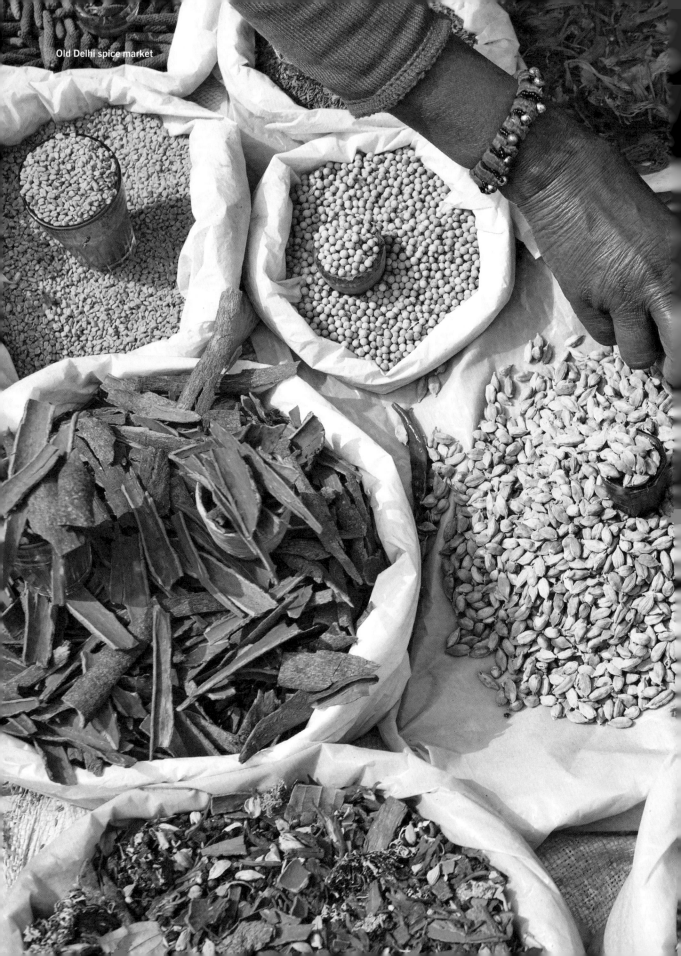
Old Delhi spice market

THE INDIAN DIET: A SYMPHONY OF SPICE

The Cardamom Hills of Kerala in Southern India are a unique eco-zone and UNESCO World Heritage Site famous for their immense biodiversity, including massive spice forests found only in this region. Throughout these forests, tangled vines of black pepper wind their way up the cinnamon, nutmeg, clove, and allspice trees, which in turn offered dappled shade to fields of turmeric, ginger, and cardamom growing below. The plants growing in these medicinal forests are a vast repository of unique and healthful compounds essential for maintaining health.

India is a great example of a country that truly reveres the power of spice. Every meal features a wide assortment of condiments and aromatic spices including all kinds of chutneys (from mint-coriander to ginger and amla berry), aromatic bowls of toasted cumin and coriander, and main courses that are legendary for their robust sauces and curry spice blends of turmeric, ginger, cumin, cardamom, fennel, and coriander. At meal's end, it's customary to sip a small cup of warm chai tea infused with still more spice: cinnamon, ginger, cardamom, or cloves. By the time the meal is done, the body is zinging with vitality and infused with unique phytochemicals and antioxidants that, over time, accumulate and provide significant benefits to our health.

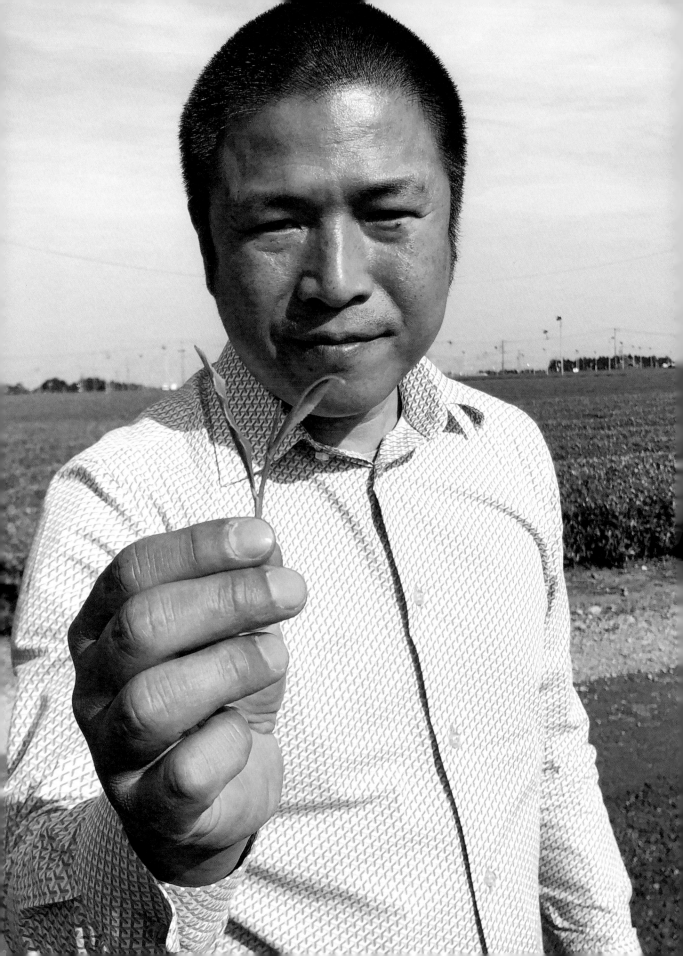

Bitters & Detoxifying Herbs | REVITALIZING PLANTS FOR DAILY RENEWAL

We've largely lost our taste for the bitter flavor in modern life, yet before they were fully domesticated, most of the plants we ate contained at least some bitter constituents. We regularly ingested small amounts of bitter plant compounds, which kept the body's digestion and detox mechanisms toned through a hormetic effect—that is, the physiologic benefit of consuming small doses of compounds that mildly stimulate our biological systems to respond. Reacquiring our appreciation for bitter-tasting plants and making a habit of adding small amounts into our daily routine are essential for optimal health.

Regular consumption of mildly bitter medicinal herbs and plants provides a gentle yet effective "daily detox" that improves the elimination of wastes, enhances digestion, and increases energy. The constituents in bitter herbs activate our detoxification mechanisms, encouraging these vital organs to more effectively process the many metabolic toxins they are responsible for removing. When we taste something bitter, it activates receptors on the tongue and triggers a reflex that increases circulation and sends currents of nerve energy to the stomach, pancreas, liver, and gallbladder. This action benefits digestion and elimination by increasing the output of saliva, enzymes, bile, and hydrochloric acid, helping the liver break down fats, stimulating peristalsis, and reducing acidity, gas, and bloating. Bitter herbs also influence important hormones that balance blood sugar, control appetite, and improve cholesterol metabolism.

Bitter herbs are most commonly consumed around mealtimes. In many European countries, they are distilled into exotic-tasting liquors to be enjoyed in small amounts as aperitifs (before meals) or digestifs (after meals). These tonics, often made from recipes passed down generation to generation, contain herbs like centaury, artichoke leaf, angelica root, wormwood, gentian root, and thistle. Many Mediterranean dishes include fresh or lightly cooked bitter greens like dandelion leaves, mustard, endives, cress, and chicory. Teas and wines made from unripe citrus peels and various fruits with both bitter and sour flavors are staples in Asia. In North America, there is a long-standing tradition of concocting springtime "purification tonics" using common herbs such as red clover, chickweed, and dandelion combined with a variety of bitter roots and barks like sarsaparilla, sassafras, and burdock root—the original root beers.

Our matcha supplier showing us a variety of green tea in Shizuoka, Japan

KEY BITTERS & DETOXIFYING HERBS

Artichoke leaf	Citrus peels	Guayusa	Sourgrass
Arugula	Coffee	Mastic resin	Tatsoi
Bitter melon	Dandelion greens	Milk thistle seed	Triphala powder
Bitters formulas	Dandelion root	Mizuna	Watercress
Burdock root	Dandy Blend	Mustard greens	Yerba maté
Cacao	Endive	Neem	
Carob	Gentian root	Olive leaf	
Chicory root	Green tea	Radicchio	

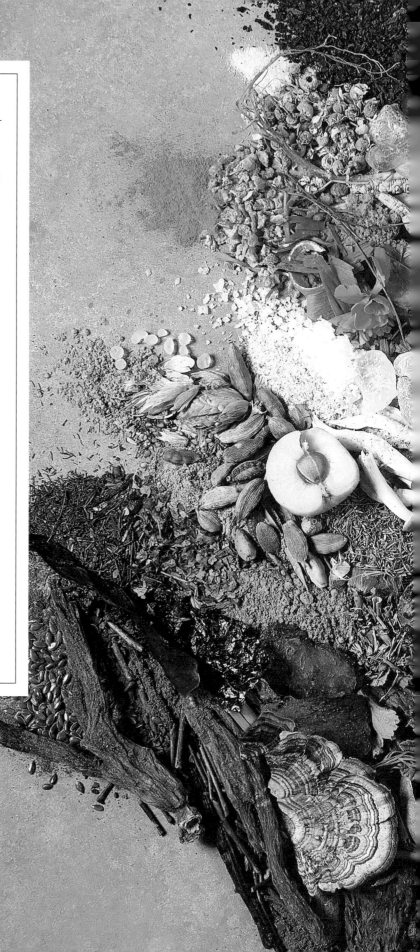

FLAVOR = ENERGY

Both Traditional Chinese Medicine and Ayurveda emphasize a diet full of flavor as a requirement for optimal health, and nowhere is diversity of flavor more abundant than in medicinal plants. TCM classically recognizes five main flavors: sweet, salty, sour, bitter, and pungent/spicy. Everything we eat is some combination of these flavors, and traditional medicine recommends ingesting some of all of them every day, ideally in each meal.

Medicinal plants get their flavors from the phytochemicals they contain. When these flavors contact receptor sites on our tongue, it generates a small electrochemical charge that transmits vital energy into our system, activating our physiology in unique and powerful ways. The more flavors we ingest, the more vital energy circulates through our physiology, enhancing the way our body functions as a whole. Adopting a diet rich in medicinal plants means expanding our palate to include a wide array of flavors—a highly enjoyable prescription for good health.

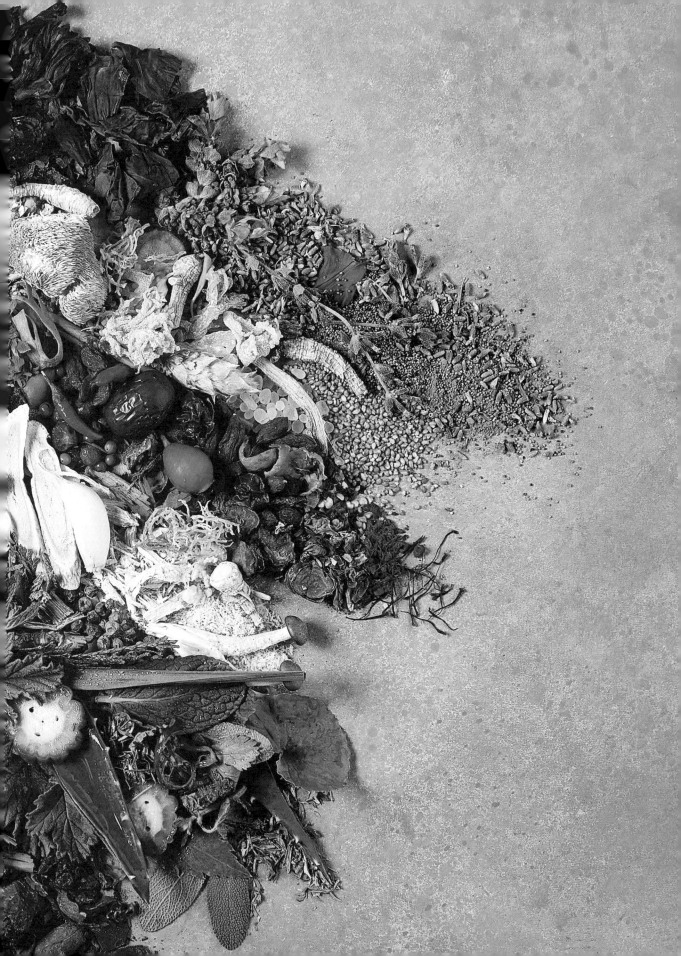

Nutritives | NUTRIENT-DENSE PLANTS THAT INVIGORATE, SUSTAIN, AND NOURISH

These days, it isn't a stretch to say that almost everyone is deficient in many of the vital micronutrients the body requires to function in an optimal way. Even small deficiencies can cause significantly diminished performance in our essential body functions. I often give new patients infusions made with nutritives (nutrient-dense herbs and berries) as a necessary first step in any health optimization protocol. These plants are invaluable reservoirs of rare and essential vitamins, minerals, trace elements, and antioxidants that are otherwise challenging to obtain solely from the plants commonly found in the Western diet.

Nutritives accumulate the micronutrients that play a crucial role in our physiology, from building the structure of bones, teeth, and connective tissue to catalyzing all of the enzymatic and biochemical reactions that are the basis of metabolism. They provide the spark that ignites all of our key health-sustaining functions, including immunity, detoxification, cognitive function, digestion, hormonal balance, and energy production. Nutritives also tend to have gentle cleansing effects: Their plentiful antioxidants and mild bitter constituents support and activate the organs of detoxification and filtration (like the liver and kidneys, colon, and skin), improving the removal of wastes and toxins.

While it's common and often beneficial to use supplements to fill our nutritional gaps, the body has evolved to absorb its nutrients best from plants. Vitamin isolates in supplements are often not well absorbed, especially if there are underlying gut issues. The nutrients in plants are packaged in an organic matrix of synergistic compounds, making them highly bioavailable and thus easy to assimilate. Regular consumption of nutritive plants fills the body's reservoirs with micronutrients, keeping it humming along like a fine-tuned machine.

Nutritive plants come in many forms and flavors. There are leafy green nettles, moringa, and gotu kola; tart antioxidant-rich superfruits like amla, goji, and acai berries; and sea vegetables dulse, nori, and kombu that contain trace elements from the ocean. You'll often find nutritives packaged as "superfoods" in the grocery store, yet in many countries they aren't expensive or considered particularly exotic—for more on this, see page 72.

Acai berry harvest in Brazil

KEY NUTRITIVES

Acai berries	Chicory root	Lingonberry	Raspberry leaf
Alfalfa leaf	Cilantro	Jujube dates	Red clover
Amla berries	Elderberries	Moringa	Rose hips
Aronia berries	Gotu kola	Nettles	Sea vegetables
Ashitaba	Hawthorn berries	Nori	Shiso leaf
Bellflower	Hibiscus	Oat tops	
Burdock root	Horsetail	Oatstraw	
Camu camu	Kombu	Parsley	

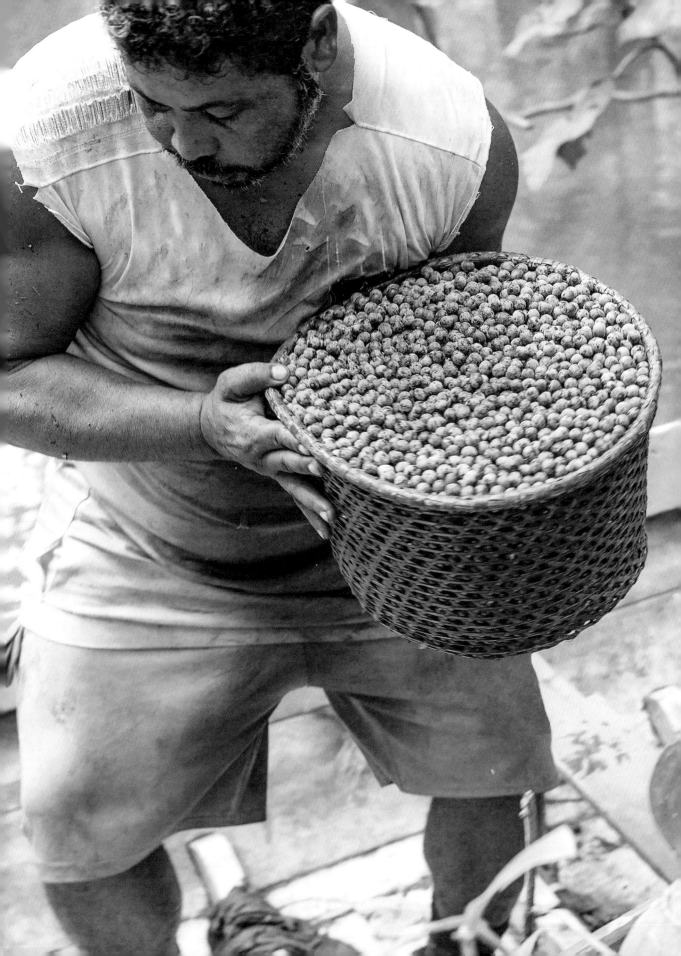

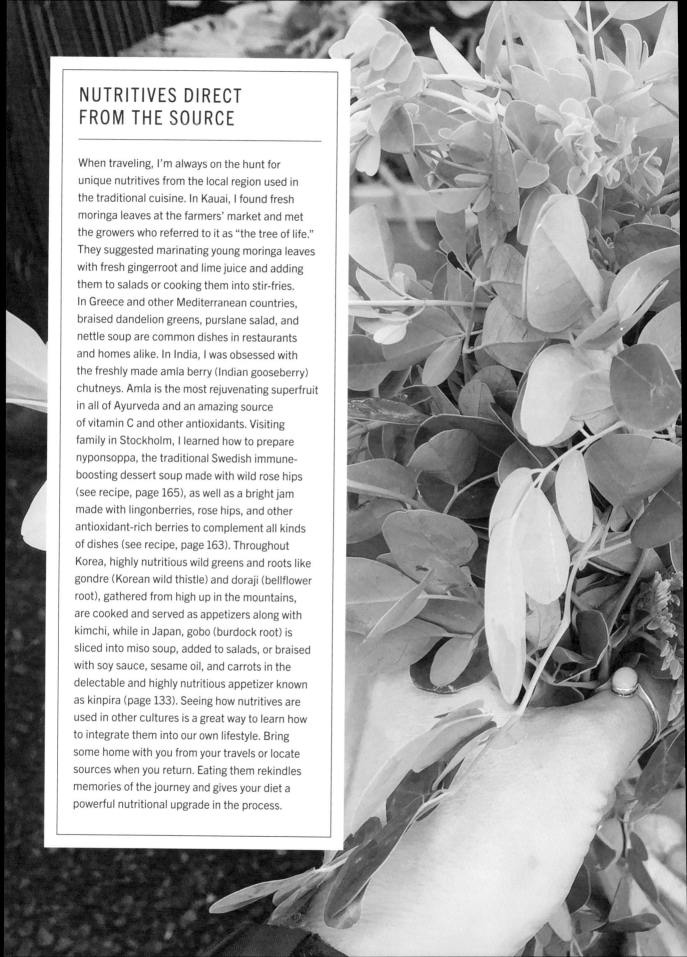

NUTRITIVES DIRECT FROM THE SOURCE

When traveling, I'm always on the hunt for unique nutritives from the local region used in the traditional cuisine. In Kauai, I found fresh moringa leaves at the farmers' market and met the growers who referred to it as "the tree of life." They suggested marinating young moringa leaves with fresh gingerroot and lime juice and adding them to salads or cooking them into stir-fries. In Greece and other Mediterranean countries, braised dandelion greens, purslane salad, and nettle soup are common dishes in restaurants and homes alike. In India, I was obsessed with the freshly made amla berry (Indian gooseberry) chutneys. Amla is the most rejuvenating superfruit in all of Ayurveda and an amazing source of vitamin C and other antioxidants. Visiting family in Stockholm, I learned how to prepare nyponsoppa, the traditional Swedish immune-boosting dessert soup made with wild rose hips (see recipe, page 165), as well as a bright jam made with lingonberries, rose hips, and other antioxidant-rich berries to complement all kinds of dishes (see recipe, page 163). Throughout Korea, highly nutritious wild greens and roots like gondre (Korean wild thistle) and doraji (bellflower root), gathered from high up in the mountains, are cooked and served as appetizers along with kimchi, while in Japan, gobo (burdock root) is sliced into miso soup, added to salads, or braised with soy sauce, sesame oil, and carrots in the delectable and highly nutritious appetizer known as kinpira (page 133). Seeing how nutritives are used in other cultures is a great way to learn how to integrate them into our own lifestyle. Bring some home with you from your travels or locate sources when you return. Eating them rekindles memories of the journey and gives your diet a powerful nutritional upgrade in the process.

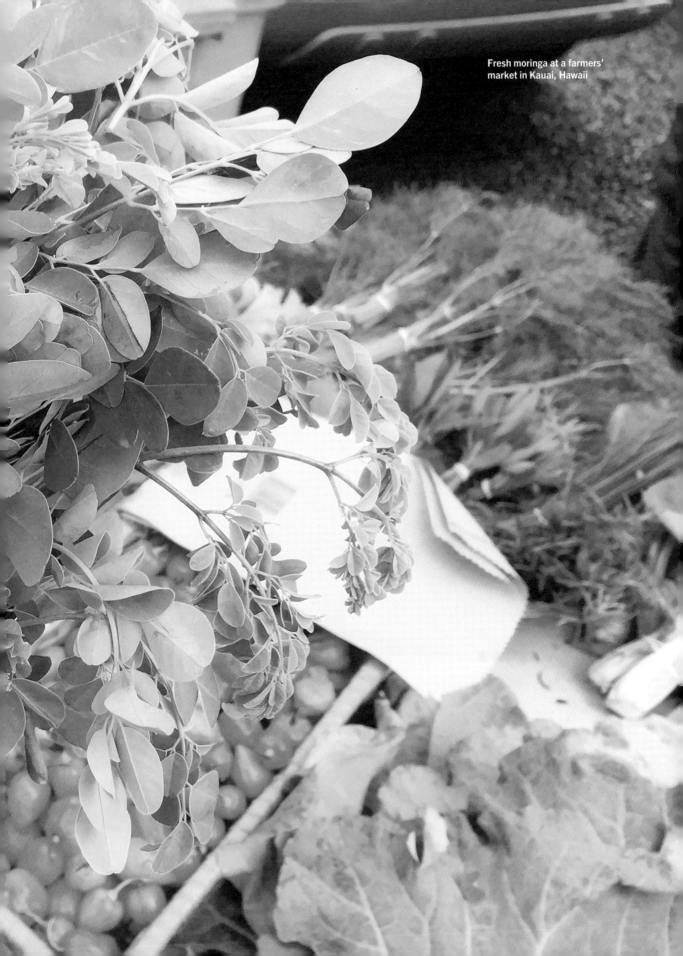

Fresh moringa at a farmers' market in Kauai, Hawaii

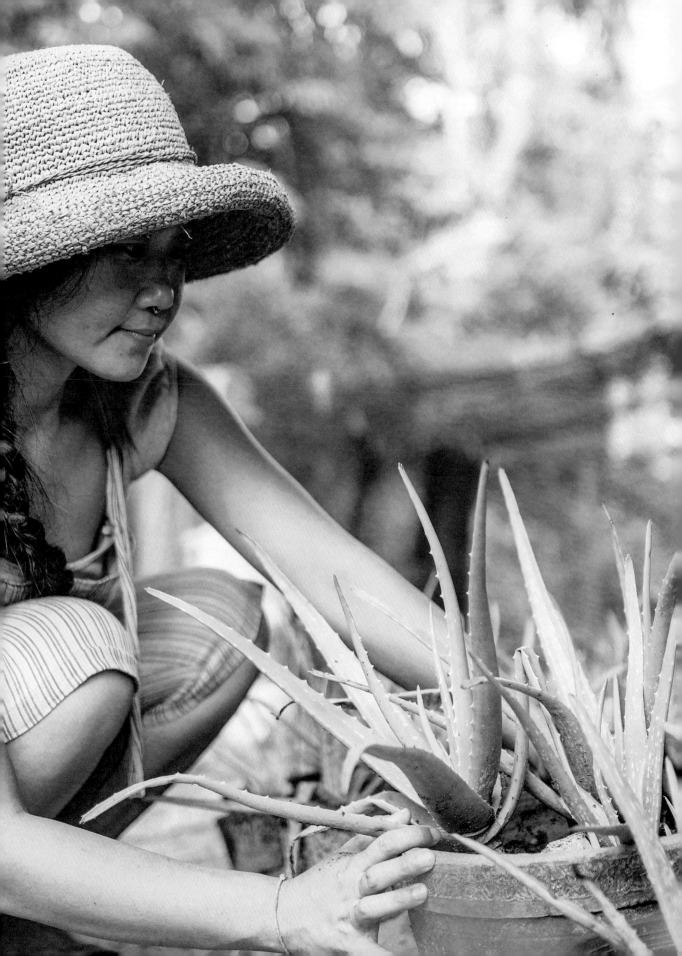

Demulcents | WATER-RICH PLANTS FOR DEEP, REPLENISHING HYDRATION

The word *demulcent* comes from the Latin *demulcere*, meaning "to caress," referring to the deeply soothing, moisturizing, and cooling effects these special plants have on the body. The gentle healing and hydrating benefits of demulcents come from their abundant content of gel, oil, and/or mucilage (a polysaccharide-rich fiber that transforms into a thick, viscous solution when mixed with water). This "plant water" acts like time-release hydration, allowing the body to fully absorb the liquid's moisture as it slowly makes its way down the GI tract—in contrast to the way it sometimes feels as if the water we drink is running right through us. Consuming demulcent beverages is more like eating water than drinking it. Adding powdered demulcents like slippery elm, marshmallow, and shatavari or seeds like chia or basil to water in small amounts throughout the day is an excellent way to enhance systemic hydration or quickly replenish lost moisture.

The delicate "inner skin" lining our respiratory system, sinuses, urinary, and GI tracts can easily become dried out and inflamed. Demulcent herbs moisten these mucous membranes and form a protective coating over them that allows healing and repair to take place underneath. This action helps reinforce the integrity and barrier function in the GI tract, preventing infiltration of pathogens and decreasing the excess permeability that occurs in conditions like "leaky gut." The mucilage and gel in demulcents act as a buffer, neutralizing excess gastric acids and inflammatory chemistry. They provide quick relief for conditions like heartburn and acid reflux while protecting sensitive tissues like the esophagus from potential damage.

Demulcents also provide our microbiome with a nourishing boost of easily digested, prebiotic-rich soluble fiber that offers a valuable source of sustenance to our friendly bacteria. You'll often find demulcents like psyllium husk, slippery elm bark, marshmallow root, Jerusalem artichoke, and licorice root at the top of the ingredient list in fiber blends for intestinal health. The mucilaginous consistency of the fiber gently lubricates and tones the lower GI tract, binding up harmful toxins and improving elimination. This unique form of fiber also helps balance blood sugar by slowing the absorption of glucose into the bloodstream.

Rehydrating with demulcents after a long night's sleep is one of the simplest and healthiest habits we can establish. Morning hydration is vital for flushing accumulated toxins, increasing energy, activating metabolism, and jump-starting the brain. Adding demulcent herbs like chia or basil seeds and a chunk of aloe gel to our morning glass of water amplifies its hydrating power.

Harvesting aloe

KEY DEMULCENTS

Aloe vera	Jerusalem artichoke	Olive oil
Basil seeds	Licorice root	Plantain leaf
Buckwheat	Linden flower	Psyllium husk
Chan seeds	Linden leaf	Shatavari root
Chia seeds	Manuka honey	Slippery elm bark
Irish moss	Marshmallow root	

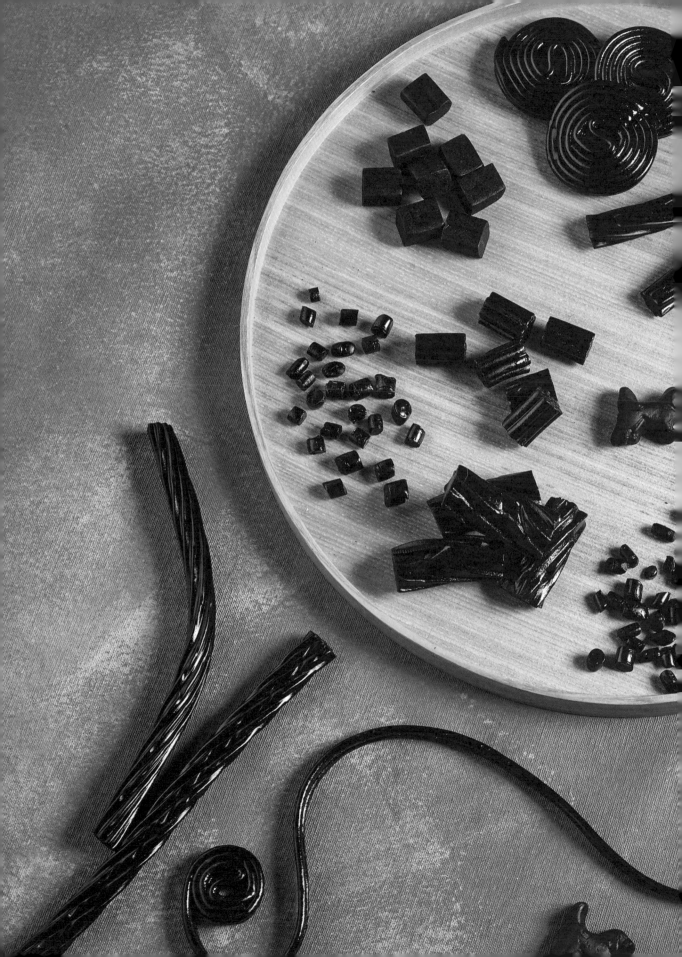

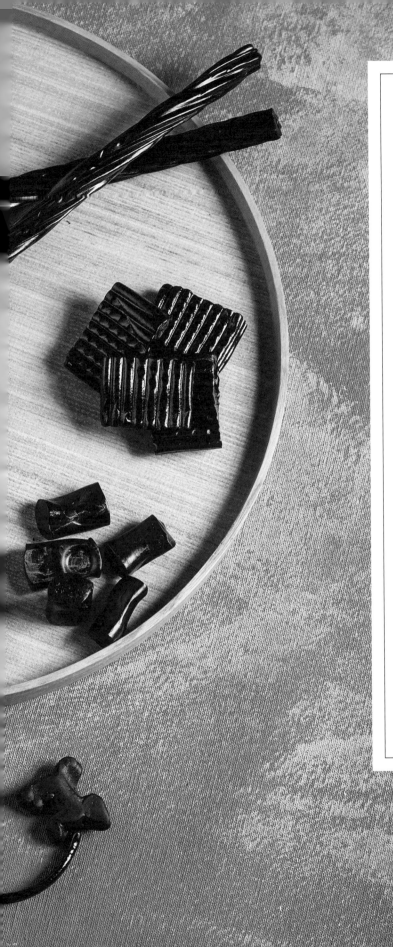

SOOTHING SWEETS: LICORICE IN SCANDINAVIA

Licorice is known as the "great harmonizer" in TCM for its soothing, moistening, and cooling properties, and because it improves the flavor and digestibility of whatever it's combined with. Black licorice candies containing real licorice have a long history of traditional use as a medicinal treat. Northern Europeans love real licorice candy, and an artisanal tradition has thrived there for more than four hundred years (it's called *lakrids* in Sweden, *lakkris* in Iceland, *lakrids* in Denmark, *lakris* in Norway, and *lakritsi* in Finland, in case you're on the lookout). In these countries, all licorice is black, and what North Americans refer to as black licorice is called "sweet licorice" to distinguish it from the salty varieties. Scandinavians prefer their licorice strong, and the salty variety is called *salmiakki*. A blend of sweet and salty, this type of licorice is an acquired taste, mostly appreciated by the intermediate to advanced licorice eater. The Dutch are the world champs of licorice eating, with each citizen eating up to 4 pounds (1.8 kg) on average per year. Take it from the residents of the happiest countries on earth, eating real licorice is a delicious and effective way to enjoy your daily dose of demulcency.

Nervines | RELAXING PLANTS FOR CREATING FREE FLOW

Nervines are medicinal plants that relax tension, calm the mind, elevate mood, improve cognitive function, deepen sleep, and generally facilitate the smooth flow of nerve impulses throughout the body. By fostering feelings of ease and calm, nervines help establish a renewed sense of mind-body integration. Their calmative actions have both immediate effects and long-term restorative benefits that create greater balance in the nervous system over time. Many nervines provide subtle relaxation throughout the day while maintaining the alertness necessary to carry on normal activity. These plants create a state of flow rather than sedation. They free up stagnant qi and, by doing so, liberate energy that was previously bound up in tension. When nerve energy flows freely, we feel more relaxed, energized, and uplifted all at the same time.

There are several groups of herbs within the overall category of nervines. Fragrant relaxants are perhaps the most widely known and commonly used. Herbs like chamomile, linden, lemon balm, peppermint, and lavender contain aromatic essential oils that gently and reliably reduce tension and elevate the mood through antispasmodic, anti-inflammatory, and circulation-enhancing actions. Drinking them as teas or infusions relaxes the dense accumulation of enteric nerves lining our gut, improving digestion and assimilation and alleviating common digestive issues such as excess gas and bloating.

Nervine calmatives are more potent in their action and stronger in their capacity to chill us out, creating a more sedative, relaxing effect that's useful in the evening or during times of heightened stress or anxiety. Herbs like skullcap, California poppy, passionflower, CBD (cannabis), kava, hops, and valerian root unravel knots in our nervous system at a deeper level. These stronger-acting nervines are especially useful for alleviating chronic stress, insomnia,

tension, and/or pain. They can be taken long term to help restore a depleted and exhausted nervous system, and are equally beneficial for easing acute pain related to tension such as headaches, menstrual cramps, sports injuries, muscular strain, and TMJ syndrome.

Finally, aromatic essential oils are an important category of nervines for soothing what Traditional Chinese Medicine refers to as our shen, or spirit. Shen corresponds to the most subtle aspects of our nervous system, the deep subconscious link between thinking and feeling. Having healthy shen means being in the present moment and not habitually reacting to our thoughts and emotions. Aromatic resins, woods, and essential oils create elevated states of mind, clearing away static and enhancing clarity, awareness, and presence. They contain a variety of compounds that, when inhaled, stimulate the production of specific neurotransmitters like serotonin, acetylcholine, dopamine, and endorphins, relaxing us and shifting our state of consciousness.

I often recommend that people diffuse their favorite floral oils throughout the day to create a background atmosphere of calm. The power of this ritual lies in the subtle way the aromatic molecules permeate the nervous system and subconsciously shift our brain wave patterns. If you're on the go, carrying a bottle of oil with you and doing some direct palm inhalations (see page 202) throughout the day creates mini-moments of space and calm and gets the good vibes going.

The more we engage in this inhalation ritual, the stronger our association with it and a sense of calm becomes. Over time, this contributes to the development of new neural networks that reinforce and strengthen the oils' effects.

Linden flowers in Provence, France

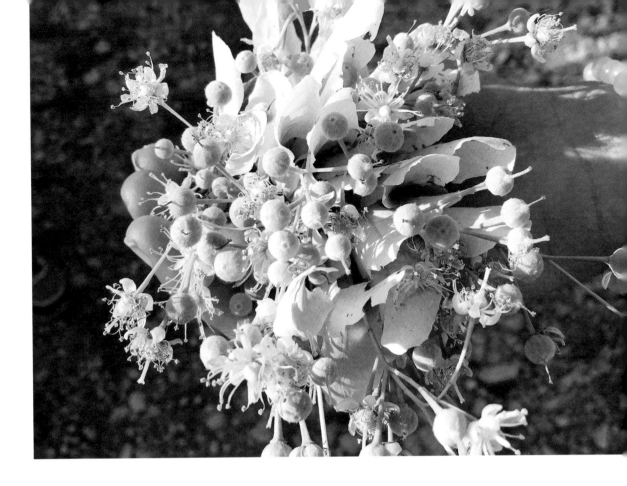

KEY FRAGRANT RELAXANTS

Chamomile

Greek mountain tea

Honeybush/rooibos

Lavender

Lemon balm

Lemon verbena

Linden flower

Linden leaf

Mint

Rose petals

Saffron

Tulsi

KEY NERVINE CALMATIVES

California poppy

Cannabis/CBD

Hops

Kava

Nutmeg

Passionflower

Poppy seeds

Skullcap

Valerian root

KEY AROMATIC ESSENTIAL OILS & RESINS

Agarwood

Citrus oils (mandarin, orange, lemon, grapefruit)

Clary sage

Frankincense

Geranium

Jasmine

Lavender

Neroli

Palo santo

Rose

Sandalwood

Ylang-ylang

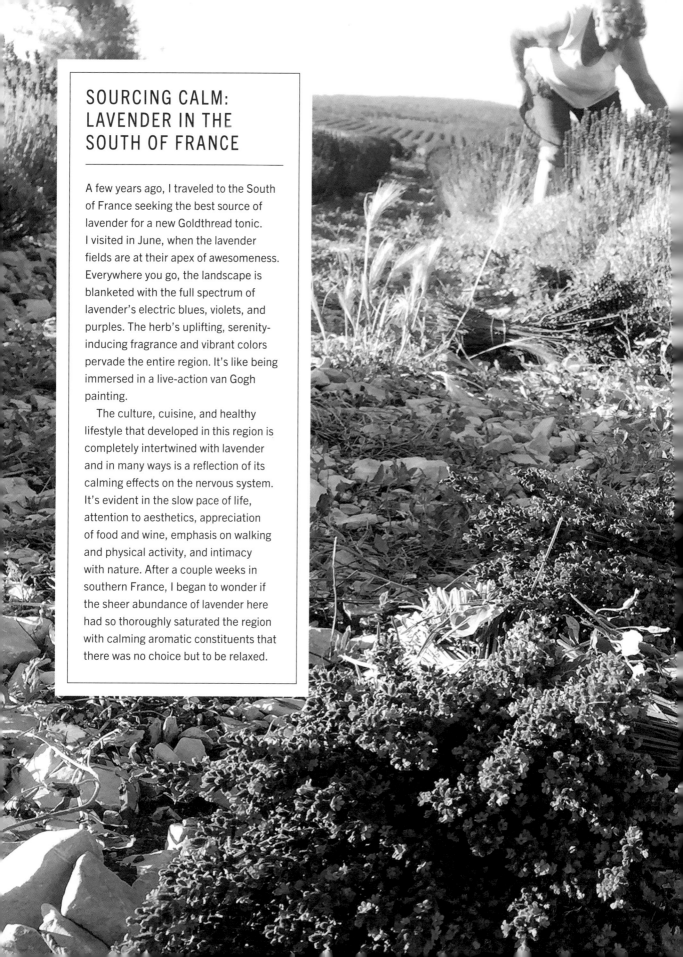

SOURCING CALM: LAVENDER IN THE SOUTH OF FRANCE

A few years ago, I traveled to the South of France seeking the best source of lavender for a new Goldthread tonic. I visited in June, when the lavender fields are at their apex of awesomeness. Everywhere you go, the landscape is blanketed with the full spectrum of lavender's electric blues, violets, and purples. The herb's uplifting, serenity-inducing fragrance and vibrant colors pervade the entire region. It's like being immersed in a live-action van Gogh painting.

The culture, cuisine, and healthy lifestyle that developed in this region is completely intertwined with lavender and in many ways is a reflection of its calming effects on the nervous system. It's evident in the slow pace of life, attention to aesthetics, appreciation of food and wine, emphasis on walking and physical activity, and intimacy with nature. After a couple weeks in southern France, I began to wonder if the sheer abundance of lavender here had so thoroughly saturated the region with calming aromatic constituents that there was no choice but to be relaxed.

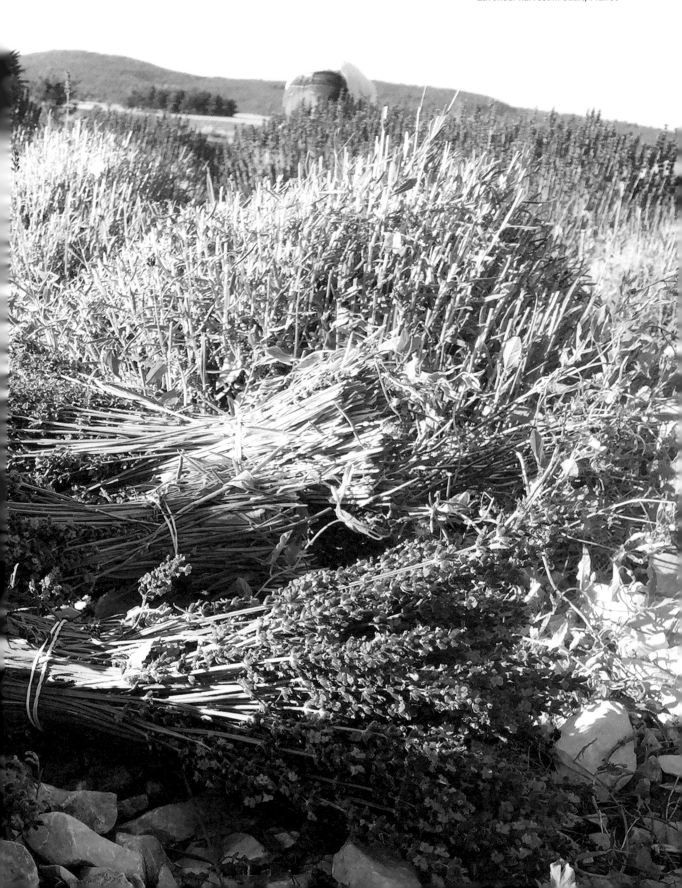
Lavender harvest in Sault, France

Adaptogens | POWERFUL PLANTS FOR RESILIENCE AND RESTORATION

Adaptogens are the superheroes of the plant medicine universe, and like all proper superheroes, they all have incredible origin stories. In China, they say the strongest ginseng roots grow where lightning strikes in the forest. In India, holy basil is considered an emanation of the goddess Lakshmi, bringer of vitality and abundance. Japanese legends talk about reishi mushroom as an enchanted spirit conveying immortality to whoever finds it growing in the wild. In India, amla berries are said to have fallen from the very first tree on earth.

The word *adaptogen* was coined in the twentieth century by scientists looking for plants that would improve the body's ability to adapt to prolonged stress and restore physiological balance. Adaptogens help regulate the stress response, reducing its toll, and ensuring more energy is available for vital body functions. Often growing in rugged environments subject to extreme conditions, these incredible plants have harnessed adversity to develop their unique powers. The same compounds that adaptogens created to thrive in challenging places also promote physical and mental resilience in us. Their broad-spectrum benefits extend to all aspects of physiology: increasing energy and endurance, sharpening cognitive function, boosting immunity, reducing cortisol levels, decreasing inflammation, deepening sleep, elevating mood, strengthening libido, and increasing fertility. And these benefits steadily accumulate the longer we consume these plants. By regularly consuming adaptogens, we become more flexible, resilient, and capable in the midst of life's daily challenges. This shows up in noticeable improvements in our capacity to maintain physical and mental composure, even in stressful circumstances.

Along with the wide range of benefits common among all the plants in this category, each adaptogen also has unique strengths and nuances. Understanding these helps us use them most effectively for specific circumstances. When colds and flus are frequent or lingering, we can fortify the immune system by simmering astragalus roots into soups or by adding powdered reishi into morning drinks as the weather starts to get cold. If the goal is enhanced athletic performance, drinking some pre-workout Korean ginseng extract or adding cordyceps to smoothies will increase endurance and speed recovery time. Drinking an infusion of tulsi (aka holy basil) or taking rhodiola tablets is a good way to improve mental energy and focus. To enhance fertility and promote hormonal balance, add some shatavari or maca root to the daily routine. To encourage deep, replenishing sleep, stir a tablespoon of ashwagandha root powder into warm oat milk with a dash of cinnamon and nutmeg at night.

Our schisandra supplier in South Korea

KEY ADAPTOGENS

Amla berries	Eleuthero	Lion's mane	Schisandra berries
Ashwagandha root	Ginseng root	Maca root	Shatavari root
Astragalus root	Goji berries	Maitake	Turkey tail
Chaga	Gymnostema	Reishi	
Cordyceps	He shou wu	Rhodiola root	

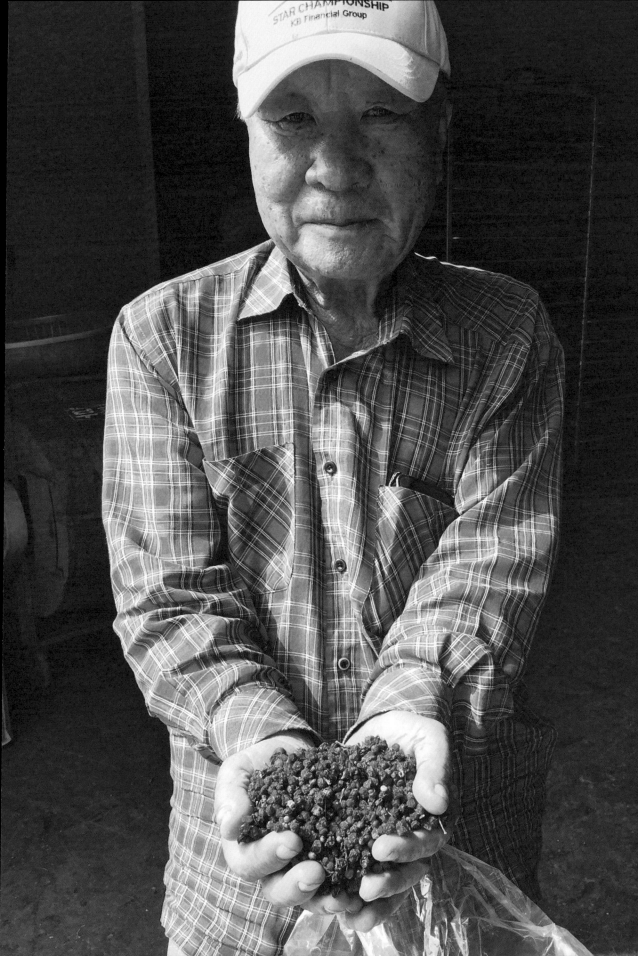

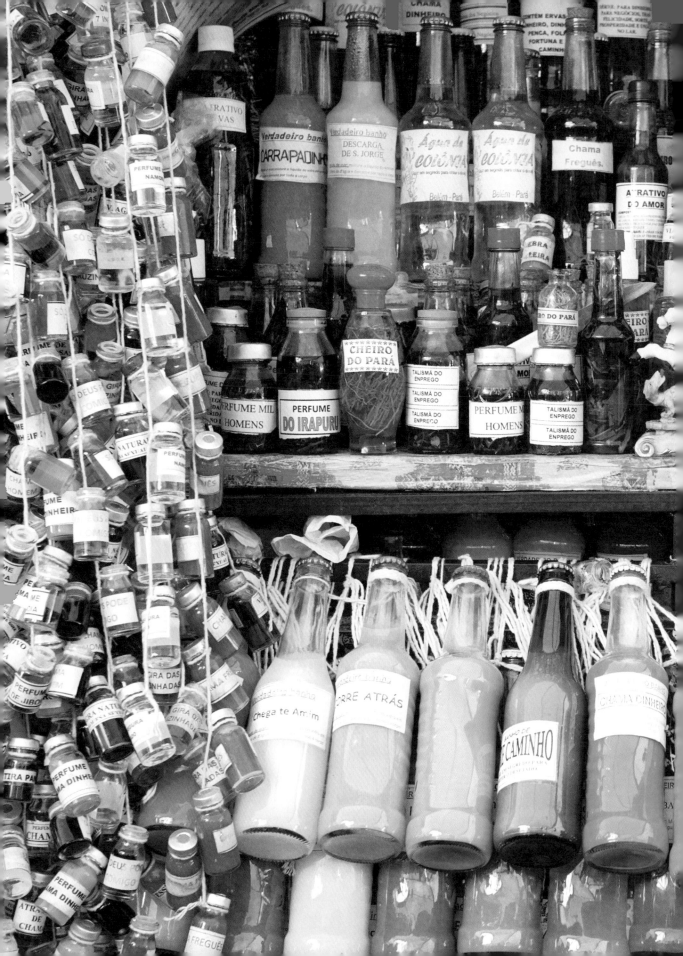

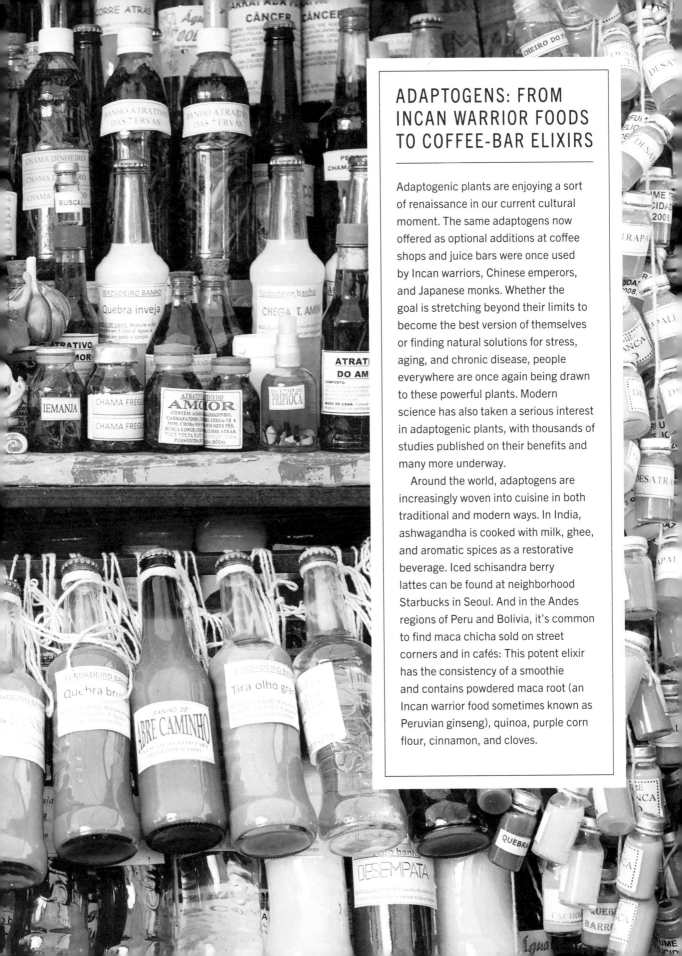

ADAPTOGENS: FROM INCAN WARRIOR FOODS TO COFFEE-BAR ELIXIRS

Adaptogenic plants are enjoying a sort of renaissance in our current cultural moment. The same adaptogens now offered as optional additions at coffee shops and juice bars were once used by Incan warriors, Chinese emperors, and Japanese monks. Whether the goal is stretching beyond their limits to become the best version of themselves or finding natural solutions for stress, aging, and chronic disease, people everywhere are once again being drawn to these powerful plants. Modern science has also taken a serious interest in adaptogenic plants, with thousands of studies published on their benefits and many more underway.

Around the world, adaptogens are increasingly woven into cuisine in both traditional and modern ways. In India, ashwagandha is cooked with milk, ghee, and aromatic spices as a restorative beverage. Iced schisandra berry lattes can be found at neighborhood Starbucks in Seoul. And in the Andes regions of Peru and Bolivia, it's common to find maca chicha sold on street corners and in cafés: This potent elixir has the consistency of a smoothie and contains powdered maca root (an Incan warrior food sometimes known as Peruvian ginseng), quinoa, purple corn flour, cinnamon, and cloves.

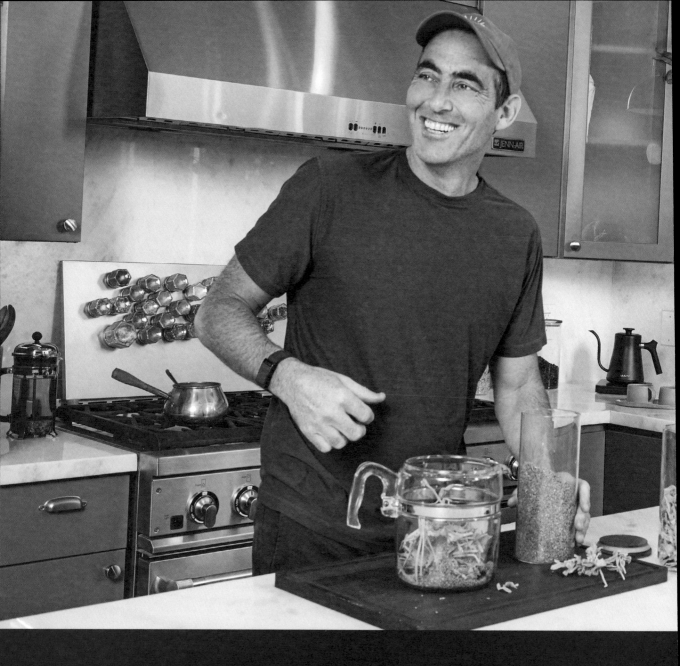

Part II

THE PLANT MEDICINE PROTOCOL

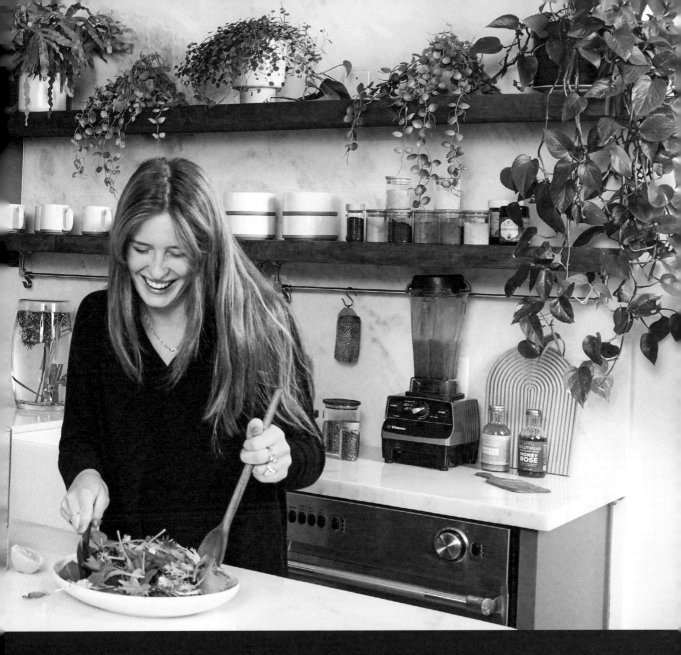

This is where we activate the power of plants to create new dimensions of vitality, energy, and resilience. The goal is to saturate our bodies with a wide range of medicinal plants each day. The design of this protocol closely mirrors the methodology I use to help patients establish a medicinal plant—powered lifestyle.

You'll be introduced to new practices, preparations, and recipes that all deliver the rejuvenating power of plants, plus all the tools and guidance you need to succeed. Move at your own pace and follow your preferences. Over time, these healthy habits will become

second nature, and the benefits will multiply. By the time you complete the protocol, you will have fully activated your own plant-powered lifestyle.

The ideal way to approach this protocol is with a spirit of curiosity, exploration, and fun. This is not a quick fix—or a slog through the mud. Think of it as an adventure and learning process that will awaken your senses and make you feel more energized, vibrant, and alive. This protocol is designed to be effective, enjoyable, and practical, and it will create a substantial upgrade to your health and well-being.

GETTING STARTED

THE PROTOCOL IS ORGANIZED INTO FIVE STEPS,
each one centered around a particular category of medicinal
plants—culinary herbs, spices, and bitters; demulcents; nervines
and relaxants; nutritives; and adaptogens—and the specific body
system(s) they benefit, as discussed in Part I. These steps build
upon one another for maximum benefits, so it's best to move
through them in order. I recommend you start by reviewing the
protocol in its entirety and begin to assemble some of the herbs
and preparations you'll need in advance so they are easily at hand.
The average amount of time to spend on a step is one to two
weeks, but feel free to go at your own pace. You'll want to be well
established and familiar with each step before you move on to
the next.

The steps are progressively layered upon one another, so that by
the end of the protocol you will be using plants from each of the
five steps simultaneously. There are two reasons for this approach:
It sustains momentum with the new habits you are building,
and it allows you to experience the synergistic health benefits of
using several plant categories at once. There's a caveat, though:
When you're on a particular step, that plant category should
be your primary focus. So don't try to continue implementing
a *full* version of the previous step(s). Instead, when you feel like
you've completed a step and are ready to dive into the next one,
choose one or two of your favorite practices or recipes to carry
forward from the previous step(s). The Minimum Daily Dose
recommendation (more on this on page 90) is a good benchmark
for how to maintain the step that you've just completed.

It's also worth saying explicitly that each protocol step is
designed to be a deep dive into a particular category of plants *for
a finite amount of time*. What a day will look like while you're in
the midst of a protocol step does not represent an average day
for a person living a medicinal plant–centric lifestyle (for more
on what that day might look like, see page 262). The idea here
is to thoroughly saturate yourself with a plant category to get a

distinct bodily impression of its effects and benefits. This method will give you a high degree of fluency, familiarity, and confidence with these plants, which will make seamlessly integrating them into your own daily lifestyle feel like second nature.

In the pages that follow, I deliberately emphasize using whole, unprocessed plants (as well as some simple preparations) over supplements, with some key exceptions. The active constituents in the medicinal plants we're working with are effective and readily accessible with minimal processing. The more you experience the flavors, textures, and aromas of the plants themselves, the more familiar and proficient you'll become with using them. It's also more economical to use whole plants, ensuring that this protocol, and the plant-powered lifestyle, are sustainable over the long term. (That said, I will always note when supplements are an option, and you should feel free to go that route if they will help ensure your consistent use of a particular plant or category.)

Try out as many options, preparations, and recipes in each step as you can to see how they make you feel, to find your favorites, and to explore the ways they might fit into your life going forward. Check out the individual plant profiles in Part IV, beginning on page 300, for detailed information on their characteristics and benefits to help you choose the best ones for you.

Lastly, we are not aiming for perfection or 100 percent adherence to the recommendations here. Success doesn't mean doing every single thing in each step, so don't be intimidated by the wide variety of options and recipes. Have fun, experiment, and remember you can always take a second pass at a step, or linger longer on one that's especially interesting to you. Sometimes you'll only be able to incorporate a few of the options in a step. As long as you're engaged and being consistent, you'll get the benefits and gain empowering new skills.

Note: The Plant Medicine Protocol is designed to fit any lifestyle regardless of where you're starting from in your pursuit of health. Remember, though, as you approach this book, that if you are taking other medications or have any health concerns, you should talk with your existing health-care providers before beginning a new health regimen or making changes to your existing treatment plans.

KEY TAKEAWAYS

- Consistency is more important than perfection.

- During each step, experiment with as many options as you can to find your favorites.

- When possible and convenient, choose whole plants over supplements.

- The steps are designed to be a more intensive deep dive than your plant-powered lifestyle after completing the protocol. Try to fully embrace the saturation effect.

- Go at your own pace and make sure you're confident in one step before moving to the next.

How Each Step Works

Each step includes the following components:

01
Plants & Other Ingredients You'll Be Using

A brief overview of the category of plants you'll be working with in the step and a list of the specific plants to use. For more on each of the plant categories, see pages 59–85. For detailed profiles of each plant, see Part IV, beginning on page 300.

02
Getting Started

Suggestions for setting up your space so that the necessary plants and tools are always at hand and ready to use.

03
How to Saturate Your Day

The basic "when" and "how" instructions for incorporating each category of plants into your day to the best effect.

04
Sample Daily Menus

Two sample days to give you a clear picture of what a protocol step could look like in practice. You can try them out as they are written, or use them as a guide to build your own personalized menu using any of the options given in the step. Don't be intimidated or limited by the sample menus: You can always include more options or do a bit less if you want to. The core tenet is Saturation + Consistency + Variety. As long as you're saturating yourself with the plant category, you're doing it right. Within these menus is also a "Minimum Daily Dose," which is meant as a baseline—for busy days when it isn't possible to engage in any other way or throughout the entire step if needed. This is also a good guide for what to carry forward once you've completed a step and are ready to begin the next one.

05
Options

A master list of all of the options, both simple and more involved, that can be incorporated into a given step. Following the framework presented in "How to Saturate Your Day," let your specific circumstances and preferences guide you toward options that work best for you.

06
Recipes

These delicious, easy-to-follow recipes show you myriad ways to integrate your favorite flavors and preparations into the protocol. Follow the instructions directly or improvise for customized variations.

07
FAQs

Beginning on page 257, I'll answer some of the most commonly asked questions for each protocol step.

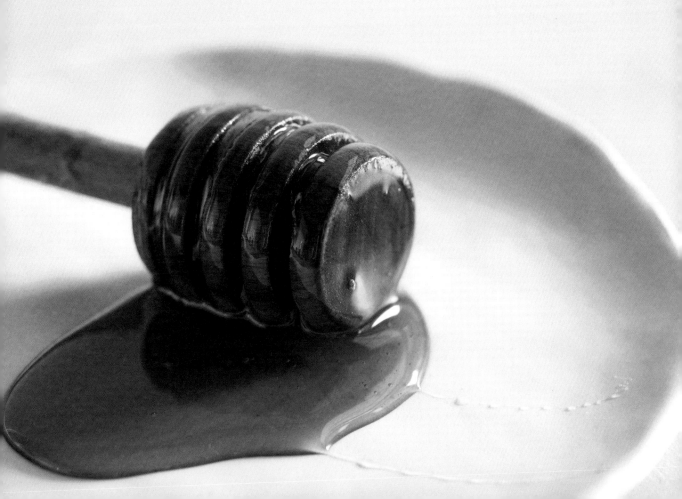

A NOTE ON SWEETENERS

Many of the recipes that follow give the option to use a natural sweetener. My overall recommendation is to limit sugar, natural or otherwise. While following the protocol, you'll be consuming several of the preparations each day, so to moderate sugar intake, consider forgoing sweetener or using zero-calorie, low-glycemic-index alternatives like monk fruit and stevia, which are better for overall metabolic health. As you progress in your new plant routines, your appreciation for the novel flavors of these herbs and spices will grow and you'll naturally require less sweetener to make things palatable.

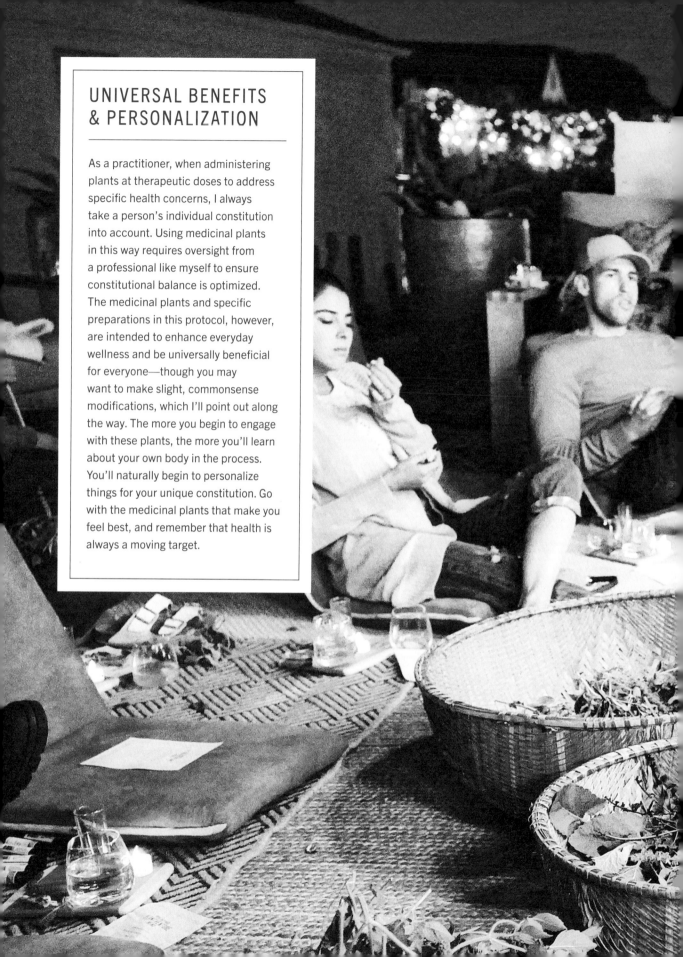

UNIVERSAL BENEFITS & PERSONALIZATION

As a practitioner, when administering plants at therapeutic doses to address specific health concerns, I always take a person's individual constitution into account. Using medicinal plants in this way requires oversight from a professional like myself to ensure constitutional balance is optimized. The medicinal plants and specific preparations in this protocol, however, are intended to enhance everyday wellness and be universally beneficial for everyone—though you may want to make slight, commonsense modifications, which I'll point out along the way. The more you begin to engage with these plants, the more you'll learn about your own body in the process. You'll naturally begin to personalize things for your unique constitution. Go with the medicinal plants that make you feel best, and remember that health is always a moving target.

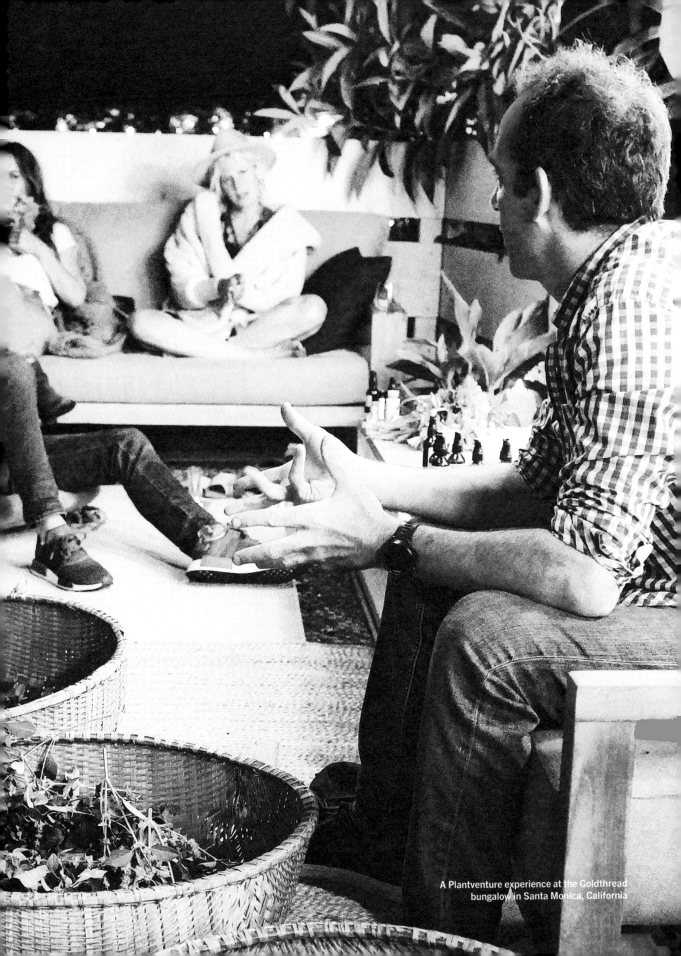

A Plantventure experience at the Goldthread bungalow in Santa Monica, California

Preparations

Medicinal plants can be consumed in many different forms that vary in potency, convenience, and expense. Below is an overview of those that appear in the protocol to follow. Most of the preparation techniques I use in this book require just a few steps and minimal effort.

Water Preparations

The preparations most frequently called for in the protocol are water based. These include teas, infusions, cold brews, and decoctions. This is because most herbs are water soluble, and the constituents in water preparations are easy for the body to absorb. You'll typically use hot water for these preparations, though certain herbs can be prepared with room-temperature or cold water.

As a general rule, the medicinal compounds in the lighter parts of plants, like flowers and leaves, are easiest to extract, meaning they require the least amount of time in water and lower temperatures. Woody and denser plant materials—like barks, stems, mushrooms, berries, and roots—require longer cooking times and, often, higher temperatures to extract their medicinal compounds. Herbs that contain a lot of essential oils, such as culinary spices and fragrant relaxants, should be covered when cooking or infusing so the oils don't escape.

TEAS

Tea is the most basic water-based preparation: Simply pour hot water over the plant material (in a tea bag or loose in an infusion basket) and steep for a relatively short period of time, 5 to 10 minutes. A general ratio is approximately 1 to 3 teaspoons dried herb (or multiple tea bags) per 1 to 1½ cups (240 to 360 ml) water. This preparation works for lighter parts of plants like leaves and flowers (and sometimes

sccds, berries, and roots) when they are finely chopped, which exposes a lot of surface area and makes the beneficial ingredients more easily extractable.

INFUSIONS

Infusions are similar to tea preparations but stronger; they are steeped for longer and use more plant material. I use approximately ½ to 1 ounce (15 to 30 g) dried herb (or tea bags in the equivalent weight) per quart (1 L) of water (with some variation depending on the herb I'm using and the relative strength and concentration I'm going for). Steeping between 20 minutes and an hour is the minimum for an infusion, but it's not uncommon to steep for 4 to 6 hours or overnight. For mineral-rich plants like nettles, alfalfa, horsetail, and moringa, for example, an overnight infusion ensures maximum extraction of all of the minerals and trace elements these plants contain.

The goal of an infusion is to achieve maximum extraction in the most convenient way—simply pour water over the preparation and leave it (as opposed to decoctions, which require you to attend to them while they simmer). A French press or canning jar is a convenient container for making infusions.

DECOCTIONS

Dense plant materials like roots, stems, bark, and mushrooms often require simmering as opposed to steeping alone. This is called a decoction, and it requires you to simmer the plant material for anywhere from 20 minutes to an hour or longer depending on the density of what you're using. (When you simmer finely cut plant material, you extract medicinal compounds more quickly than if you were to use the same amount of roughly chopped material.) Decoctions don't require fine-cut plant matter like teas and some infusions—

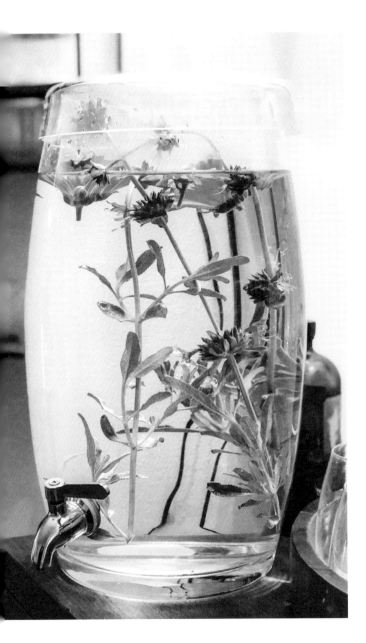

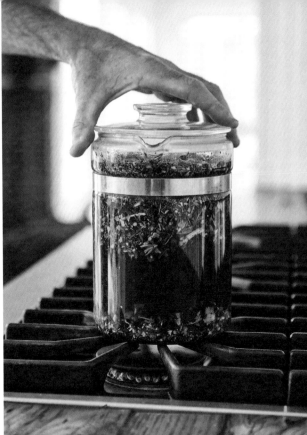

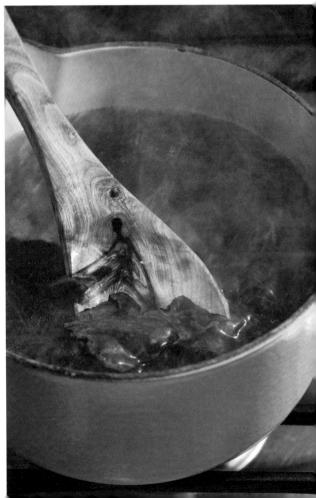

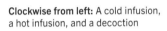

Clockwise from left: A cold infusion, a hot infusion, and a decoction

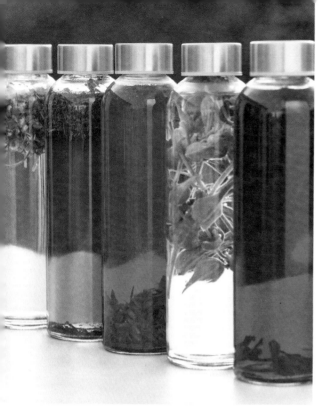

roughly chopping the material will be sufficient. The ratio of plant material to water will vary depending on the particular plant and the strength you're trying to achieve, but the average ratio is similar to an infusion: ½ to 1 ounce (15 to 30 g) dried or fresh herb to 1 quart (1 L) water.

COLD INFUSIONS

Some plants don't require heating to extract the medicinal compounds. Cold-water extraction works for fresh plants, green teas, demulcents, and lighter plant matter (such as flowers and leaves). The same ratio of plant material applies equally to cold or hot infusions (½ to 1 ounce/15 to 30 g dried or fresh herb to 1 quart/1 L water). Though most cold infusions take a minimum of 20 minutes to an hour, demulcents (such as chia seeds and basil seeds) will readily yield mucilaginous compounds in just a few minutes. Fresh herb material already contains water; account for this by adding more of it to get an equally concentrated preparation as if it were dry.

Powders, Capsules & Tablets

These are preparations that you'll be purchasing rather than making yourself. The Resources section (page 352) has all my favorite sources.

HERBAL POWDERS

Herbal powders are made up of finely ground whole plant material. Demulcents, adaptogens, nutritives, berries, and spices work well as powders and provide all the nutrients and the full complement of medicinal compounds contained in the whole plant. The powders can be added to smoothies, mixed with hot or cold water, or made into pastes.

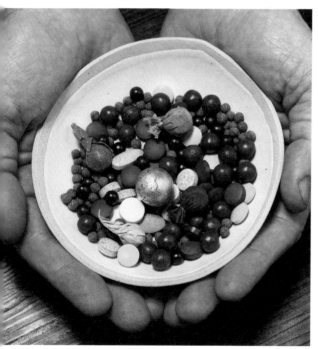

Top: Cold infusions

Bottom: Capsules and tablets

POWDERED EXTRACTS

Many herbs are available as powdered extracts, which are made by evaporating a strong, concentrated decoction of herbs until a fine powder is all that's left. Unlike herbal powders, they contain no plant fiber and will dissolve completely when added to liquid, making them easier to drink. They are often concentrated such that the potency of the extract is equivalent to several times the amount of the unprocessed herb. If 1 gram of extract equals 10 grams of the unprocessed herb, it will be labeled as 10:1 on the container.

CAPSULES & TABLETS

Capsules and tablets are made from dried herbs, powdered extracts, or specific active constituents. Capsules can be full of extracts— CO_2, liquid, or powdered extracts—or ground whole herbs in powder form. Tablets are pressed whole herbs or concentrated powdered extracts. Some are standardized to contain specific amounts of active constituents.

Other Liquid Preparations

Similar to powders, these are products you'll mostly be purchasing. Refer to the Resources on page 352 for recommended sources. If you're interested in making your own tinctures, there are great reference books in the Further Reading section on page 356 to guide you.

TINCTURES

Tinctures use a combination of alcohol and water to dissolve the active constituents in herbs and hold them in solution. The amount of alcohol in the final preparation varies depending on the specific plants used. (*Note:* Tinctures are highly concentrated, so the amount of alcohol in a dose is very low. If you wish to avoid alcohol altogether, it's possible to evaporate it off by adding your tincture dose to hot water before consuming.)

Tinctures are rapidly metabolized, so their effects tend to be fast acting. Nervine tinctures, for example, offer immediate calming and relaxing effects, particularly around bedtime. Tinctures also work well for bitter digestives and other herbs that don't taste great, because you can down them quickly.

ESSENTIAL OILS

Essential oils are the concentrated aromatic constituents in plants obtained primarily through steam distillation. Steam is passed through fresh or dried plant material to separate out the aromatic molecules in the plants. Some plants, such as citrus peels and certain fruits, yield oil through cold pressing. Essential oils are highly concentrated and are to be inhaled or applied externally (in many cases, they should be first diluted with a carrier oil); do not ingest except under the guidance of a professional.

HYDROSOLS

The water that remains after the distillation process of essential oils still contains many aromatic molecules, but in a far less concentrated form. Hydrosols are primarily used topically and in sprays. Some can be consumed in small amounts mixed into water or another beverage to create an instant aromatic formula.

HERBAL LIQUORS

Many herbs yield their constituents into less-concentrated alcohol preparations like wine or other spirits. Ayurveda has a whole category of herbal wines called *asavas*; herbs are frequently steeped in sake in Japanese medicine; and throughout the Caribbean, it's common to find "roots tonic" wines. Italian amaros and European bitter liquors distill herbs into spirits directly.

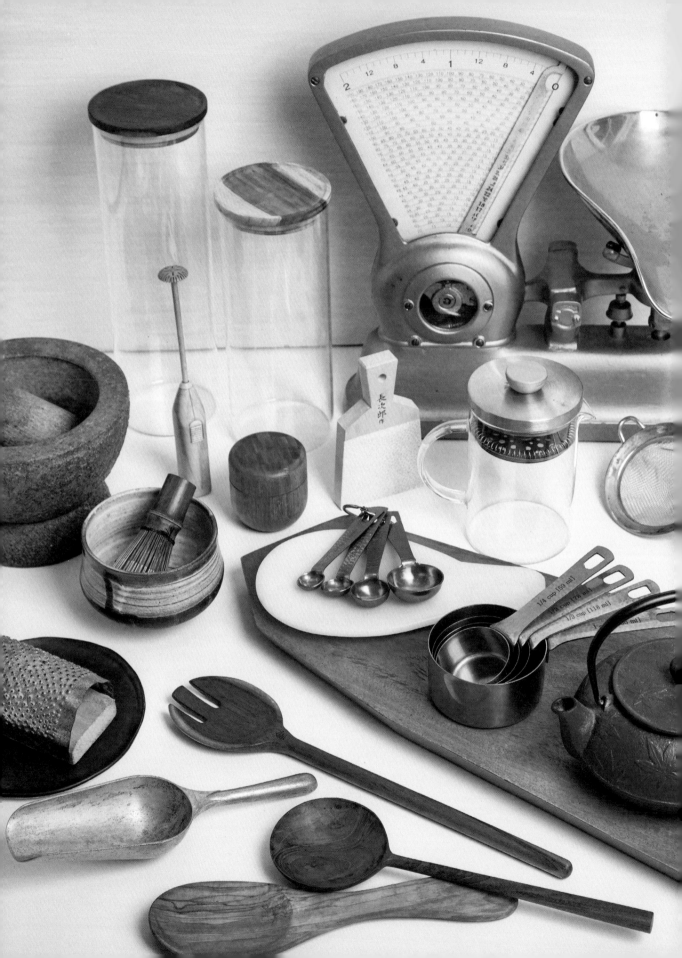

Tools

The protocol doesn't require you to buy many things beyond the herbs and other ingredients you'll be using (the Resources section beginning on page 352 directs you to the best-quality herbs and supplements). I consider the tools below indispensable to my personal plant life, however. Some tools you may already have; others you can get or make substitutions for. A digital scale quite a bit. Investing in a small digital scale will help you get the measurements just right.

- A digital scale (with the capacity to measure in both grams and ounces) is particularly essential. In the recipes that follow, you'll see that I often give measurements for plant materials in weight instead of volume. This is because herbs come in a wide variety of cuts, textures, and shapes, so their volume varies.

- Liquid and dry measuring cups

- Mixing bowls with pouring lips

- Handheld fine-mesh strainer

- Colander

- Muslin strainer bags

- High-powered blender, such as a Vitamix

- Food processor

- Electric juicer

- Electric kettle with temperature control

- Canning jars

- Milk frother with cold and hot settings

- Immersion blender, mini immersion blender, or whisk

- Traditional bamboo matcha whisk (or electric version)

- Mortar and pestle

- Regular and mini French presses

- Self-fill tea bags or removable infuser baskets for tea mugs or teapots

- Grater

- Essential oil diffusers

- Small ceramic bowl designed for burning resins and aromatic woods

- Volcanic ash/Japanese charcoals

- Tongs or tweezers, for handling charcoals and resins

STORAGE

Properly stored dried herbs and spices will retain their potency for many months. A few tips for storing your herbs and preparations:

- The main sources of degradation are heat, light, moisture, and insects. Store loose bulk herbs in airtight glass or plastic storage containers and keep in a cool, dark place.

- The more of its surface area that's exposed, the faster a substance will degrade. Powders, for example, will degrade faster than whole plant material.

- Store green teas in metal tins, away from heat and sunlight.

- Matcha powder should be stored in the fridge because it oxidizes quickly.

- Store dried fruit powders in the fridge or freezer.

- Hydrosols should be kept in the fridge.

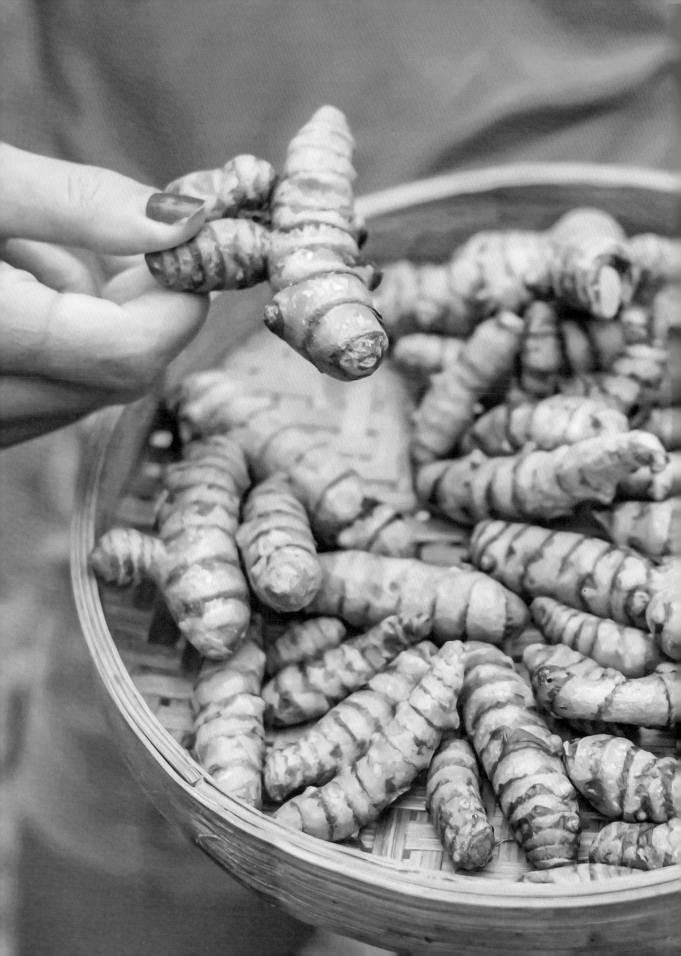

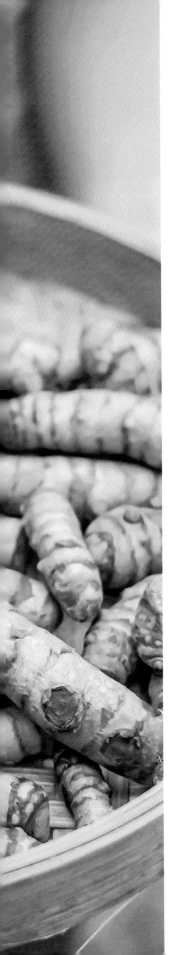

Culinary Herbs, Spices & Bitters

DIGESTION AND DETOXIFICATION ARE A DYNAMIC DUO that impact all aspects of our health—both are equally important parts of one continuous process. When our digestion is strong and healthy, nutrients from food are efficiently extracted and become the building blocks of our body structure and the energy that fuels us. Removing the residual wastes (detoxification) completes the process.

Aromatic culinary herbs, spices, and bitters help maintain and enhance our digestive and detoxification functions. The aromatic essential oils and other constituents in culinary herbs and spices kindle digestive fire, increasing the secretion of the acids and enzymes responsible for breaking down food and assimilating nutrients. Bitter compounds provide additional support for digestion and enhance the removal of wastes and toxins. Expanding our daily use of culinary and bitter herbs for optimal digestion and detoxification is the focus of Step 1.

WHAT TO EXPECT

- A balanced appetite, where you're neither ravenous before nor sluggish after meals

- An ability to distinguish between unhealthy food cravings and what the body actually requires in the moment

- Stable energy and blood sugar between meals

- Fewer digestive discomforts, such as gas, bloating, or feeling excessively full or hyperacidic after eating

- Improved elimination

- Clearer complexion

- Improved mood and clarity

Plants & Other Ingredients You'll Be Using

This step includes herbs and spices that have long been integral parts of the healthiest cuisines of the world. Many will be familiar, others less so. Familiar or not, each one of them offers the promise of optimal digestion—in addition to delicious new culinary adventures.

Culinary Herbs & Spices

This category includes the ingredients you'll find in a well-stocked spice rack and fresh culinary herbs easily sourced from the produce aisle or farmers' market.

Keep in mind that culinary spices don't always have to taste spicy to be effective. For more on this, see page 112. Draw from a broad range of herbs and spices and maintain a balanced heat profile for best results.

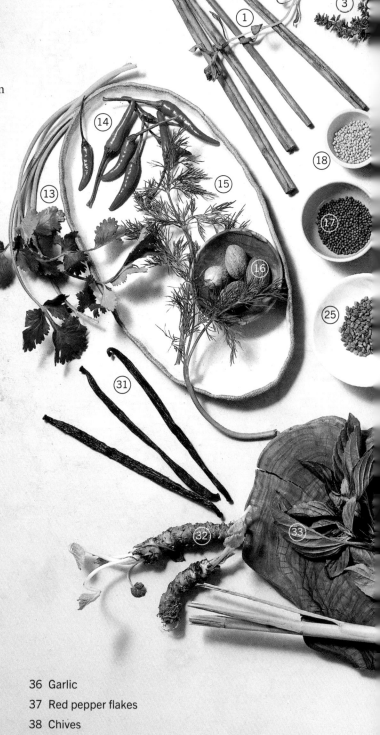

1 Cinnamon	19 Coriander
2 Tarragon	20 Red pepper
3 Thyme	22 Paprika
4 Turmeric	23 Green pepper
5 Saffron	24 Galangal
6 Bay leaf	25 Fenugreek
7 + 11 Pandan leaf	26 Cumin
8 Ginger	27 Cardamom
9 Cloves	28 Allspice
10 Oregano	29 Mace
12 Parsley	30 Rosemary
13 Cilantro	31 Vanilla
14 Chile	32 Horseradish (wasabi)
15 Dill	33 + 40 Basil
16 Nutmeg	34 Fennel
17 + 21 Black pepper	35 Star anise
18 Mustard seed	

36 Garlic
37 Red pepper flakes
38 Chives
39 Lemongrass
41 Sage

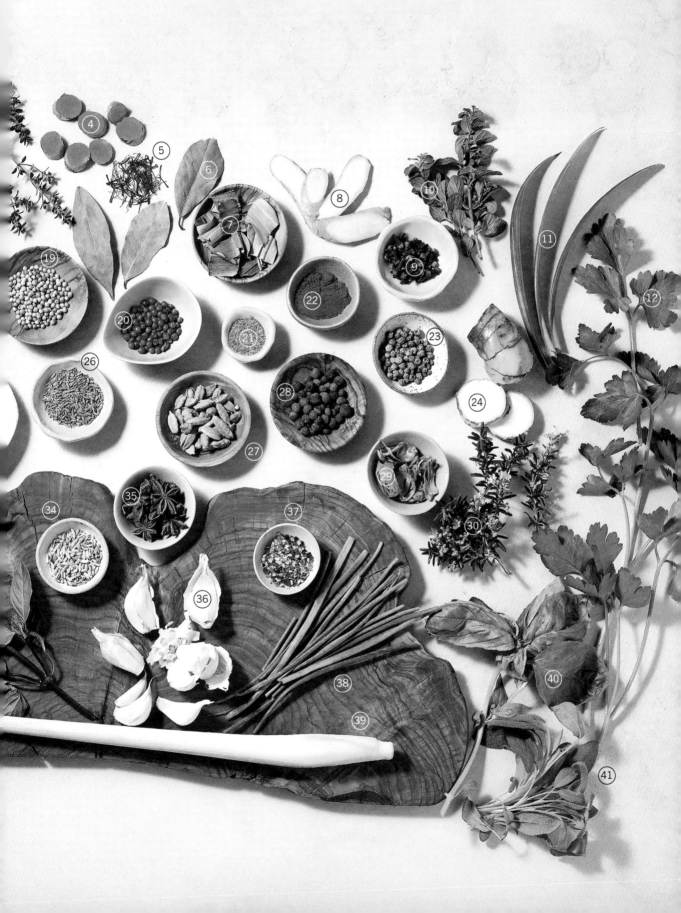

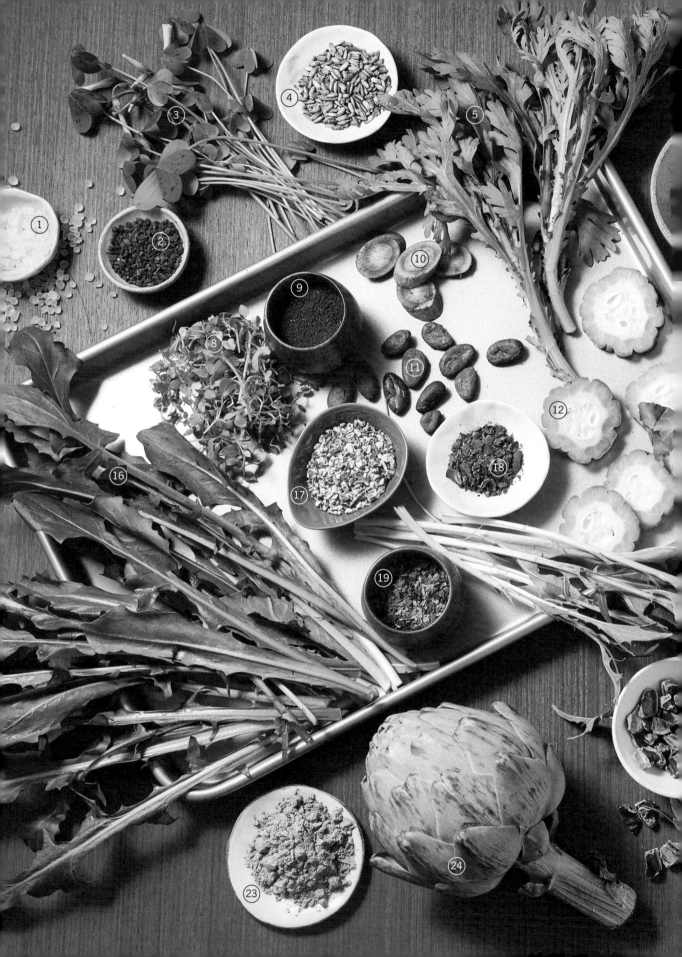

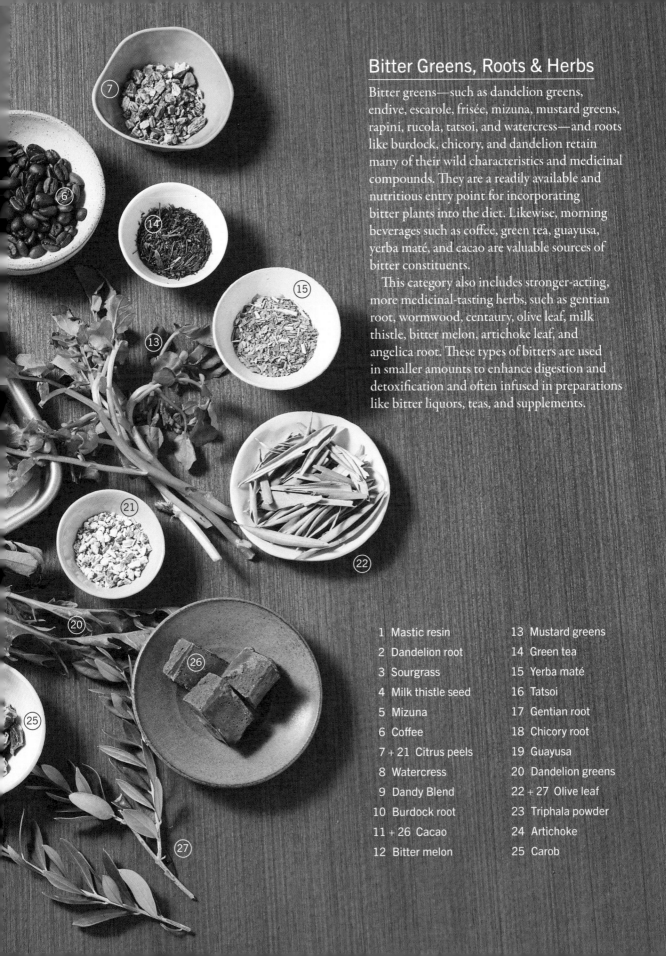

Bitter Greens, Roots & Herbs

Bitter greens—such as dandelion greens, endive, escarole, frisée, mizuna, mustard greens, rapini, rucola, tatsoi, and watercress—and roots like burdock, chicory, and dandelion retain many of their wild characteristics and medicinal compounds. They are a readily available and nutritious entry point for incorporating bitter plants into the diet. Likewise, morning beverages such as coffee, green tea, guayusa, yerba maté, and cacao are valuable sources of bitter constituents.

This category also includes stronger-acting, more medicinal-tasting herbs, such as gentian root, wormwood, centaury, olive leaf, milk thistle, bitter melon, artichoke leaf, and angelica root. These types of bitters are used in smaller amounts to enhance digestion and detoxification and often infused in preparations like bitter liquors, teas, and supplements.

1 Mastic resin
2 Dandelion root
3 Sourgrass
4 Milk thistle seed
5 Mizuna
6 Coffee
7 + 21 Citrus peels
8 Watercress
9 Dandy Blend
10 Burdock root
11 + 26 Cacao
12 Bitter melon
13 Mustard greens
14 Green tea
15 Yerba maté
16 Tatsoi
17 Gentian root
18 Chicory root
19 Guayusa
20 Dandelion greens
22 + 27 Olive leaf
23 Triphala powder
24 Artichoke
25 Carob

Around the World with Aromatic Bitters

Throughout Europe, drinking aromatic bitter liquors as digestifs after meals is an ongoing cultural tradition. These recipes are often closely guarded secrets dating back hundreds of years, with unforgettable flavor combinations: bitter, aromatic, spicy, and just sweet enough to keep you coming back for more. Many European countries have at least one bitter that's commonly known and emblematic and others that are rare regional microdistilled bitters made in small batches, available to those lucky enough to find them.

In Italy, bitter liquors are known as amaros. On a recent trip to Rome, I visited one bar that devoted an entire 20-foot (6 m) wall to bitter liquors, with upward of five hundred different bottles, most produced in and around Italy. Braulio, created in 1875 and still made by the same family, contains an assortment of herbs like juniper, yarrow, and gentian, gathered in the Italian Alps. Ramazzotti, first invented in 1815 by a young herbalist named Ausano Ramazzotti, is made using the same recipe to this day, consisting of thirty-three herbs and spices including rhubarb, rosemary, and turmeric. Fernet-Branca is perhaps the most famous of them all, created in Milan in 1845 and made with twenty-seven herbs and spices from all over the world, including myrrh from North Africa, galangal from Sri Lanka, and quinine bark from South America.

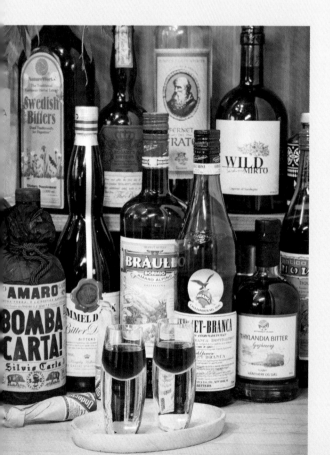

In Copenhagen, I came across Gammel Dansk (translated as "old Danish"). A relative newcomer on the bitters scene, Gammel Dansk was invented in 1964 and has since become one of the most popular bitter digestifs in Scandinavia. It contains twenty-nine herbs and spices, including angelica root, star anise, and Seville (bitter) orange. It's traditional to drink Gammel Dansk around the holidays and early in the morning during the long winter months as an invigorating body-warming digestive tonic.

Traveling through Germany, another epicenter of bitters culture, it's impossible

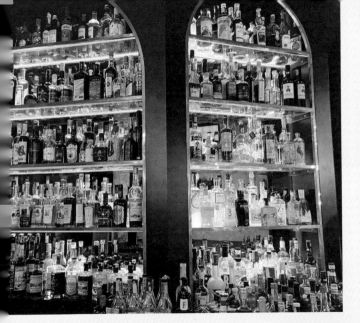

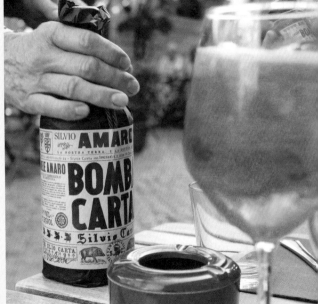

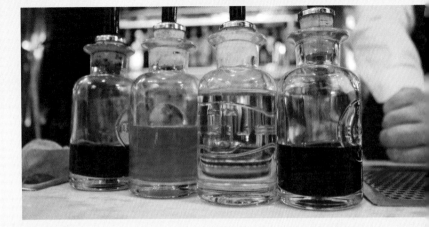

Opposite page: A collection of bitters

Top left and right: Il Marchese
bitters bar and osteria in Rome, Italy

Right: Sardinian bitters at a café
in Rome

to miss Underberg, the ubiquitous national bitters brand. Originally formulated in 1846 in Rheinberg by Hubert Underberg, this potent bitter contains forty-three different herbs and spices from all over the world distilled into a secret recipe known to only five people to this day. Unique among bitters, Underberg comes in distinctive little bottles individually wrapped in kraft paper and apportioned for the perfect dose—a precursor, perhaps, to bitter supplements.

Swedish bitters is arguably the bitter with the most name recognition in the world; at very least, it is among the oldest in continual use. The original formula is said to have come from a recipe invented by Paracelsus, the famous sixteenth-century Swiss physician. It was rediscovered and distilled by the eighteenth-century Swedish doctor Klaus Samst and is now produced in Norway. Swedish bitters contain thirteen herbs including cape aloe, carline thistle, and camphor. It has a far more bitter taste than most bitter liquors and medicinal action that gets right to the point. One sip after meals is all it takes with this "cure-all"— a valuable one to have in your collection.

Collecting these digestifs for your own bitters bar (see page 109) is half the fun. For a list of recommended bitter liquors and where to find them, go to the Resources on page 352.

Getting Started

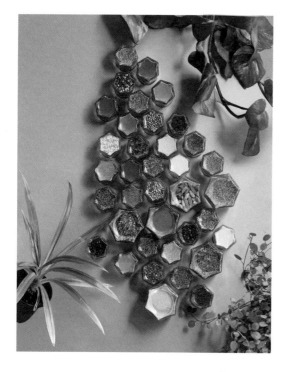

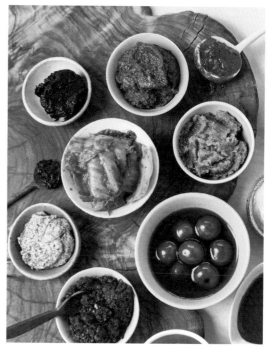

Spice Rack

Free your spices from the cupboards and drawers where they never get used and put them center stage where they belong! Keeping spices at hand means you'll use them more often and encourages spontaneous experimentation when you're preparing meals. To give your spice collection an upgrade, start by finding a rack that's easy to use and organize; avoid those that come with prefilled bottles, which are likely to contain old spices whose potency has degraded. Start with a collection of seven to ten spices you know you like and use often and build from there. As you discover new spices and blends, add to the collection. Purchase your staples in bulk and store in airtight containers nearby to make refilling the rack simple.

Condiment Collection

Condiments, too, are an excellent vehicle for getting the benefits of culinary herbs and spices into your daily routine. Make some space in your fridge for a varied collection of digestive-enhancing condiments saturated with culinary spices. Alongside staples like Dijon mustard and horseradish, consider harissa spread, chutneys, chimichurri, kimchi, wasabi, pickled gingerroot, and umeboshi plum paste. Keeping a collection of culinary condiments on hand and using them regularly will turn any dish into a delicious, healthful experience.

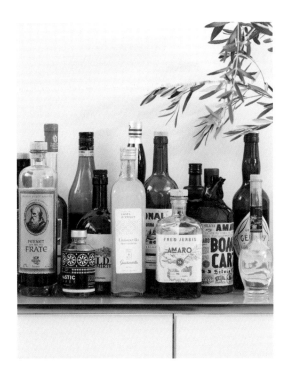

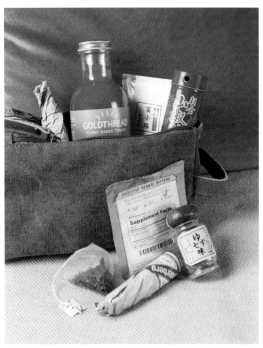

Bitters Bar

Keeping a collection of bitters close by where you eat your meals makes it easy and fun to develop a ritual of journeying to the "bar" for an after-meal digestif. Your bitters bar could be as simple as a tray or cabinet with a handful of bitter liquors. Or you could go all-in with dozens of varieties (a bottle of Italian amaro, another of Greek mastiha, perhaps some Scandinavian bitters), creating an opportunity to experience all sorts of interesting and nuanced botanical flavors and fragrances.

On the Go

Don't be shy about carrying a favorite spice blend or two with you when you're on the go—having it on hand means it's right there when you need to get your sprinkle on. It may feel a little awkward at first to be packing condiments, but in no time everyone will be asking for a shake or two. Supplements for kindling digestive fire, especially from the Ayurvedic tradition, are also an easy and convenient option for traveling, and premade shots containing culinary herbs and spices—especially ginger and turmeric—are readily available in grocery stores these days. They make handy aperitifs to kindle the digestive system when you're on the go (see the Resources on page 352 for recommended options).

How to Saturate Your Day

Culinary spices are best consumed just prior to (or cooked into) major meals. Their strength is kindling the digestive fire during the initial stages of digestion. Bitters enhance the downward movement of food through the GI tract and specifically activate the liver and other organs involved in the latter stages of digestion. Milder-tasting bitter greens and roots can be treated like food and thus incorporated into meals. Stronger, more medicinal bitters are traditionally reserved for after meals to complete the digestive process and initiate post-digestive detox. Keep in mind that these are not hard-and-fast rules—culinary spices and bitters often have overlapping functions. Many bitter herbs have some digestive fire–kindling benefits, and culinary spices like ginger are very good in a post-meal digestif. All herbs contain a complex mixture of hundreds of active constituents, giving them a wide range of functions. That's the nature of herbalism.

When it comes to specific amounts and dosages of plants in this category, there's no need to overthink it—what's most important is expanding your usage of culinary herbs and spices in variety, quantity, and consistency. Ideally, that means eating more meals infused with aromatic culinary herbs, spices, and bitter greens; consuming more condiments; sprinkling dried spices and blends onto food as seasoning; and incorporating special shots, elixirs, and teas as aperitifs and digestifs into your daily routine.

Aperitifs

Consume aperitifs (options are given on pages 114–115) 15 to 20 minutes before the major meals of the day, to allow your body enough time to kindle appetite and rev digestion. Suggested dosages for preparations vary depending on the individual, so treat them as approximations.

Mealtime

Enhance the major meals of the day by incorporating your choice of sprinkles, toppers, sides, condiments, culinary spices, fresh herbs, or any other options given on pages 115–117.

Digestifs

After the major meals of the day, enjoy a digestif option from pages114–117, to support complete digestion and initiate a post-digestive detox.

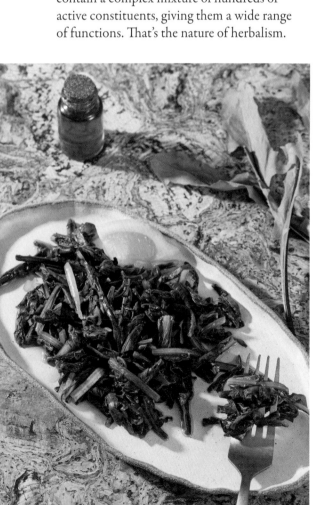

Horta Vrasta (page 133)

SAMPLE DAILY MENUS

MINIMUM DAILY DOSE

At a minimum, incorporate one culinary spice and/or bitter option into each mealtime. If you've cooked with spices or sprinkled some on a dish, taken a ginger shot prior to eating as an aperitif or a sip of bitters afterward, you're headed in the right direction. If you can't go the extra mile on a given day, rely on a few familiar favorites to make sure you get at least some digestive and detox support each time you eat.

MENU 1

Upon waking:
Ginger-Turmeric Shot (page 124)

At breakfast:
Herbes de Provence omelet with some extra fresh basil on top; Dandelion, Chicory, and Carob Latte (page 127) post-meal

Before lunch:
Lemon-ginger tea

At lunch:
Pasta with basil pesto and olive oil, Kalamata olives, and minced fresh garlic on top; a bitter greens salad; green tea post-meal

Before dinner:
Sparkling Rosemary Limeade (page 126)

At dinner:
Tacos seasoned with a Mexican spice blend and topped with fresh cilantro; Fernet-Branca or other bitter liquor post-meal

Before bed:
Triphala tablets

MENU 2

Upon waking:
Lemon-ginger tea

At breakfast:
Cinnamon-spiced chia pudding with nuts and berries; green tea post-meal

Before lunch:
Chai tea

At lunch:
Arugula salad with Milk Thistle Detox-Enhancing Dukkah (page 135); espresso shot post-meal

Before dinner:
Sip of draksha

At dinner:
Kitchari (page 134) and amla chutney with a side of cooked dandelion greens; bitter liquor shot and Coriander, Cumin, and Fennel Tea (page 128) post-meal

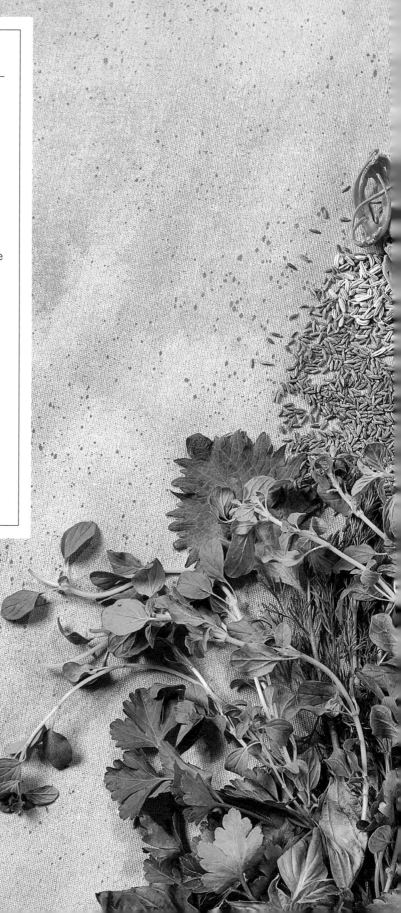

SOME LIKE IT HOT

Spices don't necessarily have to taste hot to be beneficial. To some extent, heat tolerance is based on individual constitution, with the overall goal being a slow, sustainable simmer in the digestive system rather than a quick raging boil. In Ayurveda this is referred to as *sama*, or balanced agni. Having balanced agni allows us to efficiently digest the widest range of foods possible without adverse symptoms. Think of the heating capacity of spices on a scale of one to ten, with ten being the hottest. Spices like cayenne pepper, wasabi, black pepper, and horseradish are up around ten; a little goes a long way on the hot end of the scale, so no need to overdo it with these. Cumin, fennel, and coriander occupy somewhere in the middle, and saffron, cilantro, and parsley sit close to the low end of the heat scale. Using spices primarily from the middle of the spectrum works best for everyday kindling.

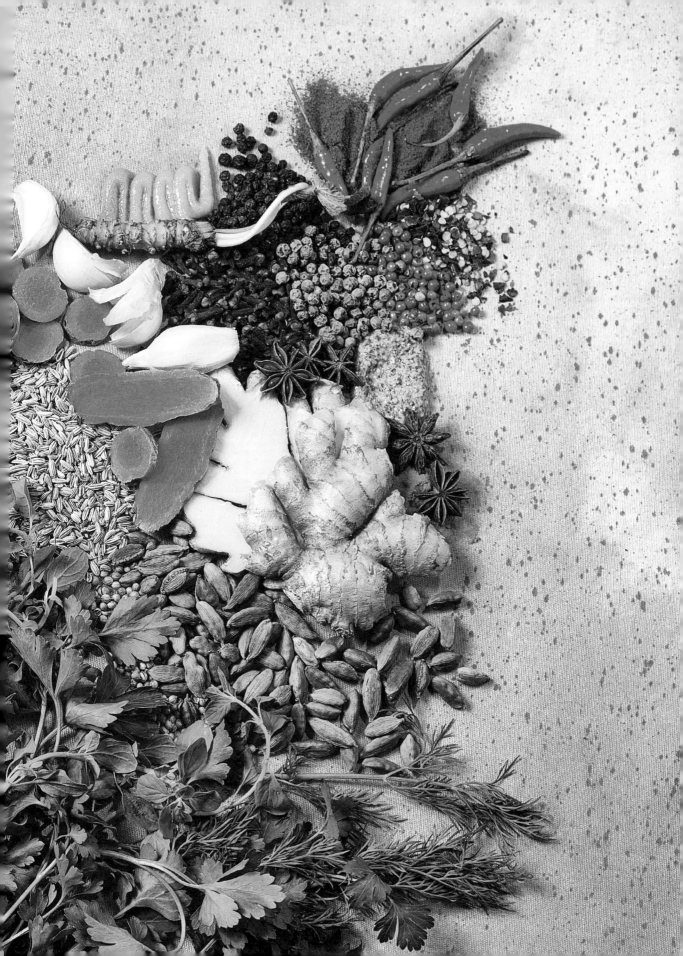

Agni-Kindling Honey
APERITIF

This recipe (page 123) combines honey with cinnamon, ginger, cardamom, and fennel for an effective and delicious aperitif. Take a small spoonful on its own, or melt it into ½ cup (120 ml) warm water and drink 15 to 20 minutes before meals.

Ginger "Pizza"
APERITIF

Another agni kindler from the Ayurvedic tradition. Take 1 thinly sliced piece of fresh gingerroot and add a squeeze of lime juice and a dash of sea salt. Eat 15 to 20 minutes before meals.

Turmeric Balls
APERITIF • DIGESTIF

This simple recipe (page 123) makes for a convenient, great-tasting delivery mechanism for getting a daily dose of anti-inflammatory, antioxidant-rich turmeric. Eat two or three a day, preferably 10 to 15 minutes prior to or after meals, to kindle digestion and metabolism.

Ginger and Turmeric Shots
APERITIF • DIGESTIF

These could be premade or one of my recipes on page 124 (Ginger Shots, Turmeric-Orange-Lime Shots, Ginger-Turmeric Shots). Whichever option you choose, drink 2 ounces (60 ml) 10 to 15 minutes before or after meals to fire up the digestive system and ensure maximum absorption of nutrients.

Draksha
APERITIF • DIGESTIF

A delicious Ayurvedic herbal wine (produced from grapes and an assortment of digestive-enhancing herbs and spices, such as cinnamon, ginger, and cloves), draksha contains very little alcohol (5 to 10 percent). Drink 2 ounces (60 ml) 10 to 15 minutes prior to or after meals.

Bitter Liquors
APERITIF • DIGESTIF

These aromatic digestive liquors are distilled formulations containing bitter roots, barks, and leaves, with hints of aromatic spices and citrus peels. With a relatively low alcohol content (between 15 and 40 percent), bitter liquors are commonly consumed in small amounts after meals as digestifs.

If alcohol is a concern, pour a small amount (as little as ¼ to ½ shot glass) and sip slowly. It's also nice to enjoy bitters over ice or mixed with sparkling water. Sip on bitters 30 minutes before or after a meal for best results.

Bitters Formulas and Supplements

APERITIF • DIGESTIF

Bitters can be found in liquid or tablet preparations in the supplement aisle or online. These supplements tend to be more concentrated than liquors, formulated primarily for their medicinal action rather than enjoyment. The best ones are formulated by herbalists with expertise in blending herbs and spices together for a balanced effect. Take 10 to 15 minutes before or after a meal.

Avipattikar, Hingvastak, or Trikatu

APERITIF • DIGESTIF

These three classic Ayurvedic formulas contain blends of spices and herbs used for digestion. Avipattikar is the coolest of the three in terms of spiciness level/heat factor, and trikatu is the hottest. These formulations come in tablet or powder form, making them portable and convenient for those times when you're traveling or don't have access to the kitchen. Take two tablets or stir 1 or 2 grams powder into ½ cup (120 ml) warm water 10 to 15 minutes before or after meals.

Turmeric Golden Milk Latte

APERITIF • DIGESTIF

This digestive-enhancing latte (page 127) makes for a nourishing beverage between meals. Its golden color and agni-enhancing qualities come from a combination of turmeric, cinnamon, and gingerroot, and its creaminess from coconut milk.

Sparkling Rosemary Limeade

APERITIF • MEALTIME

Drink this tart, aromatic elixir (page 126) 15 to 20 minutes before or during meals.

Chai Tea

APERITIF • MEALTIME • DIGESTIF

There are lots of great chai blends to try. See page 127 for a Tulsi Rose Chai recipe that was a favorite on the Goldthread farm.

Coriander, Cumin, and Fennel Tea

APERITIF • MEALTIME • DIGESTIF

Also known as CCF tea, this legendary Ayurvedic beverage (page 128) regulates and increases digestive fire. It's equally beneficial before, during, or after meals.

Cinnamon Tea

APERITIF • MEALTIME • DIGESTIF

Cinnamon is lightly kindling to digestive fire, and studies also confirm it has a positive effect on maintaining stable blood sugar levels when consumed after meals. See page 128 for a recipe for a tea using fresh cinnamon sticks—it smells as good as it tastes.

Vietnamese Artichoke Elixir

APERITIF • MEALTIME • DIGESTIF

This recipe (page 129) is my personal take on the refreshing Vietnamese beverage nước khổ qua lá dứa, famous for hydrating and cooling one down on hot days. It is full of essential nutrients and antioxidants, benefits digestion and liver function, and provides a daily detox.

Mukhwas

MEALTIME

These are sweetened fennel seeds you'll often find at Indian restaurants on the way out the door. Mukhwas enhance digestion, freshen breath, and reduce feelings of bloating and excess gas. Eat a teaspoonful or so right before or after a major meal. You can buy these premade online or make your own with the simple recipe on page 135.

Spice Blends and Toppers

MEALTIME

Add fresh or dried culinary spices into your recipes while cooking, sprinkle them on dishes as a topper, or garnish meals with fresh herbs once prepared. Citrus zest is another excellent accompaniment to meals. You can also chew on cardamom pods or toasted cumin or fennel seeds on their own as a quick-and-easy digestive aid. For a few of my favorite spice blends and toppers, see pages 118–120.

Milk Thistle Detox-Enhancing Dukkah

MEALTIME

Nuts, seeds, and spices are combined in this versatile topper that works with all kinds of savory dishes. See page 135 for the recipe.

Condiments

MEALTIME

Condiments that contain culinary spices make excellent additions to meals, giving them some agni-boosting power. Try Dijon mustard, horseradish, harissa, umeboshi, chutneys, sriracha, Cholula, pesto, Parsley Chimichurri (page 164), and herb-infused olive oil.

Gremolata

MEALTIME

This bright and zesty condiment (page 130) featuring parsley, garlic, and lemon zest is fresh, quick, and easy to prepare. Use it to liven up all kinds of dishes, including dips like hummus.

Pickled and Fermented Foods

MEALTIME

Choose from a variety of traditionally fermented plants that are rich in digestive-enhancing probiotics for promoting gut health—options include kimchi, sauerkraut, pickled gingerroot, pickle relish, and assorted pickled veggies like daikon radish and burdock root.

Spring Salad with Wild Greens

MEALTIME

Wild greens include dandelion greens, purslane, lamb's-quarters, sorrel, chickweed, wild amaranth, and shiso leaf. I like to mix them with traditional lettuce varieties, other fresh veggies, and aromatic culinary herbs for a delicious and nutrifying side or main dish (see recipe on page 130).

Wild Bitter Greens

MEALTIME

Bitter greens (a category that includes dandelion greens, chicory greens, amaranth, mustard greens, tatsoi, mizuna, purslane, shepherd's purse, garlic mustard, wild fennel, sheep sorrel, nettles, chickweed, and lamb's-quarters) can be incorporated into a variety of meals, fresh or cooked. They work well in salads, or try the common Mediterranean side dish Horta Vrasta (page 133).

Shiso, Shiitake, and Burdock Kinpira

MEALTIME

See page 133 for my take on this delicious Japanese side dish, made with nutrient-dense and detox-enhancing burdock root, shiso leaf, shiitake mushroom, and dulse flakes.

Kitchari

MEALTIME

This famous healing dish from the Ayurvedic tradition is a combination of dal, rice, and agni-kindling spices: cumin, coriander, fennel, onion, garlic, turmeric, cardamom, oregano, and black pepper. It's both nourishing and easy to digest. It gives the digestive system a rejuvenating rest, thus freeing up energy needed for healing and renewal. See page 134 for the recipe.

Spring Cleaning Tonic

MEALTIME • DIGESTIF

This unique tonic has a flavor reminiscent of root beer. It's traditionally used to enhance detoxification and support proper elimination with a combination of sassafras, sarsaparilla, licorice, burdock, dandelion, yellow dock, chamomile, and red clover. Drink 1 to 3 cups (240 to 720 ml) a day, hot or iced. See page 128 for the recipe, or seek out another detox tea blend that uses similar ingredients.

Traditional Caffeinated Plants

DIGESTIF

Yerba maté, green tea, oolong tea, guayusa, coffee, and espresso all contain mild bitter constituents that promote digestion and detoxification.

Dandelion, Chicory, and Carob Latte

DIGESTIF

This satisfying post-meal latte (page 127) enhances digestion and detoxification. Versions of this blend are available at health food stores and online. For those who wish to avoid caffeine, these are great coffee alternatives made from plants with similar flavor and aroma, such as carob powder or roasted dandelion and chicory roots that are loaded with nutrition and prebiotic fiber, and support the functioning of our liver and kidneys.

Triphala Tablets

One of the most effective detoxification formulations, triphala is a blend of three bitter fruits: amalaki (amla berry), bibitaki, and haritaki. It should be taken 2 hours after eating dinner or an hour or so before breakfast (it's best on an empty stomach). See the profile on page 346 for in-depth info on its uses and benefits.

Spice It Up

Global cuisines are often defined by the spices that give them their distinct flavors and aromas. Give these delicious blends a prominent place in your kitchen or on your table to encourage their frequent use. Mix up your own blends and toppers or purchase premade varieties. Below are some of the all-stars to get things started, but the list isn't comprehensive, so continue to explore and experiment with the many varieties of spice blends available.

Spice Blends

- **Caribbean curries.** These curry blends are considered the taste of the Caribbean, the foundation for the distinctive flavor of jerk chicken and fish. Many of these curries' ingredients overlap with other countries' curry blends (turmeric, coriander, cumin, black pepper, ginger, mustard seeds), but there are a few standout flavors specific and local to the region, including allspice, star anise, nutmeg, and dried Scotch bonnet chiles.

- **Cinnamon spice blends.** A blend of some combination of cinnamon, nutmeg, clove, allspice, ginger powder, anise seed, and vanilla powder is excellent in hot cereals, desserts, sauces, baked goods, and smoothies.

- **Furikake Japanese spice blends.** You'll find dozens of variations of this popular spice blend in any Japanese market, and just about every restaurant or kitchen table in Japan has a shaker or two. This blend is designed to convey the famous umami flavor to any dish. Most blends include toasted sesame seed, nori flakes, red pepper flakes, dried shiso leaf, shiitake powder, bonito flakes, sea salt, and a pinch of sugar.

- **Greek spice blends.** These combine all of the famed aromatics that make Mediterranean cuisine so healthy and delicious. Make your own by mixing dried basil, oregano, thyme, granulated garlic, rosemary, marjoram, dill leaf, ground black pepper, sea salt, lemon peel, and onion flakes.

- **Indian curries.** It seems as if every family in India has its own special recipe for Indian curry, and blends vary from region to region. The spices are often lightly toasted (which releases aromatic properties) and immediately ground into powders to preserve freshness. If you're making your own, you can toast your spices or—for simplicity's sake—combine pre-ground powders. The most common spices in curry powders are turmeric, coriander, cumin, fennel, chile pepper, ginger, mustard, cardamom, and black pepper.

Left to right: Mexican, Japanese furikake, Indian curry, North African, cinnamon, Thai, and Greek spice blends

---

- **Mexican spice blends.** Mexican cooks have perfected the art of combining different varieties of chile peppers to make dangerously delectable spice blends. In addition to hot peppers, Mexican seasonings often contain spices such as garlic powder, coriander, cumin, Mexican oregano, allspice, anise seed, cacao powder, onion flakes, black pepper, and epazote (an aromatic herb).

- **North African spice blends.** The Arabic phrase *ras el hanout*—translated as "best of the shop"—refers to spice blends containing the best spices available. Ras el hanout generally consists of a dozen or so spices, among them cumin, coriander, cardamom, clove, cinnamon, nutmeg, mace, allspice, ginger, chile pepper, black pepper, paprika, fenugreek, saffron, and turmeric. (Ras el hanout spice blends found in Tunisia, Algeria, and Morocco use many of the same herbs but in varying proportions and built around local preferences.)

- **Thai spice blends.** Thai cuisine is light and fragrant, with a spicy edge. Most Thai spice blends build from a combination of lemongrass, ginger, makrut lime leaves, peppercorns, galangal, chile pepper, garlic powder, and star anise.

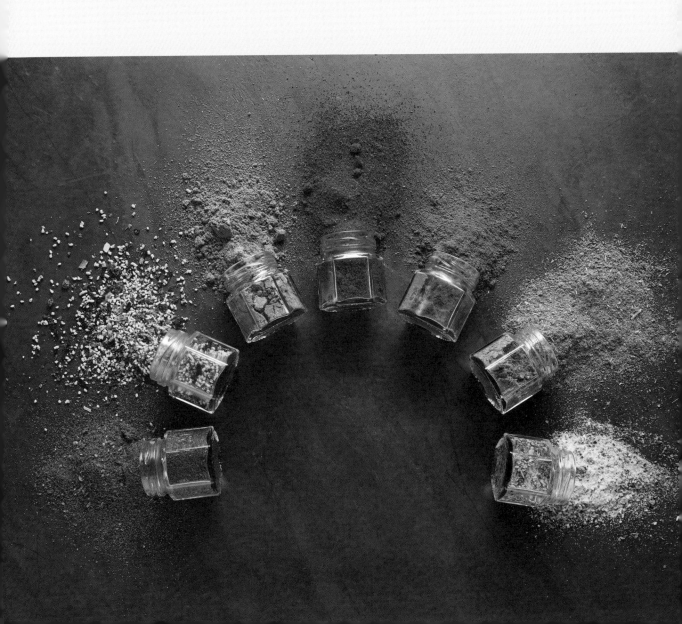

Sprinkles & Toppers

Salt and pepper have had a monopoly on the dinner table for far too long. In many countries I have visited, it's common to see tables and trays laden with a far greater variety of tasty, health-enhancing spice blends and toppers. Sprinkling culinary spices onto dishes is an easy and enjoyable way to kindle digestive fire. Organize your spice blends in shakers or small jars in a tray or rack of some kind. Put them in a prominent place on the dining room or kitchen table, and rotate the contents of the tray from time to time to keep things interesting. Here are a few of my favorites.

- **Dukkah.** Milk Thistle Detox-Enhancing Dukkah (page 135) is a variation on this nutritious North African spice-and-nut blend, combining agni-enhancing culinary spices with detox-enhancing milk thistle seeds in one easy recipe.

- **Gomasio.** Sprinkle this Japanese blend on soups, rice dishes, and stir-fries. It contains toasted white or black sesame seeds, sea salt, nori flakes, garlic powder, dried basil leaf, dried oregano, red pepper flakes, and dried parsley.

- **Gremolata.** A traditional topper from the Mediterranean, gremolata has only three ingredients: chopped fresh parsley, finely minced garlic, and fresh lemon zest. It's perfect as a garnish for a pasta dinner or as an appetizer mixed with olive oil. Turn to page 130 for a recipe.

- **Yuzu kosho.** This famous Japanese condiment is made from the zest of the aromatic citrus fruit yuzu, which is similar to lemon but stronger and more tart, blended with small amounts of fermented chile peppers and salt.

- **Za'atar.** This traditional spice topper from the Middle East blends sesame seeds with savory dried herbs such as oregano, thyme, marjoram, cumin, coriander, and dried sumac.

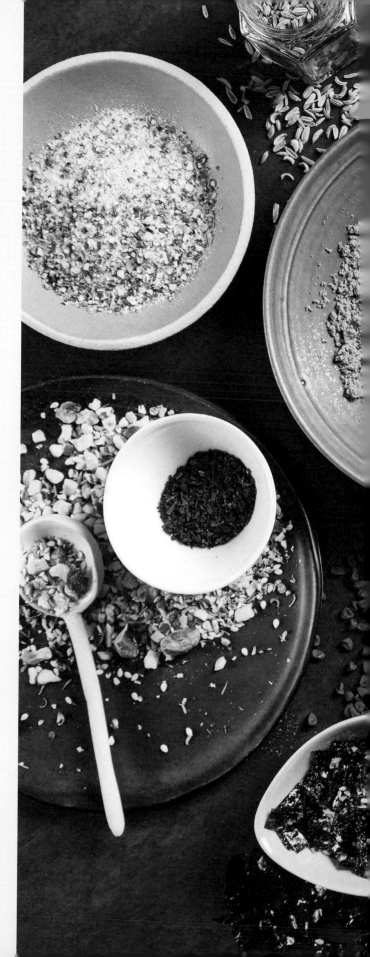

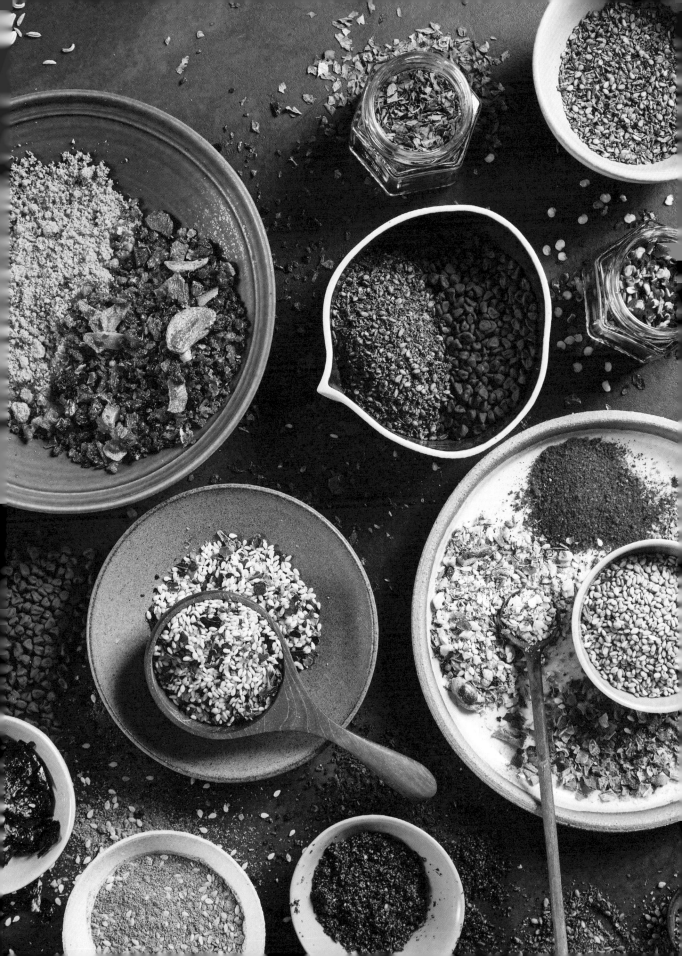

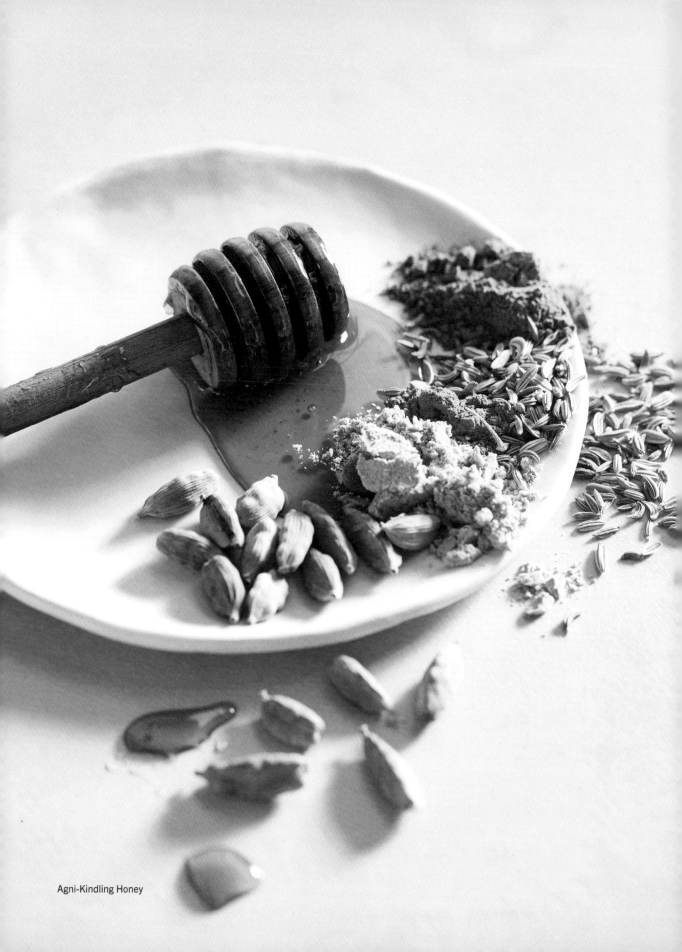

Agni-Kindling Honey

Agni-Kindling Honey

Thoroughly mix **1 teaspoon cinnamon powder, 1 teaspoon ginger powder, ½ teaspoon cardamom powder,** and **½ teaspoon fennel powder**. Stir the powder blend into **1 cup (240 ml) manuka honey or other honey of your choic**e until completely combined. Take a small spoonful on its own, or melt it into ½ cup (120 ml) warm water and drink 15 to 20 minutes before meals. Store in a glass jar in the fridge; because honey is naturally anaerobic (oxygen-free), this preparation will stay good for 2 weeks. Makes 1 cup (240 ml).

Note: Feel free to swap in other culinary spice powders as desired; keep ratios approximately the same for optimal consistency.

Turmeric Balls

Combine **½ cup (120 ml) liquefied honey, 2 tablespoons coconut butter, 1 teaspoon coconut oil,** and **⅛ teaspoon ground black pepper** in a mixing bowl. Gradually add **¾ cup (85 g) turmeric powder** until it is fully incorporated and the mix has a dough-like consistency. Sprinkle a thin layer of **dragon fruit powder** on a small plate. Form the dough into approximately 12 gumball-size balls and roll each one in the dragon fruit powder until fully covered. Place the balls on a parchment paper–lined plate, cover, and refrigerate for an hour or so until they firm up. Stored in a sealed container in the fridge, they'll be good for up to 2 weeks. Makes 12 balls.

Ginger Shots

Use approximately **5 ounces (140 g) organic fresh gingerroot** and **6 large lemons** (enough to make 1 cup/240 ml juice each). Wash the ginger with a vegetable brush (no need to peel); peel the lemons before juicing. Juice the ginger and lemons.

Combine the ginger juice, lemon juice, and **1 cup (240 ml) coconut water**. Spoon in **2 tablespoons manuka honey or a natural sweetener of your choice to taste** and mix well with a mini immersion blender. Store in the fridge; it will last up to 1 week. Makes 3 cups (720 ml).

Ginger-Turmeric Shots

Use approximately **2 to 3 ounces (60 to 85 g) organic fresh gingerroot, 2 to 3 ounces (60 to 85 g) fresh turmeric rhizome**, and **6 large lemons** (enough to make 1 cup/240 ml juice each). Wash the roots with a vegetable brush (no need to peel); peel the lemons before juicing. Juice the ginger, turmeric, and lemons.

Combine the three juices and **1 cup (240 ml) coconut water**. Spoon in **2 tablespoons manuka honey or a natural sweetener of your choice to taste** and **1/16 teaspoon ground black pepper** and mix well with a mini immersion blender. Store in the fridge; it will last up to 1 week. Makes 1 quart (1 L).

Turmeric-Orange-Lime Shots

Use approximately **5 ounces (140 g) fresh turmeric rhizome** (enough to make 1 cup/240 ml juice), **2 to 3 oranges** (enough to make ½ cup/120 ml juice), and **2 to 3 limes** (enough to make ¼ cup/60 ml juice). Scrub the turmeric with a vegetable brush (no need to peel); peel the oranges and limes before juicing. Juice the turmeric, oranges, and limes.

Combine the three juices and **½ cup (120 ml) coconut water**. Stir in **2 tablespoons manuka honey or a natural sweetener of your choice to taste** and **1/16 teaspoon ground black pepper** and mix well with a mini immersion blender. Store in the fridge; it will last up to 1 week. Makes 2¼ cups (540 ml).

Notes: Take 2 ounces (60 ml) of any of these recipes in a shot glass, 10 to 15 minutes before or after meals. To sip on this drink, rather than taking it as a shot, dilute 2 to 4 ounces (60 to 120 ml) ginger shot with an additional 1½ to 1¾ cups (360 to 420 ml) coconut water and/or water, mix, and pour over ice. Add a slice of lemon for garnish. Also, a teaspoon or two of fresh basil, cilantro, or shiso juice make nice boosts in terms of both flavor and medicinal benefits to any of these shots. If you feel a cold or flu coming on, add a pinch of cayenne pepper or fresh or dried oregano.

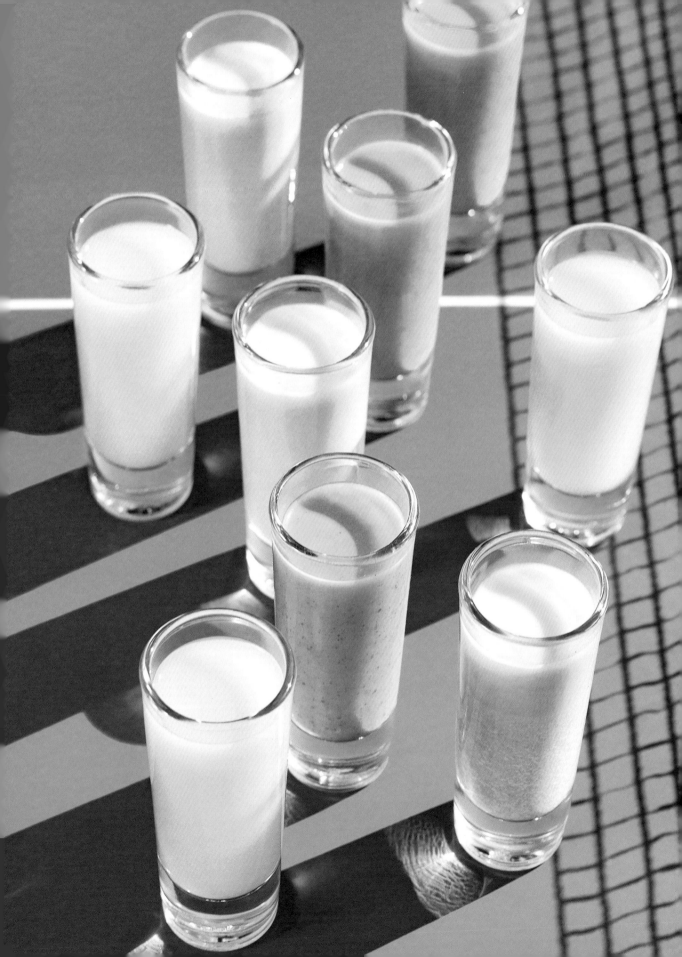

Sparkling Rosemary Limeade

Combine **1 teaspoon finely chopped fresh rosemary** and **1 tablespoon fresh lime juice** in a bowl. Let sit for 10 minutes, then strain and discard the needles. Pour into a glass with **a natural sweetener of your choice** to taste, if desired, and **1½ cups (360 ml) sparkling water**. Mix well and serve over ice, garnish with **fresh rosemary sprigs** and **lime wheels**, if desired.

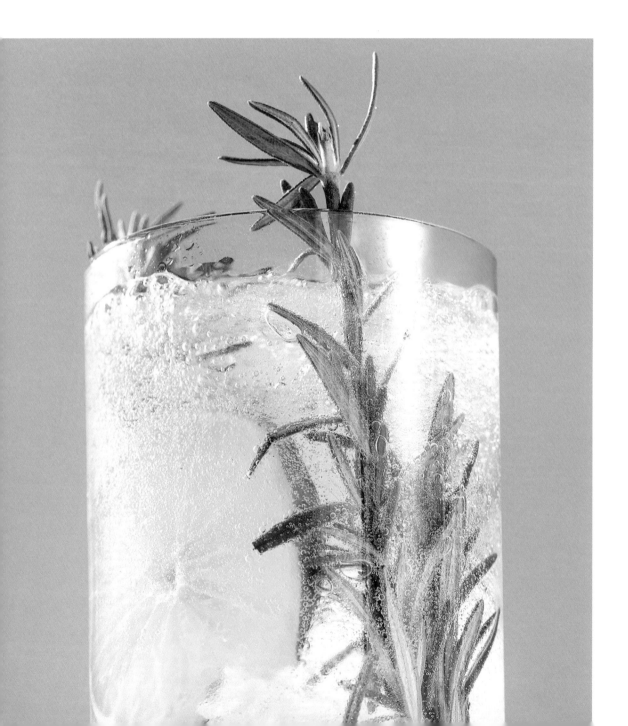

Turmeric Golden Milk Latte

Combine **½ teaspoon turmeric powder**, **¼ teaspoon ginger powder**, **¼ teaspoon cinnamon powder**, and **½ teaspoon vanilla extract** in a cup. Pour **1 to 1¼ cups (240 to 300 ml) hot water** over while stirring. Add **a natural sweetener of your choice** to taste and **a small pinch of ground black pepper** and blend. Froth **½ cup (120 ml) coconut milk** and pour over. Add **a dash of cinnamon powder** on top.

Tulsi Rose Chai

Combine **1½ teaspoons dried tulsi leaf, ½ teaspoon rose petals, ½ teaspoon dried orange peel, ¼ teaspoon cinnamon powder, ¼ teaspoon ginger powder**, and **½ teaspoon vanilla extract** in a bowl. Spoon the mixture into a French press or a self-fill tea bag or removable infuser basket in a mug. Pour **1¼ to 1½ cups (300 to 360 ml) boiling water** over; let steep for 10 minutes. Plunge the press or press on the tea bag or loose tea to squeeze out any additional liquid. Sweeten with **1 teaspoon honey or maple syrup**, if desired. Add **½ cup (120 ml) warmed cashew or coconut milk**.

Note: For an iced chai, use half to two-thirds the amount of water. Chill the mixture and pour over ice cubes.

Dandelion, Chicory, and Carob Latte

Combine in a mug **½ teaspoon each roasted and powdered dandelion root, roasted and powdered chicory root**, and **powdered carob root; ¼ teaspoon cinnamon powder;** and **½ teaspoon vanilla extract** and mix with a spoon. Pour **1 cup (240 ml) hot water** into the mug and mix thoroughly with a spoon or mini immersion blender. Add **½ cup (120 ml) warm cashew or oat milk** along with **a dash of cinnamon powder**.

Note: For an iced latte, use half to two-thirds the amount of water. Chill the mixture and milk, pour over ice cubes, and garnish with the cinnamon.

Coriander, Cumin, and Fennel Tea

Add **1 tablespoon each coriander, cumin, and fennel seeds** to **1 quart (1 L) water in a saucepan.** Gently simmer, covered, for 10 minutes. Strain. Drink 1 cup (240 ml), sweetened with **a natural sweetener of your choice** to taste, if desired, before or with meals. The remaining tea can be stored in the fridge for a few days; it's best to drink it warm or at room temperature. Makes 4 servings.

Note: You can adjust these ratios slightly to strengthen or dilute the flavor based on your preference. You can also add 1 teaspoon grated fresh gingerroot or 1 teaspoon dried peppermint, if desired.

Cinnamon Tea

Break up **1 small cinnamon stick** and simmer in **1½ cups (360 ml) water** for 5 to 10 minutes. Strain. (Alternatively, simply add **1 teaspoon cinnamon powder** to hot water.) Add **1 teaspoon natural sweetener of your choice**, or to taste, and **a squeeze of lemon juice**.

Spring Cleaning Tonic

This tea uses dried loose herbs. Mix together **2 parts each sassafras and sarsaparilla bark**; **1 part each licorice root, burdock root, dandelion root, and yellow dock**; and **½ part each chamomile and red clover** in a bowl. (Convert parts to whatever form of measurement you choose depending on how much you would like to make.) Store in an airtight container out of light and away from heat. Dry tea mixes last for many weeks this way.

To make a cup of tea, use **1 to 2 tablespoons dry tea mix** per **1½ cups (360 ml) hot water**. Infuse in a removable infuser basket for 10 minutes. To make a larger quantity of tea, use a French press or a quart (1 L) canning jar.

Vietnamese Artichoke Elixir

Halve **2 medium artichokes**. Place them in a large saucepan with **8 cups (2 L) water** and bring to a boil. Reduce the heat to low, cover, and simmer for 30 minutes. (Alternatively, use 1 or 2 ounces/30 or 60 g dried artichoke leaf tea.) Add in **1 cup (30 g) chopped fresh or dried pandan leaves, ¼ cup (35 g) fresh lemongrass,** and **¼ cup (55 g) chopped fresh gingerroot.** Simmer for an additional 30 minutes. Strain through a fine-mesh strainer into a heat-resistant bowl. Add **2 to 4 tablespoons natural sweetener of your choice, ¼ cup (60 ml) fresh lemon juice,** and **2 teaspoons vanilla extract.** Gently stir and let cool. Once cooled, stir in **1 to 2 tablespoons liquid chlorophyll** to give it a deep emerald-green color and additional nutritional benefits. Pour into a glass serving pitcher and chill in the fridge for an hour or two. Serve over ice, if desired. Makes 4 to 6 servings.

Note: Pandan leaves can be found fresh or frozen at most Asian grocers; dried leaves are available online.

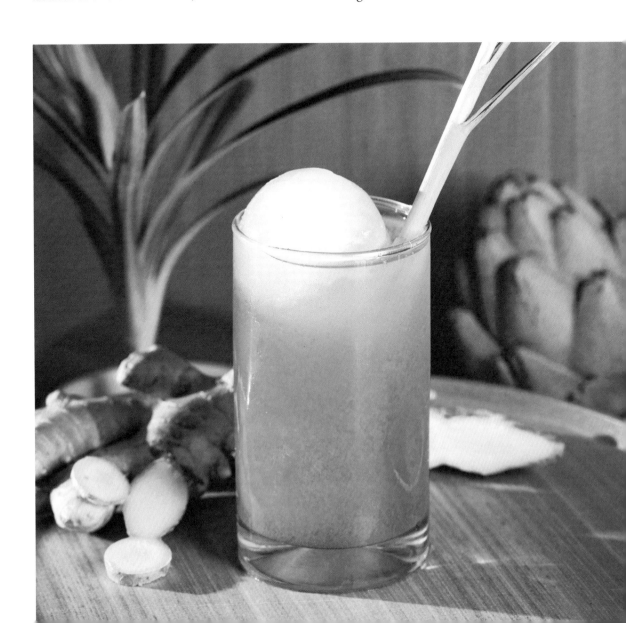

Gremolata

Mince the leaves of **1 medium bunch fresh flat-leaf parsley** and put in a small bowl. Add **1 finely chopped garlic clove** and the **zest from 1 medium lemon** and mix thoroughly. Use immediately, as a topper on a main dish, or as an appetizer spread mixed with olive oil. The gremolata can be kept in the fridge for a day or two. Makes about 1 cup (240 ml).

Note: You can substitute fresh mint for the parsley and use other types of zest, like orange or grapefruit.

Spring Salad with Wild Greens

This salad uses a ratio of **1 cup (20 g) wild greens**, **1 cup (15 g) culinary herbs**, and **2 cups (80 g) traditional lettuces (red leaf or your favorite variety)**. For wild greens, choose from the following: dandelion greens, purslane, lamb's-quarters, sorrel, chickweed, and wild amaranth. For the fresh culinary herbs, choose from the following: shiso leaf (red or green), basil, cilantro, parsley, spearmint or peppermint, and small amounts of oregano and/or rosemary. Wash and dry the herbs and lettuces thoroughly. For the dressing, cut **1 garlic clove** into big slices and, with the back of a spoon, press the garlic into the bottom of a bowl. Add **½ cup (120 ml) extra-virgin olive oil**, **2 tablespoons balsamic vinegar**, **1 tablespoon mustard**, **1 teaspoon fresh lemon juice**, and **sea salt and ground black pepper** to taste. Whisk the dressing until thoroughly mixed and drizzle over the salad. **Edible flowers**, like nasturtium or dandelion flowers, can be used as garnish. Makes 2 servings.

Note: Wild greens are most common in springtime (though some can be enjoyed year-round). When it comes to peak flavor, look for younger plants.

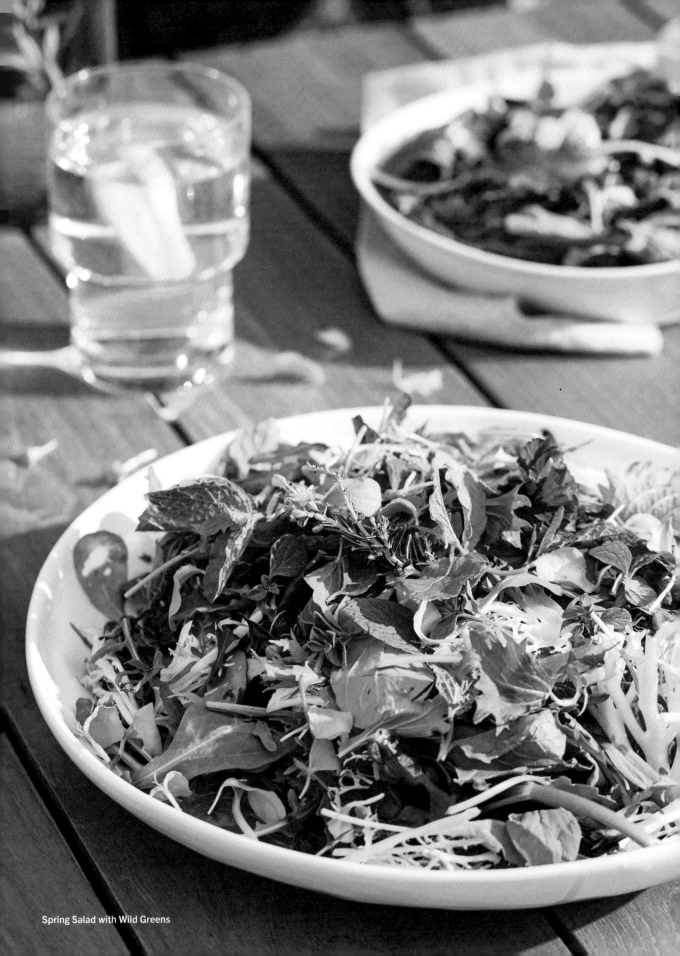

Spring Salad with Wild Greens

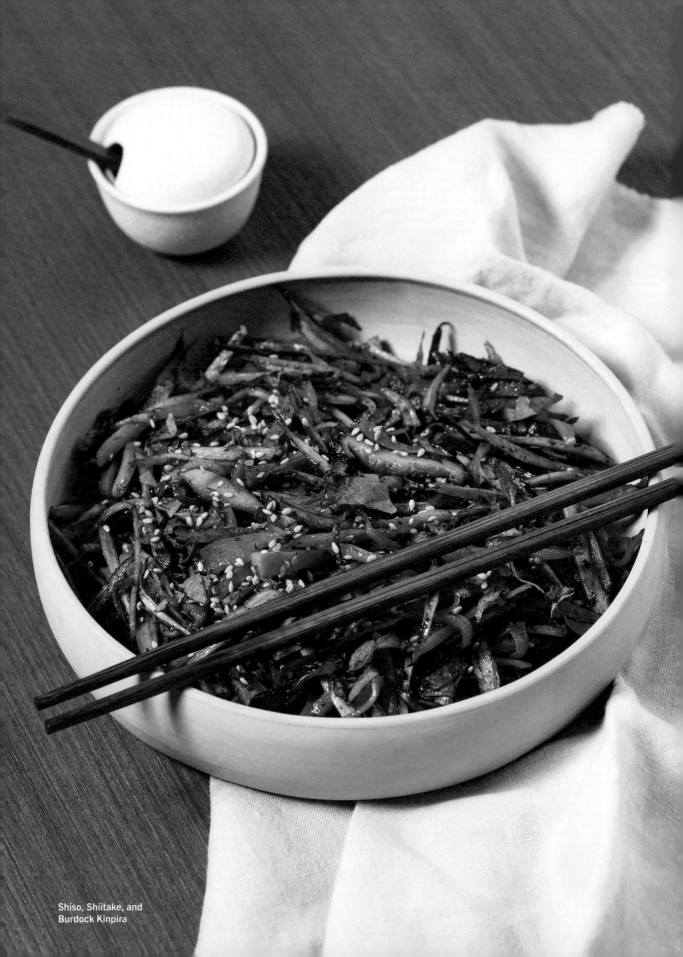

Shiso, Shiitake, and
Burdock Kinpira

Horta Vrasta

The traditional Greek dish horta vrasta is an easy and delicious way to cook wild greens. In my version, I blanch rather than boil the greens, to retain their vibrant color and nutrients. Wash and roughly chop **1 bunch dandelion greens** and **1 bunch spinach** with stems removed. Cover the greens with water and soak for a few minutes, rinse, and drain in a colander to remove any grit. Bring a large pot of water to a boil and add **1 tablespoon salt**. Prepare a large bowl of ice water. Add the greens to the boiling water and cook for 1 to 2 minutes, then remove with a handheld strainer and immediately submerge in the ice water. Drain and toss with a dressing made of **1 minced garlic clove, 2 tablespoons extra-virgin olive oil**, the **juice of 1 lemon**, and **salt and ground black pepper** to taste. Makes 2 to 4 servings.

Note: Any of the following can be substituted for the greens called for here: chicory greens, amaranth, mustard greens, tatsoi, mizuna, wild fennel, nettles, and lamb's-quarters.

Shiso, Shiitake, and Burdock Kinpira

In a bowl, make a sauce with **½ cup (120 ml) water, 2 tablespoons mirin, 2 tablespoons tamari, 2 tablespoons sake, 1 teaspoon powdered shiitake mushroom**, and **½ teaspoon powdered dulse flakes**; set aside. Warm **2 to 3 tablespoons toasted sesame oil** in a skillet over medium heat and add **1 thinly sliced burdock root**. Sauté for 5 to 7 minutes, until the root starts to get tender. Pour in the sauce and cook for an additional 5 to 7 minutes, stirring frequently. Transfer to a serving bowl. Add **2 teaspoons white sesame seeds** and **3 minced shiso leaves** and stir. Garnish with additional sesame seeds and shiso leaves, if desired. Makes 2 to 3 servings.

Kitchari

Place **2 tablespoons ghee** in a saucepan with **1 teaspoon each whole cumin, coriander, and fennel seeds**. Sauté over low heat for 1 to 2 minutes, until the seeds start to turn golden brown. Add **1 cup (200 g) split yellow dal or red lentils** and **½ cup (90 g) basmati rice** and continue to sauté for another minute or two. Add **6 cups (1.4 L) water**, **1 teaspoon dried oregano**, **½ teaspoon onion powder**, **½ teaspoon garlic powder**, **½ teaspoon turmeric powder**, **¼ teaspoon cardamom powder**, **a pinch of ground black pepper**, and **a pinch of asafoetida powder**. Cover and bring to a boil, then reduce the heat and simmer for 30 to 45 minutes, until tender—the consistency is more stew than soup, but feel free to add more water to thin as desired. Garnish with **parsley**, **cilantro**, and/or **coconut flakes** before serving. Makes 3 to 4 servings.

Note: This recipe goes big on spices, but feel free to adjust to suit your taste. It's fine to play around with the ratio of rice and dal as well. In fact, kitchari has many possible variations. You can sprinkle on some toasted sesame or sunflower seeds or roasted buckwheat hulls. A teaspoon or two of Sea Vegetable Sprinkles (page 164) gives it a nutritional boost. Veggies, like carrots, onions, yams, and leafy greens, also make a nice addition to the basic recipe.

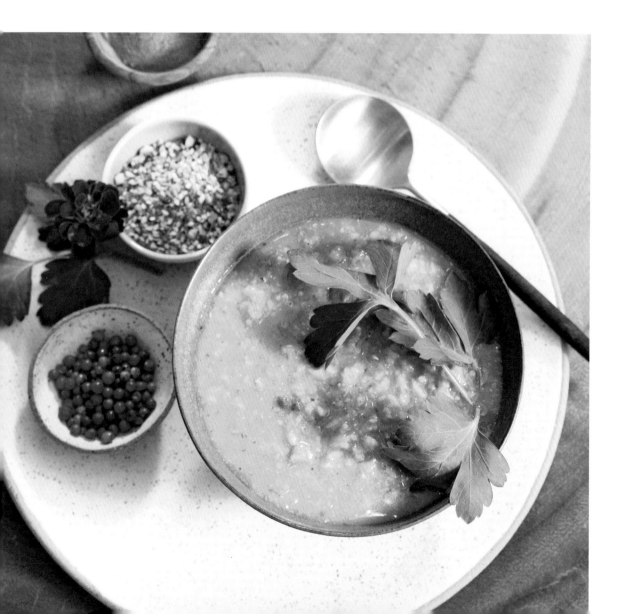

Milk Thistle
Detox-Enhancing Dukkah

Toast **½ cup (70 g) hazelnuts**, **3 tablespoons almonds**, **3 tablespoons hulled pistachios**, and **1½ tablespoons milk thistle seeds** in a skillet over medium heat, tossing regularly until the nuts turn golden brown. Transfer the nut mixture to a food processor or blender and pulse until the mixture is coarsely ground. Add **2 tablespoons sesame seeds** and **1 teaspoon each fennel seeds, coriander seeds, cumin seeds, and dried lemon peel** along with **1 teaspoon salt** and **a pinch each of cayenne pepper and ground black pepper** and pulse again until the mixture is evenly blended and the consistency of fine powder. Be careful not to overmix to a nut butter–like texture. Store in an airtight container. Sprinkle the dukkah on anything you like, eat a spoonful on its own, or mix a spoonful with olive oil and use as a spread. Makes 1¼ cups (120 g).

Mukhwas

Combine in a bowl **¼ cup (25 g) each fennel seeds, coriander seeds, and dill seeds**; **2 tablespoons anise seeds**; **½ teaspoon sea salt**; and **1 tablespoon fresh lemon juice**. Mix thoroughly and let sit for an hour. Transfer to an unoiled nonstick (preferably cast-iron) pan and toast for 2 to 3 minutes. Remove from the heat and let cool slightly. Add **1 teaspoon coconut or date sugar** and mix thoroughly. Let cool completely and store in an airtight container for up to a week. Makes 1 cup (110 g).

Japanese Green Tea:
Mindfulness & Mastery

For thousands of years, green tea has been the Japanese elixir of longevity and a significant reason the people of Japan are among the healthiest and most long-lived on earth. The tea comes from the leaves of *Camellia sinensis*, a small shrub native to China, now widely cultivated throughout Asia. Once a coveted treasure reserved for the wealthy, green tea found a larger audience when monks drinking it for increased energy and alertness during early-morning meditations spread the word about its innumerable benefits for health and well-being. Today green tea is second only to water in beverages consumed in Japan.

After harvesting, green tea leaves undergo a minimal steam-processing method that locks in antioxidants, vitamins, minerals, and other important constituents such as L-theanine, an amino acid that increases the levels of GABA, serotonin, and dopamine in the brain. (L-theanine also contributes to the tea's unique umami flavor.) These neurotransmitters are responsible for calming the nervous system, improving cognitive function, and elevating mood. The steam process also gives the tea its vibrant green color and relatively low caffeine content in comparison with black tea or coffee, making it far more sustainable to drink throughout the day. The clarity and alertness green tea produces enhance awareness without causing jittery overstimulation.

The average age of green tea farmers in Japan has been steadily going up over the past few decades as fewer and fewer young people are taking their place. The farmers I hung out with in Japan were all in their seventies yet had the physical vitality and stamina of twenty-year-olds. They drank upward of ten cups of green tea per day during the intensive labor of

harvesting and processing plants, and invariably had smiles on their faces as they worked. (I know that sounds like a lot of caffeine! Each serving is quite small, and the varieties of green tea they drink, such as bancha, have a relatively low caffeine content and are enjoyed for their refreshing and hydrating qualities.) When asked what they attribute their obviously vibrant health to, all agreed that drinking green tea was an essential element.

More than two thousand years ago, Kampo, the traditional herbal medicine system of Japan, characterized green tea as "an elixir that brightens the eyes of those who drink it," a reference to its ability to promote extraordinary health and vitality. Copious research has since backed this up: Green tea has proven medicinal benefits for the cardiovascular and immune systems, improving metabolism, lowering certain cancer risks, and reducing inflammation. The concentrated amount of nutrients and unique antioxidants in green tea make it one of

A green tea plantation in Utogi, Japan

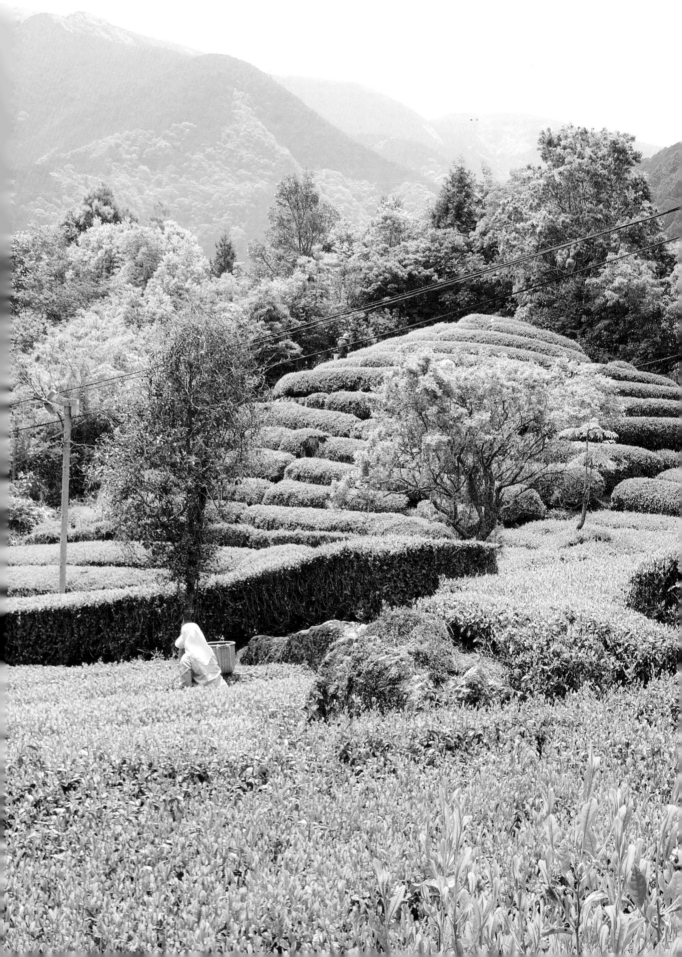

the healthiest beverages on earth. It's as if the Japanese farmers have been drinking an extra ten servings of vegetables all day long, for decades.

In Japan, green tea is much more than a healthy beverage, however; it's a way of life, and drinking it in a traditional context brings a whole different dimension to the experience. Preparing and serving tea in Japan is serious business. The process is infused with precision and attention to detail—there's no multitasking going on when making tea. Green tea is served in a refined and aesthetically pleasing manner. The teapot and cups are often beautiful artisanal pieces. The water temperature, steeping time, and amount of tea used per cup are all precisely measured to arrive at the desired result. Tea shops and restaurants even provide customers with little sand hourglasses or digital timers so they don't mess it up.

In an otherwise hectic and technologically advanced society, the ritual of drinking green tea remains a portal into a more intentional and simpler frame of mind. In contrast to the way people rely on coffee in our culture, as a way to amp up and fuel productivity, drinking green tea in Japan is an opportunity to relax and create spaciousness in the mind.

The tea itself becomes a vehicle for creating a moment outside of the normal, busy flow of time, to be present and appreciate the people we're with and what's around us. In my visits to Japan, I've shared green tea with people in thousand-year-old temples, in bonsai gardens while butterflies flittered about, in the middle of ancient tea fields, and from street carts in Tokyo. In each instance, the essential spirit of the occasion and the great care that goes into preparing and serving green tea as a gesture of respect and gratitude feel the same.

Drink green tea for its health benefits and amazing flavors, and as you do, remember the deeper context for an even richer experience.

Opposite: Matcha grown in the shade of solar panels in Shizuoka, Japan

Below: Green tea farmers delivering their harvest to be processed in Uji, Japan

---

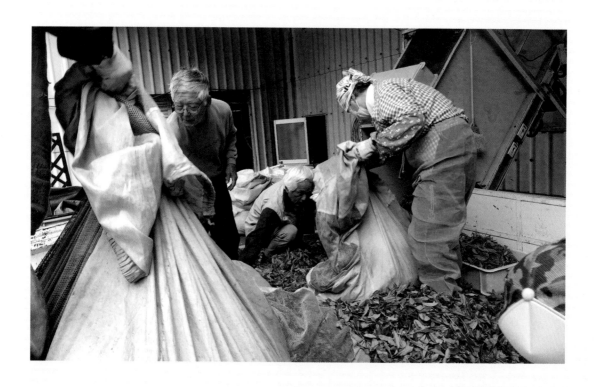

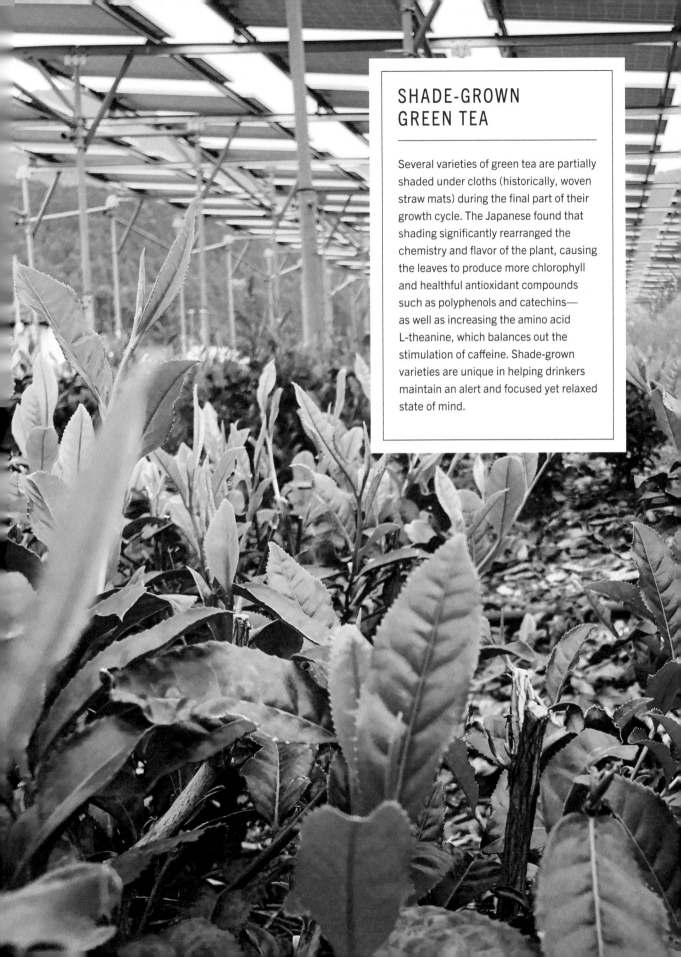

SHADE-GROWN GREEN TEA

Several varieties of green tea are partially shaded under cloths (historically, woven straw mats) during the final part of their growth cycle. The Japanese found that shading significantly rearranged the chemistry and flavor of the plant, causing the leaves to produce more chlorophyll and healthful antioxidant compounds such as polyphenols and catechins—as well as increasing the amino acid L-theanine, which balances out the stimulation of caffeine. Shade-grown varieties are unique in helping drinkers maintain an alert and focused yet relaxed state of mind.

hojicha

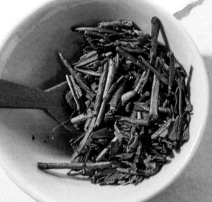

Tencha

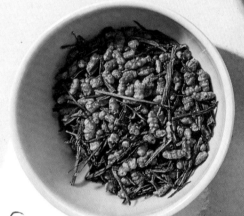

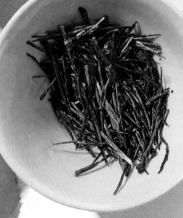

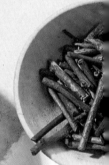

Genmaicha

Sencha

kukicha

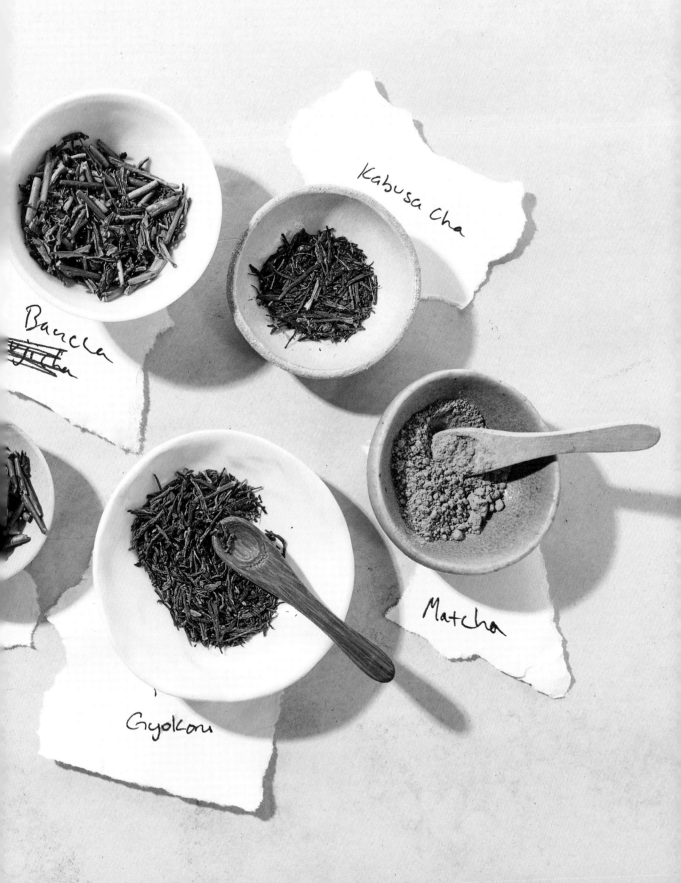

Kabusa Cha

Bancha

Gyokoru

Matcha

Brewing Green Tea

Japanese green tea comes in hundreds of varieties, each with different flavors and characteristics depending on how it is grown, harvested, and processed (more on this below). No matter which variety you choose, proper brewing technique ensures extraction of the widest variety of health-enhancing constituents and peak flavor, color, and aroma.

Each variety has a different optimal temperature (between 140°F / 60°C and 185°F / 85°C). If the tea you purchase doesn't come with specific instructions, seek out guidance from the seller or a reputable site. If the water is too hot, it can result in a tea with an overly bitter and astringent taste and degrade green tea's delicate medicinal compounds.

Likewise, brewing time can vary between 1 and 3 minutes. Once your pot is brewing, set a timer for 1 minute. Once the timer goes off, take a small sip every 30 seconds until you reach the desired flavor and color.

Note: For a more refreshing version of green tea that can be sipped on throughout the day, try cold infusion. Cold-water brewing doesn't liberate nearly as many of the bitter tannins in green tea even when left for a longer brewing time (10 to 30 minutes) compared to hot water.

Popular Green Tea Varieties

• **Sencha** ("simmered tea") accounts for over 80 percent of all green tea consumed in Japan. Sencha is characterized by needle-shaped leaves, a deep green color, a fresh aroma, and a grassy, vegetal flavor. The tea is harvested three times throughout the season, and each harvest (known as a flush) is considered to be somewhat sweeter and fresher tasting as the season continues.

• **Bancha** ("last tea") comes from the fourth and final tea harvest in the autumn. It is often pan-roasted to remove any remaining moisture and to create a sweet, nutty flavor and golden-colored infusion. Bancha is thirst quenching and nourishing and a nice option for cold infusions (see page 94). It has half the caffeine content of sencha and is a rich source of iron and other trace elements and minerals.

• **Kukicha** ("twig tea") is made from the stems and young twigs of green tea plants. A staple of the macrobiotic diet, kukicha has a nutty fragrance and a mildly sweet flavor. It comes in both green and brown varieties depending on whether or not it has been roasted. Though kukicha is made exclusively from the stems, it's no afterthought—many artisanal producers specialize in kukicha.

• **Hojicha** ("roasted tea") is made from green tea that has been roasted in porcelain pots over charcoal, creating a rich, reddish-colored brew with a distinctive earthy flavor, very little bitterness, and the lowest caffeine content of any green tea. This makes hojicha a good choice for afternoon and evening.

• **Genmaicha** ("brown rice tea") is made from combining sencha with toasted or puffed brown rice in equal proportions, creating a toasted, nutty-flavored tea similar to Japanese rice crackers. The mild starches from the rice give genmaicha a uniquely nourishing quality, good for drinking between meals.

- **Gyokuro** ("jade dew"), so named for its neon green color when brewed, is considered one of the highest-quality varieties of green tea, and is thus among the most expensive and sought after. It is one of several unique green teas shaded beneath cloth for some part of its growing cycle to produce a rich, sweet umami flavor with a seaweed-like aroma. Gyokuro is handpicked only once a year and consumed in small quantities in a deliberate manner to preserve the subtle nuances of flavor and aroma.

- **Kabuse cha** ("covered tea") is a variety of sencha that is shaded for the final seven to ten days before harvest, resulting in a tea that could be considered a hybrid between sencha and gyokuro. It has characteristics of both: the fresh bright aroma of sencha and some of the sweet umami of gyokuro. It's less expensive than gyokuro, and thus a good option if you want to drink a shaded variety on a regular basis.

- **Matcha** ("ground tea") is perhaps the world's most popular green tea variety and is used in the famous Japanese tea ceremony. Shade-grown during the final three to four weeks before harvest, matcha then undergoes an elaborate multistage processing method whereby the stem and midveins of the leaf are removed before the leaves are steamed, dried, and stone ground by massive granite wheels (designed to handle delicate constituents without too much heat) into a fine jade-green powder. Matcha has the highest content of L-theanine of all green teas, making it the best variety for calming the mind and enhancing cognitive function. And by consuming the whole leaf as powder, you're getting the plant's entire spectrum of nutritional benefits. Matcha typically comes in three varieties (ceremonial, premium, and culinary), each one denoting quality and flavor characteristics. For a matcha latte recipe, see page 220.

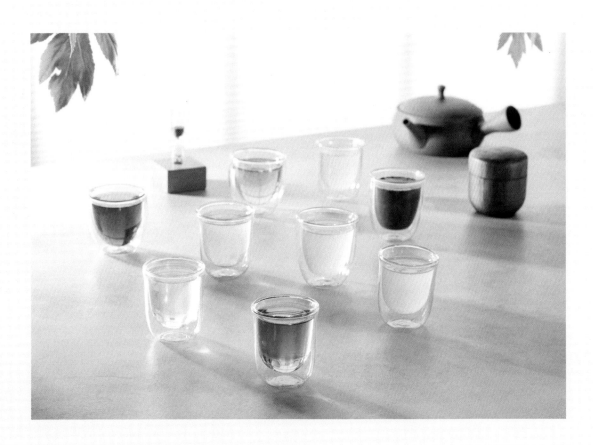

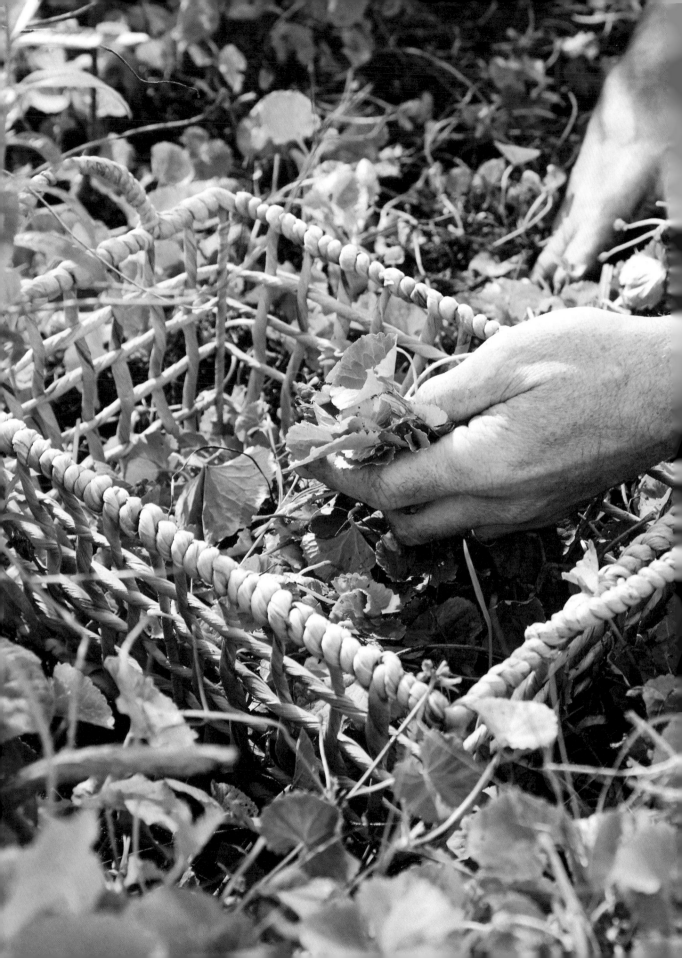

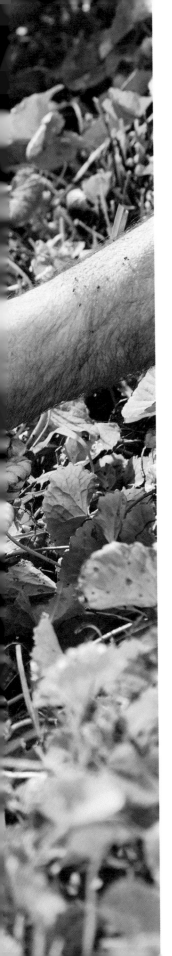

step 2 | Nutritives

NO MATTER HOW HEALTHY OUR DIETS ARE, IT CAN STILL BE A challenge to get enough of all the essential nutrients we require for optimal health. The focus of Step 2 is supercharging our body with nutritives: true superfoods that provide us with a powerful and unparalleled source of essential vitamins, minerals, trace elements, and antioxidants to fuel our metabolic and cellular functions. When we integrate nutritives into our daily routines and begin replenishing the body's reservoirs of essential nutrients, we start feeling healthier and more resilient. Vital physiological functions get tuned up and become more responsive, giving us the stability and balance required to meet the challenges of the day.

WHAT TO EXPECT

- A sensation of being more grounded and resilient

- A calmer and more centered disposition

- Deeper sleep

- Improved blood sugar stability

- Stronger and more lustrous skin, hair, and nails

- Increased energy and endurance

- Clearer, sharper thinking

Plants & Other Ingredients You'll Be Using

All plants in this category—from nutritive herbs to superfruits to sea vegetables—contain essential vitamins, minerals, trace elements, and antioxidants in varying proportions.

Green and leafy herbs like nettles, moringa, dandelion leaves, ashitaba leaf, and gotu kola contain copious amounts of important minerals like magnesium, calcium, iron, phosphorus, and potassium. Many of these nutritives are used as ingredients in traditional recipes or consumed as liquid infusions or powdered additions to smoothies and beverages.

Tart-tasting superfruits such as rose hips, acai, camu camu, amla, and goji are packed with vitamin C and immune-enhancing antioxidants. They make bright and flavorful additions to jams and chutneys, and when powdered can be blended into smoothies, teas, and other beverages.

Veggies from the sea, such as nori, dulse, wakame, and kombu, contain more rare trace elements (like iodine, phosphorus, manganese, copper, and selenium), and at far greater concentrations, than those grown on land. Incorporate them into soups and broths, salads, and condiments.

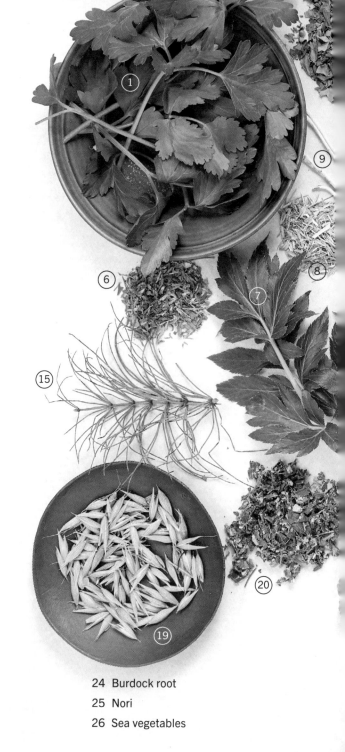

1 Parsley	12 Elderberries	24 Burdock root
2 Moringa	13 Jujube dates	25 Nori
3 Rose hips	14 Nettles	26 Sea vegetables
4 Super berries	15 Horsetail	
5 Cilantro	16 Chicory root	
6 Alfalfa leaf	17 Hibiscus	
7 + 20 Ashitaba	18 Amla berries	
8 Oatstraw	19 Oat tops	
9 Bellflower	21 Gotu kola	
10 Shiso leaf	22 Red clover	
11 Camu camu	23 Acai berries	

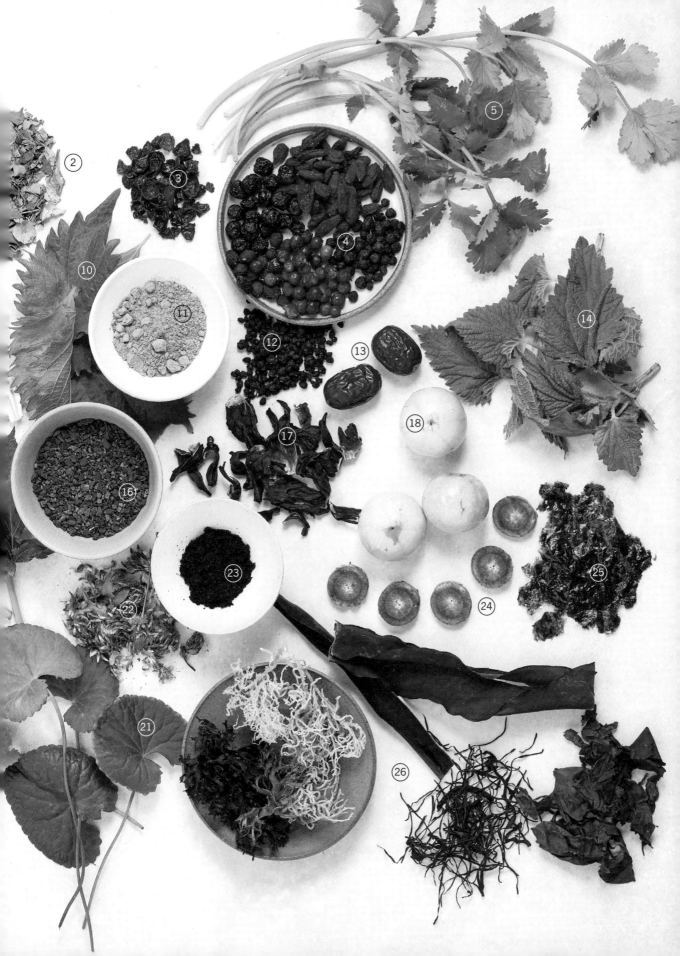

Getting Started

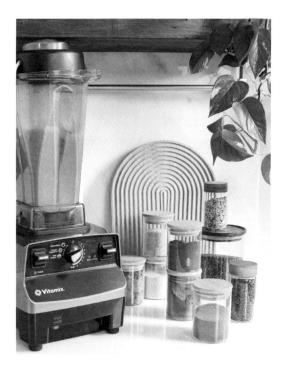

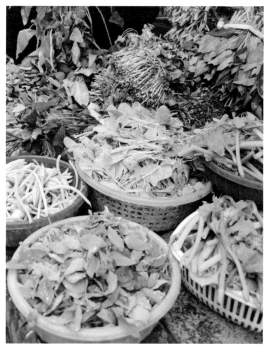

Smoothie Setup

Relying on store-bought smoothies of decent quality can get pricey, and inexpensive ones are often sugar bombs with few health benefits. It's more economical (and beneficial) to make your own power smoothies, with just a few basic ingredients and tools.

Be sure to have the following ingredients on hand as a base around which to build your smoothies: healthy fats, like coconut oil; quality nut butter (I like raw almond butter, but go with your favorite); frozen berries and bananas; and unsweetened nut or oat milk.

Farmers' Markets & Produce Aisles

Farmers' markets are great places to discover exotic nutritives you won't find anywhere else, especially when you're traveling. Many of these nutritive herbs have a brief window of seasonality and rarely find their way into grocery stores. That said, you may be surprised how many nutritives are hiding in plain sight in the produce aisle. Common garnishes like parsley, cilantro, and fresh culinary herbs will often be the most nutritious items on your plate. Asian markets are a good source of fresh nutritives like shiso leaf, ashitaba, and burdock root that are difficult to find elsewhere.

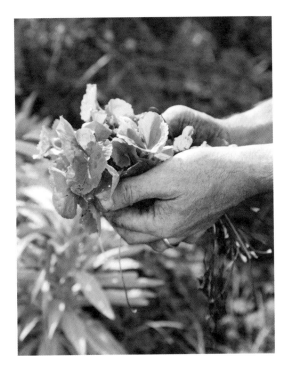

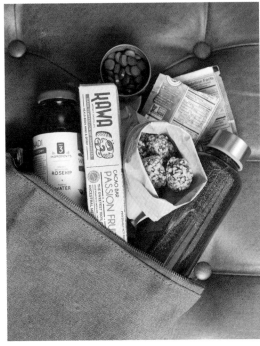

Backyard Garden

Backyards and gardens are another potential source for nutritive plants. Many grow as common weeds and take up residence in a well-fed garden plot, where they help replenish lost nutrients from the soil, protect against erosion, enhance microbial diversity, and attract beneficial insects. They are uniquely capable of drawing up minerals from deep within the soil and transferring that rich source of essential nutrients directly to us when we consume them.

Purslane, chickweed, lamb's-quarters, sorrel, wild mustard, and dandelion are all reliable visitors to backyard gardens—when harvesting tomatoes and cukes, keep an eye out for these nutritional gems. Toss them in salads, cook them into soups and stir-fries, or use them as garnishes.

On the Go

It can be challenging to stay properly nourished when your schedule is hectic. Luckily, many nutritives are available in supplement form. I frequently carry nutritive powder blends with me to add to my water bottle during travel or on hikes, or for pre-workout energy and post-workout replenishment. Both the Super Berry and Green Power Powder Blends (see page 158) work well for this purpose. There are also many excellent store-bought green blends, tablets, and capsules available. See the Resources (page 352) for recommendations.

How to Saturate Your Day

A key to getting the full benefits of nutritives is variety: Strategically adding these medicinal plants in different forms throughout the day ensures that we saturate our bodies with as complete an assortment of essential micronutrients as possible. For this step, aim for three or more servings of nutritives daily. See below for three suggested opportunities for fitting nutritives into your day. And if you're short on time or traveling, a wide range of supplement options are available to provide a quick hit of nutrition.

Between Meals

Nutritives can be consumed between meals in tonics, elixirs, smoothies, or jams for an energizing boost. Add them to the snacks you already enjoy. Choose one of the options on the following pages, or just mix the powder blends with a couple ounces (60 ml) of water for a nutritious shot.

Performance & Recovery

Nutritives are an excellent way to improve performance and recovery during and after all kinds of physical activities. This can be defined broadly, including everything from running errands all day to traveling, gardening, or working out.

Mealtime

Many nutritives can be incorporated into meals. Add goji berries to breakfast cereal, fresh purslane leaves to a spring salad, or dried sea vegetable flakes to a stir-fry. Others, like steamed dandelion leaves with lemon and olive oil or rose hips soup, are satisfying dishes on their own.

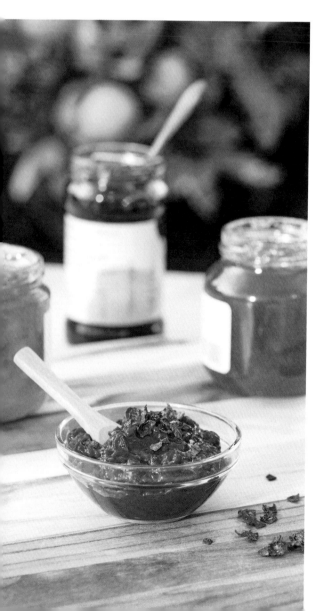

Rose Hips Super Berry Antioxidant Jam (page 163)

SAMPLE DAILY MENUS

MINIMUM DAILY DOSE

Drink three servings of a nutritive beverage of your choice per day. You can use a powder blend—ideally one that includes several of the all-stars from this category—or a strong infusion made with nettles, moringa, oatstraw, ashitaba, and/or alfalfa.

MENU 1

Upon waking:
Green Power Powder Blend (page 158) added to a Chia-Aloe-Lime Rehydrator (page 193)

At breakfast:
Super Berry Power Smoothie
(page 159)

In the afternoon:
Rose Hips Super Berry Antioxidant Jam
(page 163) and a nettles infusion (page 156)

At dinner:
Super Seed Topper (page 164) on a stir-fry
and a seaweed salad

MENU 2

Upon waking:
Moringa infusion (page 156)

At breakfast:
Oatmeal mixed with Super Berry Power Powder Blend (page 158) and topped with goji berries

In the afternoon:
Nori sheets as a snack and a Mint Chocolate Chip–Green Power Smoothie (page 159) post-workout

At dinner:
Nettles Soup (page 167)

step **2** | Options

Strong Infusion

BETWEEN MEALS • PERFORMANCE & RECOVERY

Infusing nutrient-dense herbs in water is an efficient way to extract the vitamins, minerals, and trace elements they contain. Drinking infusions allows the body to absorb nutrients without requiring a lot of digestive energy. You can drink an infusion all in one serving or sip on it throughout the day. See page 156 for a nutritive-specific infusion recipe that you can use with nettles, oatstraw, alfalfa, moringa, or a homemade nutritive blend (page 156).

Nutritive Tea

BETWEEN MEALS • PERFORMANCE & RECOVERY

Many nutritive herbs, including nettles, red clover, moringa, gotu kola, oatstraw, alfalfa, raspberry leaf, horsetail, dandelion leaf, ashitaba, hibiscus, and rose hips, are available in tea bags either on their own or as part of a blend. For an average cup of tea, start with 3 tea bags per cup. The end result should be dark and nutritious tasting. You can also use a pitcher of water and 10 to 20 tea bags to cold-brew several servings in the fridge. To make a nutrient-dense infusion from a blend of your own, see page 156.

Nutritive Powder Boost

BETWEEN MEALS • PERFORMANCE & RECOVERY • MEALTIME

Combine 1 or 2 tablespoons Green Power Powder Blend or Super Berry Power Powder Blend (page 158) with ½ to ¾ cup (120 to 180 ml) water or your favorite juice.

Mint Chocolate Chip–Green Power and Super Berry Power Smoothies

BETWEEN MEALS • PERFORMANCE & RECOVERY

Use the Green Power Powder Blend or Super Berry Power Powder Blend (page 158) as a base for a nutritious and delicious smoothie.

Microalgae Supplements and Powders

BETWEEN MEALS • PERFORMANCE & RECOVERY • MEALTIME

Spirulina and chlorella are popular and highly nutritious microalgae. Both are available in supplement form—tablets, powders, and liquids—at natural food stores and online. You can add them to smoothies and other beverages; see Green Power Powder Blend (page 158). For more on the nutritional benefits of microalgae, turn to page 311.

Fresh Juice

BETWEEN MEALS • PERFORMANCE & RECOVERY • MEALTIME

Juicing is a potent option for consuming fresh nutritives such as cilantro, parsley, wheatgrass, gotu kola, moringa, and purslane. Moisture content and strength vary in fresh nutritive herbs; 2 to 4 ounces (60 to 120 ml) of liquid is a sufficient serving, either on its own or as an addition to other beverages such as smoothies or tonics.

Gotu Kola and Lime Clarity Elixir

BETWEEN MEALS • PERFORMANCE & RECOVERY

A refreshing citrusy drink to improve focus and clarity, this elixir (page 162) is an easy alternative to juicing and retains all the benefits of using fresh leaves. Learn more about the many benefits of gotu kola in the plant profile on page 319.

Goji-Chrysanthemum-Pomegranate Eye-Brightening Elixir

BETWEEN MEALS • PERFORMANCE & RECOVERY

This nourishing elixir (page 157) is based on a traditional recipe used for centuries in China to improve vision and ease eye irritation and strain. Chrysanthemum is very good at cooling inflammation and clearing away excess heat in the eyes from overuse—particularly beneficial when staring at digital screens all day. Goji and pomegranate also nourish the eyes and provide a host of antioxidants such as luteolin, beta-carotene, and zeaxanthin as well as many trace elements and minerals.

Heart Health Tea

BETWEEN MEALS • PERFORMANCE & RECOVERY

This delicious tea blend (recipe page 158), which contains hawthorn leaf, hawthorn berry, oatstraw, rose hips, and hibiscus, has a refreshing tartness. These antioxidant-rich herbs are beneficial for nourishing and enhancing the cardiovascular system, supporting healthy cholesterol levels, calming the nerves, and gently easing blood pressure. Drink 1 to 3 cups (240 to 720 ml) a day, hot or iced.

Nutritive Green Power Balls

BETWEEN MEALS • PERFORMANCE & RECOVERY

These are an excellent, nutritious snack and a great way to get a delicious dose of nourishing nutritive greens any time of day: pre- and post-workout, between meals as a healthy snack, and on hikes. See page 163 for the recipe.

Nutritious Toppers
MEALTIME

A flavorful way to enhance the nutritional content of your meals, hemp seeds, sesame seeds, ground milk thistle seeds, and poppy seeds as well as toasted nori, dulse flakes, and shiso powder can be used individually or mixed together into nutrient-dense blends (see page 120 for two of my favorite combinations). Place in small spice bottles or jars, label, and store in your spice rack or right on the dining-room table for easy accessibility.

Emphasize the Garnish
MEALTIME

Go big on fresh, nutrient-dense herbs, and treat them like you would a serving of vegetables. That sprig of parsley or watercress garnishing your dinner platter may be the most nutrient-dense item on the plate. I almost always add a big handful of chopped fresh herbs like parsley, mint, basil, watercress, cilantro, shiso leaf, or daikon to a main course, either on the side or as a hefty garnish atop the dish.

Sea Seasonings, Snacks, and Salads
BETWEEN MEALS • PERFORMANCE & RECOVERY • MEALTIME

Sprinkles, flakes, and snacking sheets are a convenient, ready-made way to get the benefits of sea vegetables. Nori sheets are a commonly available option for snacking that are delicious on their own. Small servings of fresh sea vegetables make great salads and side dishes. For more on these nutrient-dense vegetables, see page 339.

Parsley Chimichurri
MEALTIME

Parsley is a superfood hiding in plain sight, with an extremely high allotment of micronutrients and minerals. The recipe on page 164 uses it in combination with cilantro to make a nutrient-dense chimichurri: a famous Argentine sauce that can be used as a condiment or in cooking.

Eat Your Weeds
MEALTIME

Here are some ways to make common nutritive weeds shine on your dinner table: The crunch and lemony flavor of raw purslane makes it an ideal ingredient in salads (just wash thoroughly and remove the thick stems before eating). Use wild dandelion greens to make the Greek classic horta vrasta (page 133). Roast stems of lamb's-quarters like you would any green vegetable: Dress with oil, season with salt and any favorite spices, place on a roasting pan, and bake in a 350°F (175°C) oven for 10 minutes, or until crispy. Ashitaba leaves work well in stir-fries and pesto. Other nutritious weedy plants to try include garlic mustard, chickweed, and sorrel.

Nettles Soup
MEALTIME

This delicious and deeply nutritious classic spring soup (recipe page 167) is made with young nettle tops packed with revitalizing nutrients. It has a vibrant green color and a silky texture.

Rose Hips Super Berry Antioxidant Jam

BETWEEN MEALS • PERFORMANCE & RECOVERY • MEALTIME

This flavorful antioxidant- and vitamin C–rich jam (recipe page 163) uses rose hips as a base, combined with Super Berry Power Powder Blend (page 158). The pectin content in rose hips creates a simple and quick jam-like texture when combined with water and is a great source of prebiotic fiber. I like to use this jam to spread on toast and eat it by the spoonful in between meals. Add a dollop on breakfast cereals or blend into smoothies. It also makes a nice chutney or relish.

Nyponsoppa: Scandinavian Rose Hips Soup

MEALTIME

Rose hips are the fruits produced by various species of roses. In Scandinavia, where fresh vitamin C–rich fruits are scarce, rose hips are celebrated for their high vitamin C content and abundant antioxidants. In Sweden, fresh, wild rose hips are made into the traditional fruit soup nyponsoppa that's often served as a dessert or eaten for breakfast. The dried rose hips used in my take on the recipe (page 165) are equally beneficial and delicious. It's common to eat this tart soup during the colder months to boost immunity. Top it with whipped cream or vanilla ice cream.

Strong Infusion

Extracting minerals and nutrients from herbs takes some time. Make nourishing infusions using nettles, oatstraw, alfalfa, and moringa individually, or use a homemade nutritive blend (see recipe below).

Place ¾ **to 1 ounce (20 to 30 g) dried herbs** in a 1-quart (1 L) canning jar. Pour enough hot water over the herbs to cover. Screw the lid on the jar and let steep. I recommend a minimum infusion time of 1 to 4 hours, but the longer, the better. Strain the liquid into an empty jar, pressing the herbs with a wooden spoon to squeeze out all the liquid. What you strain out is the daily dose I recommend—try to get a minimum of 12 ounces (360 ml) a day. Any remainder can be left in the fridge for a couple days.

Note: You can infuse nutritives overnight to get the maximum amount of nutrients out of them. Simply follow the instructions for steeping above and, when the mixture has cooled down, place the jar in the fridge overnight. The next day, strain and enjoy.

Homemade Nutritive Tea Blend

Combine **1 cup (20 g) each nettles, oatstraw, and raspberry leaf**; **½ cup (10 g) each moringa and red clover**; **¼ cup (25 g) dried rose hips**; **¼ cup (10 g) dried hibiscus flowers**; and **2 tablespoons orange peel** in a small bowl. The tea blend can be stored in an airtight container in a cool, dark place for several weeks.

To make a cup of tea, measure **2 tablespoons dry tea blend per 12-ounce (360 ml) cup** into a self-fill tea bag or a removable infusion basket. Pour in hot water and infuse for 10 to 15 minutes. To make a larger quantity, use a French press or 1-quart (1 L) canning jar.

Note: If you want to give the blend a little extra flavor, add more herbs and spices (such as cinnamon, ginger, lemon verbena, or lemongrass) and/or a small amount of a natural sweetener of your choice to the infusion before drinking.

Goji-Chrysanthemum-Pomegranate Eye-Brightening Elixir

Put **1 tablespoon goji berries** and **1 tablespoon dried chrysanthemum flowers** into a mug with a removable infuser basket or into a small teapot. Pour **1½ cups (360 ml) hot water** over the mix and swish around with a spoon to fully saturate and submerge the herbs. Let steep, covered, for 10 to 15 minutes, then remove the infuser or strain the liquid into a cup. Add **2 teaspoons unsweetened pomegranate juice** and **a natural sweetener of your choic**e to taste, if desired.

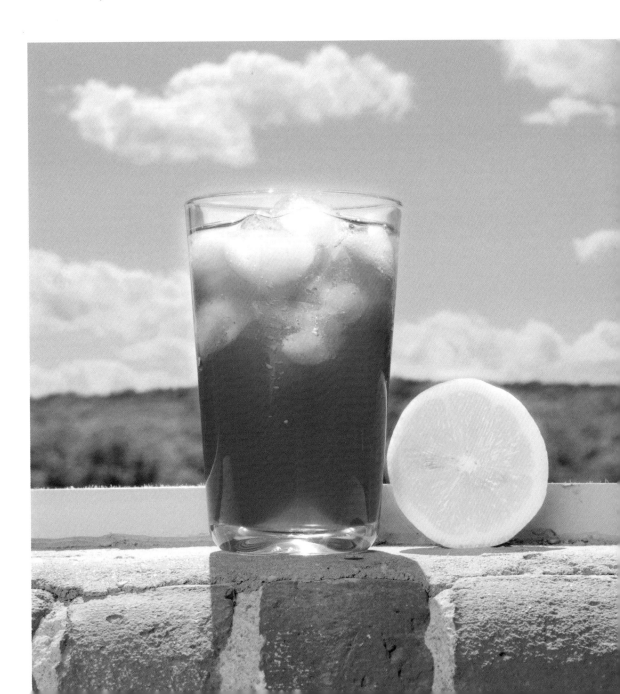

Heart Health Tea Blend

This tea blend uses dried loose herbs. Mix together **2 parts hawthorn leaf and flower; 1 part each hawthorn berry, oatstraw, rosebuds, rose hips, and hibiscus**; and **½ part each linden leaf and flower and lavender flowers**. (Convert parts to whatever form of measurement you choose, depending on how much you want to make.) Store in an airtight container in a cool, dark place; dry tea blends will last for many weeks this way.

To make a cup of tea, measure **2 tablespoons dry tea blend per 12-ounce (360 ml) cup** into a self-fill tea bag or a removable infusion basket. Pour in hot water and infuse for 10 to 15 minutes. To make a larger quantity, use a French press or 1-quart (1 L) canning jar.

Super Berry Power Powder Blend

Mix together equal parts of the following powders: **acai berry, raspberry, pomegranate, lingonberry, wild blueberry, dragon fruit, black cherry, cranberry, camu camu,** and **goji berry** (for sourcing information, see page 352). Blend thoroughly; if the mixture is clumpy, put it into a coffee grinder or high-powered blender and pulse for a few seconds. Stir **1 to 2 tablespoons powder** into **¾ to 1 cup (180 to 240 ml) water or juice** of any kind.

Green Power Powder Blend

Mix together equal parts of the following powders: **nettles, ashitaba, alfalfa, barley grass, and parsley**. Add **½ part each chlorella and spirulina powders** and **3 parts pineapple powder**. Blend thoroughly; if the mix is clumpy, put into a coffee grinder or high-powered blender and pulse for a few seconds. Stir **1 to 2 tablespoons powder** into **¾ to ½ cup (180 to 240 ml) water or juice** of any kind.

Super Berry Power Smoothie

Using a high-powered blender, combine **2 cups (480 ml) plant-based milk, 1 cup (155 g) frozen blueberries, 1 cup (140 g) frozen raspberries, 1 cup (240 ml) coconut-milk yogurt, 1 fresh or frozen banana, 4 tablespoons (16 g) Super Berry Power Powder Blend** (page 158), **2 tablespoons cacao nibs, 1 or 2 tablespoons almond butter, 1 tablespoon Irish Moss Gel** (page 188), and **½ teaspoon vanilla extract**. Blend until you reach the consistency you desire. Add more milk or water as needed to make the beverage thinner or smoother. Makes 2 or 3 servings.

Mint Chocolate Chip– Green Power Smoothie

Using a high-powered blender, combine **2 cups (480 ml) plant-based milk, ½ cup (80 g) frozen spinach, ½ cup (75 g) frozen banana, ½ avocado, 1½ tablespoons cacao nibs, 2 teaspoons Green Power Powder Blend** (page 158), **10 fresh mint leaves**, and **a natural sweetener of your choice** to taste. Add more milk or water as needed to reach your desired consistency. Pour into glasses or cups and garnish each with a few extra **cacao nibs** and **a fresh mint leaf**. Makes 2 servings.

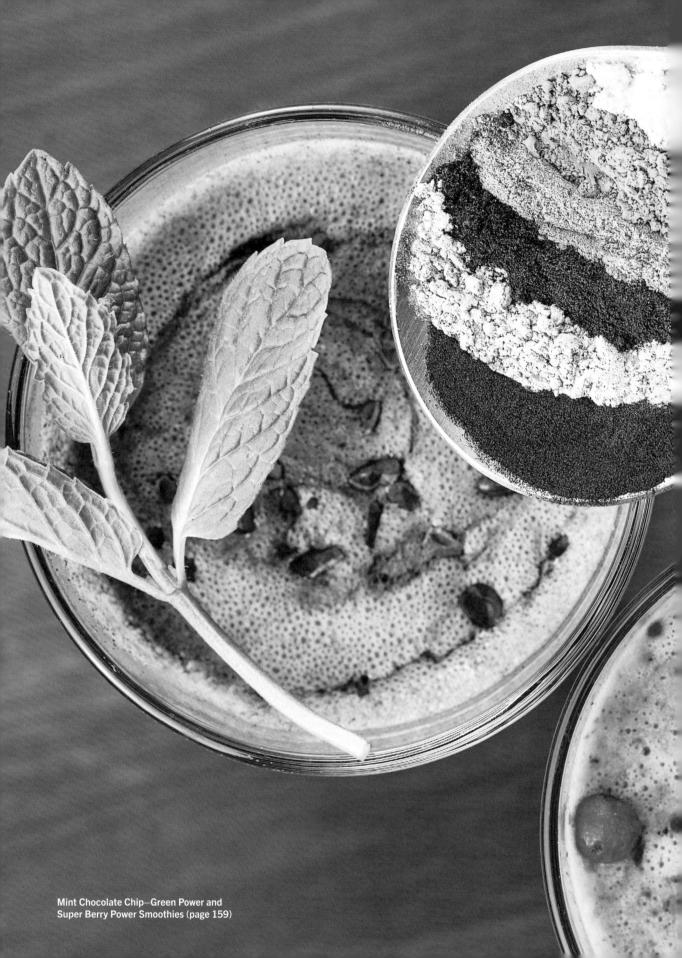

Mint Chocolate Chip–Green Power and
Super Berry Power Smoothies (page 159)

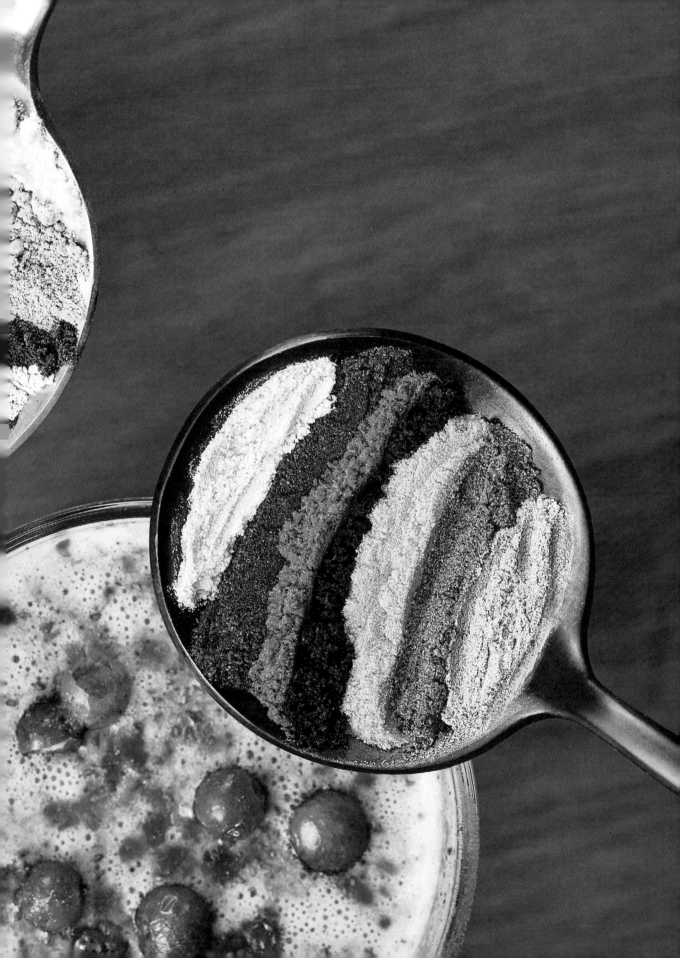

Gotu Kola and Lime Clarity Elixir

Thoroughly wash **1 ounce (30 g) fresh gotu kola leaves** in a colander and pat dry. Put the leaves in a blender with **1½ cups (360 ml) coconut water (or half water/half coconut water)** and **1¼ teaspoons fresh rosemary**. Blend the ingredients at medium speed until thoroughly mixed. Strain the liquid. Add **2 teaspoons fresh lime or lemon juice** and watch the color immediately turn to vibrant green. Add **a natural sweetener of your choice** to taste. The ingredients oxidize quickly, so immediately store any leftovers in an airtight jar in the fridge—the elixir will last for a few days. Makes 1 or 2 servings.

Note: Asian markets are a great source for fresh gotu kola leaves. Or grow your own—the plant is a perennial and a member of the parsley family.

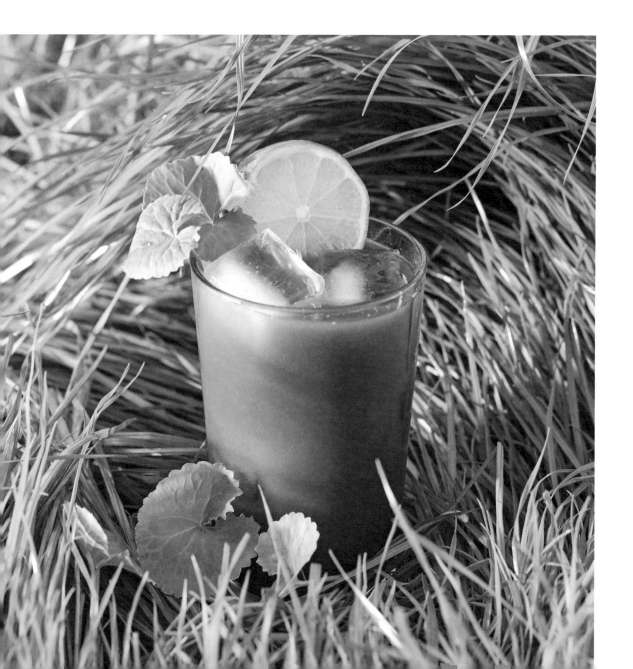

Rose Hips Super Berry Antioxidant Jam

Place **1 cup (100 g) dried rose hips** in a bowl. Add **½ to 1 cup (120 to 240 ml) water** and stir (adjust the amount of water to your desired consistency). Let sit for an hour or so, stirring occasionally, until the rose hips soak up most of the water and soften. Stir in **6 tablespoons (24 g) Super Berry Power Powder Blend** (page 158) and **2 teaspoons natural sweetener of your choice**. Thoroughly blend with an immersion blender into a smooth puree. Store in the fridge, covered, for up to 5 days. Makes 1 cup (240 ml) jam.

Note: This recipe calls for incorporating Super Berry Power Powder Blend, but you can use any individual super berry powders, together or in combination, if you choose.

Nutritive Green Power Balls

Soak **10 dates** in water for 5 minutes to soften, then finely chop. In a food processor, grind **½ cup (50 g) walnuts or cashews** until they reach a fine texture. Add **2 to 3 tablespoons semisweet chocolate chips**, **2 teaspoons hemp seeds**, **2 teaspoons coconut butter**, **1½ teaspoons coconut oil**, and **1 teaspoon matcha powder**. Add the dates and process, stopping occasionally to scrape the mixture into the center of the bowl with a flexible spatula, until the mixture reaches a fine, doughy consistency that you can form into balls without it breaking apart. If the texture is too dry, add a bit more coconut oil; if it's too moist, a bit more of the ground nut mixture. Spread a fine layer of **raspberry powder** on a small plate. Form the dough into approximately 12 gumball-size balls and roll each one in the raspberry powder until fully covered. Place the balls on a parchment paper–lined plate, cover, and refrigerate for an hour or so until they firm up. Stored in a sealed container in the fridge, they'll be good for up to 2 weeks. Makes about 12 balls.

Parsley Chimichurri

Combine **1 cup (50 g) finely chopped fresh flat-leaf parsley,** **¾ cup (180 ml) extra-virgin olive oil, ½ cup (30 g) minced scallions, ⅓ cup (20 g) finely chopped fresh cilantro, 4 finely chopped garlic cloves, 3 tablespoons red wine vinegar, 2 tablespoons fresh lemon juice, 2 teaspoons red pepper flakes,** and **salt and ground black pepper** to taste in a bowl. Mix well. The chimichurri should be kept refrigerated and is best if used within 48 hours, but it will last in the fridge for up to 1 week.

Note: Add any other fresh herbs you wish, such as thyme, basil, or oregano.

Super Seed Topper

Mix **⅓ cup (55 g) each hulled hemp seeds, whole black and white sesame seeds, chia seeds,** and **poppy seeds** with **¼ to ½ teaspoon sea salt.** Store in an airtight jar in the fridge; the topper will keep for at least a few weeks. Bring out at mealtime as a condiment to sprinkle liberally on salads, soups, and stir-fries.

Sea Vegetable Sprinkles

Take **1 or 2 sheets toasted nori** (depending on your preference), **⅓ cup (50 g) toasted sesame seeds, ¼ cup (10 g) dulse flakes,** and **a pinch of salt** and pulse-grind in a food processor until the ingredients are blended and a condiment texture is achieved (aim for a texture you can sprinkle on food). Transfer to a bowl and add **wasabi powder and/or red pepper flakes** to desired taste and spice level. Store in an airtight container in the fridge for up to 2 weeks.

Nyponsoppa: Scandinavian Rose Hips Soup

Place **4 cups (1 L) water** and **2 cups (200 g) dried rose hips** in a medium pot or saucepan. Let soak for at least 1 hour. Add an additional **4 cups (1 L) water** and cook at a low simmer for 20 minutes, or until the rose hips are pulpy and soft. Remove from the heat and blend with an immersion blender. Working in batches, pass the blended rose hips through a fine-mesh strainer into another container, using a wooden spoon to smush the rose hip mash through the strainer and intermittently rinsing the strainer to speed up the process. Once all of the puree has gone through the strainer, return the puree to the saucepan. In a separate bowl, whisk together **2 tablespoons organic potato flour** with **½ to ¾ cup (120 to 180 ml) cold water**. Slowly add the flour mixture to the rose hips liquid and whisk. Add **2 to 4 tablespoons natural sweetener of your choice**. If the soup is too thick, add a cup or two of water to reach your desired consistency. Warm the soup, add **a small to medium-size dollop of vanilla-flavored nondairy coconut ice cream or whipped cream**, and serve. Makes 2 to 3 servings.

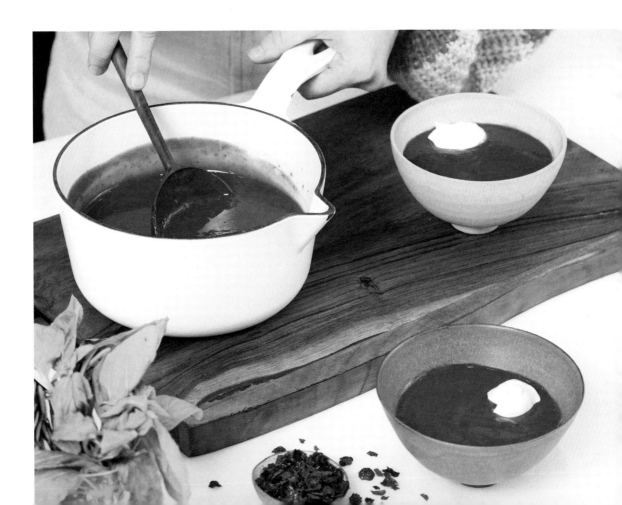

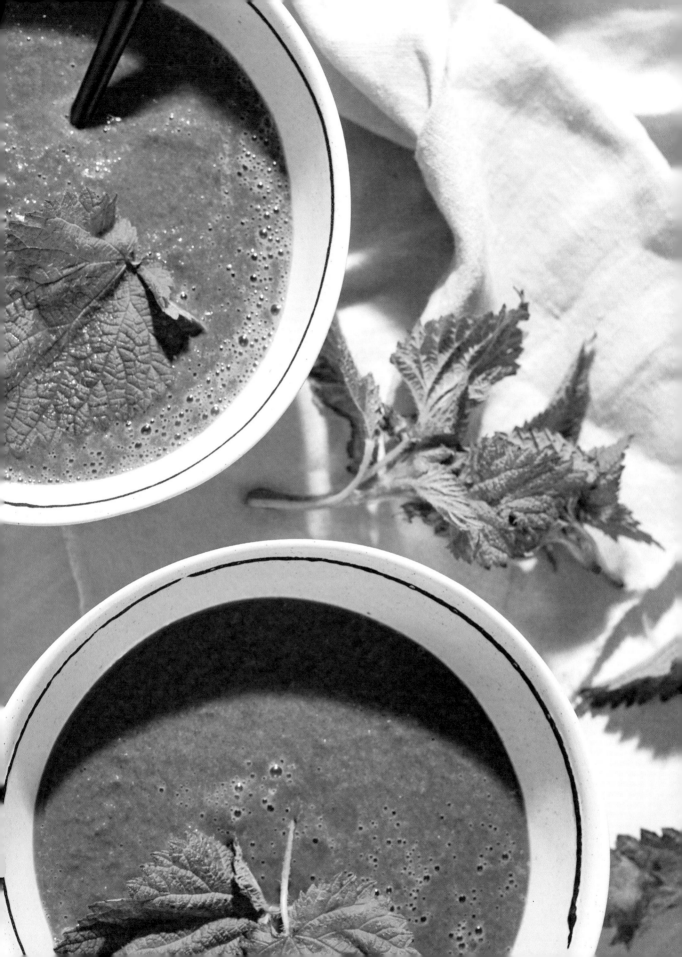

Nettles Soup

Fill a small bowl with ice water. Bring a pot of water to a boil and blanch **4 cups (80 g) washed nettle leaves** for 1 to 2 minutes. Strain in a colander; place the nettles in the ice-water bath for a few seconds and then back in the colander. Lightly heat **2 tablespoons olive oil** in a medium to large saucepan. Add **1 medium chopped leek, 3 cloves finely chopped garlic**, and **½ cup (50 g) diced celery**. Sauté for 5 to 7 minutes, until translucent. Stir in **6 to 8 cups (1.4 to 2 L) water** (depending on your desired consistency), **2 cups (280 g) diced potatoes, 2 teaspoons vegetable bouillon, 1 teaspoon dried oregano, 1 teaspoon dried thyme, ½ to 1 teaspoon ground black pepper, 1 bay leaf**, and **salt to taste**. Cover and simmer for 10 to 15 minutes, until the potatoes are soft. Add the blanched nettle leaves and cook for another minute, until the leaves have wilted; scoop out and discard the bay leaf. Add **1 tablespoon fresh lemon juice** and **½ can (approximately 6 ounces/180 ml) coconut cream** and blend with an immersion blender until smooth. Garnish with **a sprig of fresh thyme**, if desired. Makes 4 to 6 servings.

Cacao: Food of the Gods

Cacao is among the world's healthiest and most delicious superfoods. To the ancient Mayans and Aztecs, it was considered a gift from the gods. Xocoatl, or "bitter drink," was the name of the original Aztec elixir made by cooking roasted cacao paste, chile peppers, and cornmeal in hot water, then pouring the mixture back and forth between special pots to create a spicy, chocolaty drink with a thick layer of foam on top. The echo of this ancient technique still exists in a traditional Oaxacan beverage called tejate, made with cacao, cornmeal, mamey fruit seeds, and a unique flower called the rosita de cacao (*Quararibea funebris*); a special tool called a *molinillo* creates a frothy layer on top of the beverage.

The Aztecs preferred to drink their cacao cold, combining it with herbs and spices like vanilla, allspice, cinnamon, and cayenne (this was reportedly the favorite after-dinner drink of Montezuma II). The first sweetened version of cacao appeared in Spain in the 1500s, and once cacao met sugar and became chocolate, it was game over. Today, with worldwide consumption approaching three million tons per year, cacao has become as ubiquitous as its fellow plant staples coffee and tea.

Cacao comes from a medium-size tropical tree (*Theobroma cacao*) native to the jungles of Central and South America. Pods growing directly from the trunk contain twenty-five to fifty cacao beans, enveloped in a sweet pulpy fruit known as baba. Harvested by hand, the pulp-covered cacao beans are then separated and left to ferment for five to ten days. Afterward, they are spread onto tarps and dried in the sun. The final stage involves light roasting and either cracking the beans into small pieces called nibs or grinding them into a paste, which is used as the basis for making chocolate.

Cacao is a nutritional powerhouse. It's among the highest sources of magnesium in the plant world and contains substantial amounts of iron, zinc, phosphorus, selenium, and a host of other trace elements. A powerful tonic for the cardiovascular system, the beans are packed with hundreds of potent antioxidants, including a wide range of polyphenolic flavonoids that increase nitric oxide production, relaxing and dilating blood vessels, improving blood flow, and lowering blood pressure. They're also rich in unique constituents known to increase our internal supply of feel-good chemicals: Compounds such as theobromine, caffeine, and anandamide (the so-called bliss molecule) improve clarity, elevate mood, and generate feelings of contentment by increasing the amounts of serotonin, dopamine, and endorphins flowing in our system.

Cacao puro, a traditional drink of the Kuna people in Ustupo, Panama

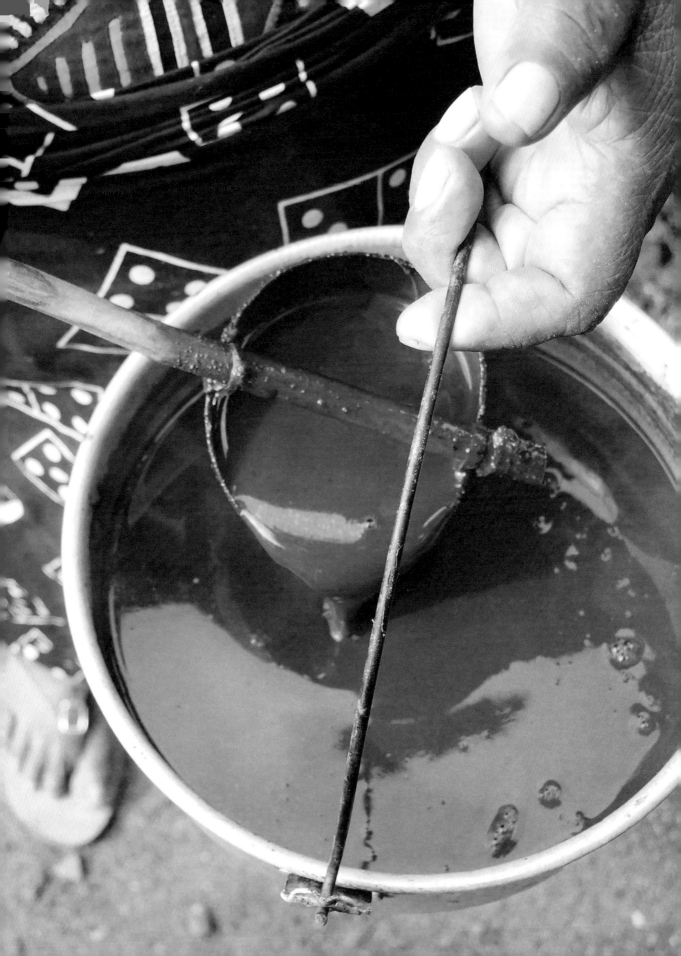

On several sourcing trips, I've made a point of visiting some of the places and people that know cacao best to get an understanding of how it is traditionally used. The Kuna people, indigenous to the Caribbean coast of Panama, have a profound connection to cacao and an intimate knowledge of its health-enhancing powers. These incredibly rugged and resilient people subsist primarily on the fish they catch and the fruits, vegetables, and nuts they harvest from permaculture jungle plots. They are famously healthy and have been the focus of numerous scientific studies, including one conducted by Harvard researchers that concluded that their low incidence of chronic disease, especially cardiovascular disease, can be attributed in part to the copious quantities of cacao they drink.

Each morning I spent with the Kuna began with several cups of freshly prepared cacao shared in a communal hut before the group set out to work for the day. Cacao promotes increased circulation, oxygenation, and cardiovascular endurance and is also a rich source of nutrients. The Kuna drink two types of cacao: one blended with ripe bananas to sweeten it and give it a smoothie-like texture, and the other a simple preparation of roasted beans combined with chiles—a blend they call *puro*— that's potent, bitter, and spicy. A few small cups of cacao puro enhance blood flow throughout the entire body, generating feelings of increased energy and vigor bordering on euphoria. The Kuna believe blood to be the vehicle for life force and an open heart the place from which it flows. They gather their cacao beans from the same species the Mayans used, which gives this magical elixir a deep magenta color, like blood itself.

Drinking pure cacao affects our physiology and consciousness in a far more powerful way than, say, eating a chocolate bar. Beyond its innumerable physical benefits, the concentrated number of powerful compounds ingested when drinking cacao combined with synergistic herbs and spices produces a tangible feeling of joy, vitality, and openness. Sharing cacao with friends accentuates its expansive effects and amplifies all that good brain chemistry.

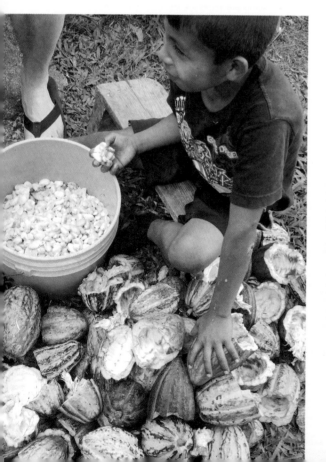

Preparing cacao for fermentation and drying (left) and roasting it for use in bars and beverages (below) in the Maya Mountains of Belize

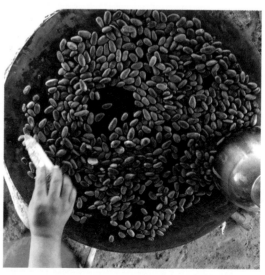

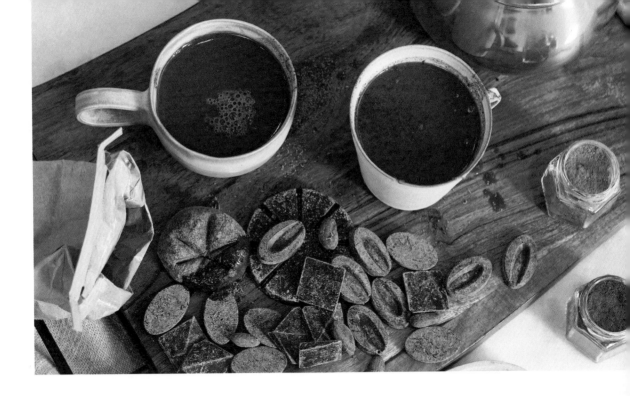

Blissful Beverage:
Making the Perfect Cup of Xocoatl

This recipe is strong—and it's supposed to be. We are looking to make a potent and authentic cacao elixir here. The addition of cinnamon, vanilla, and cayenne pepper increases cacao's mood-elevating effects and enhances absorption of all of its healthy nutrients and compounds. Cayenne varies quite a bit in terms of heat level—and a pinch means different things to different people—so adjust accordingly. The goal is to harmonize the spiciness of the pepper with the bittersweet notes of the cacao without letting any one flavor dominate.

Heat **1 to 1½ cups (240 to 360 ml) water** (depending on your preferred concentration) and **1 ounce (30 g) unsweetened cacao chunks** in a saucepan over low heat. Melt the cacao, stirring frequently with a whisk so it doesn't stick to the bottom of the pan. When the cacao is semi-melted (within a few minutes), add **1 teaspoon cinnamon powder**, **1 teaspoon vanilla extract**, and **a pinch of cayenne pepper or chili powder**. Add a **dash of a natural sweetener of your choice**, if desired. Remove from the heat. Using an immersion blender or a whisk, blend everything thoroughly until a significant froth appears, then immediately pour into one to three cups. If you like, use a milk frother to form a bit more froth on top of each cup.

Notes: You can substitute the unsweetened cacao chunks for semisweet chunks (no less than 70 percent cacao) or even chips, if that's all you've got. To give your xocoatl an adaptogenic boost, add 1 teaspoon powdered extract of reishi and/or cordyceps mushrooms. You can also let the drink cool slightly and pour it over ice cubes (or blend with ice to make a frappé).

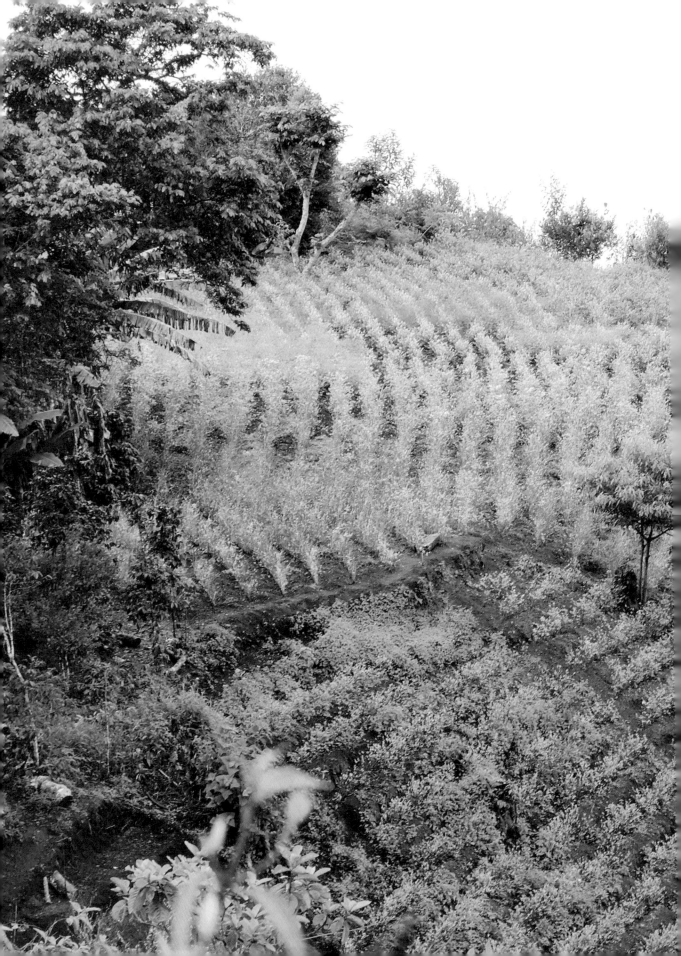

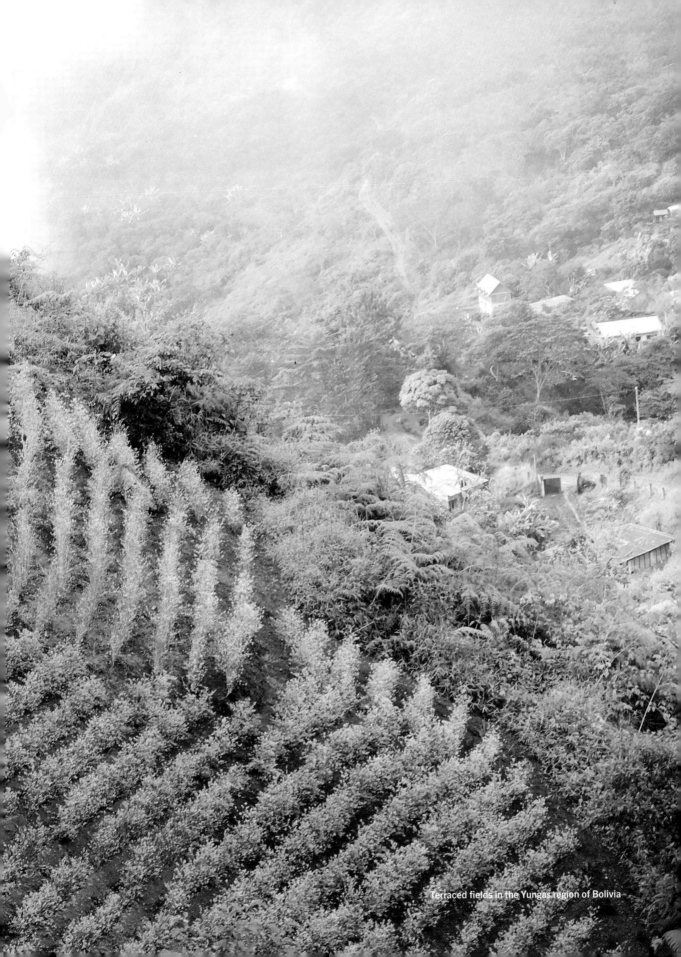
Terraced fields in the Yungas region of Bolivia

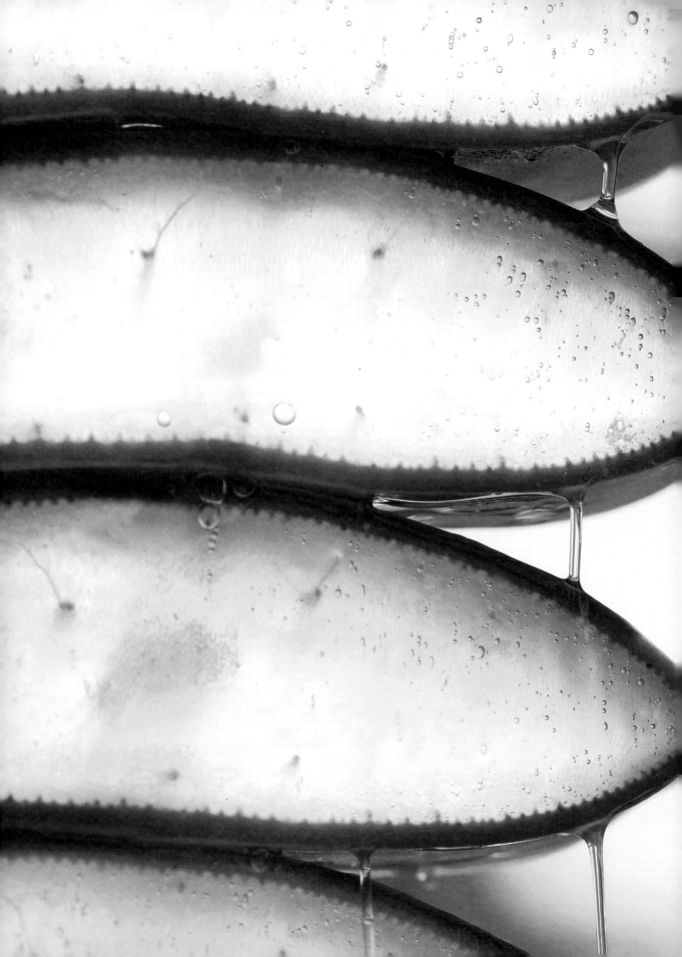

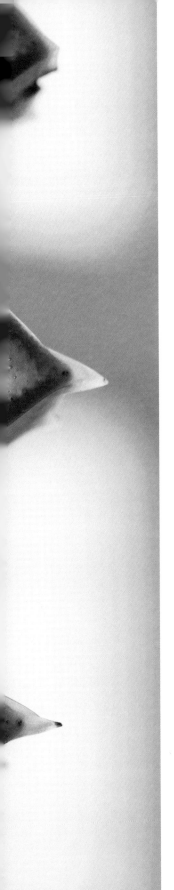

step 3 | Demulcents

THE FAST PACE OF MODERN LIFE CAN REALLY DRY US OUT, making it common to exist in a state of chronic low-level internal dehydration, sapping vitality and accelerating aging. In this step, you'll harness the power of demulcents to achieve a state of deep hydration down to the cellular level and experience the supple resilience that happens when the body is thoroughly quenched.

WHAT TO EXPECT

- More radiant and supple skin and hair

- Deeper and more restorative sleep

- Sharper thinking and greater clarity and concentration

- Less irritability and more stable moods

- Better digestion and elimination; diminished hyperacidity and inflammation

- Greater physical energy and endurance, with faster recovery and recuperation after injury or exertion

Plants & Other Ingredients You'll Be Using

All demulcents share similar attributes and benefits: They replenish moisture, promote healing, and cool inflammation—especially in the GI tract. All are rich sources of prebiotic soluble fiber and nutrients. Some, such as slippery elm and marshmallow, are high in mucilage content and therefore ultra-soothing, especially for the mucous membranes in the GI tract. Others, like linden leaf and hibiscus, have a lighter mucilage content and other beneficial constituents. They taste delicious, help improve digestion, and lightly hydrate. Chia and basil seeds are somewhere in the middle in terms of mucilage content but include omega-3 and omega-6 fatty acids, vitamins, and minerals, combining demulcency with nutrient density. Irish moss is the source of a soothing gel and prized as a comprehensive tonic, containing practically every mineral and trace element the body requires. Licorice and aloe vera are the most cooling and anti-inflammatory of the bunch, making them indispensable for healing overheated GI conditions. This step is intended to familiarize you with these and other essential demulcents, so you can zero in on the right ones for your needs and circumstances.

It's worth noting that a number of foods also contain demulcent properties and can be included in our diet. Examples include okra, yams, oats, nopal cactus, and kelp.

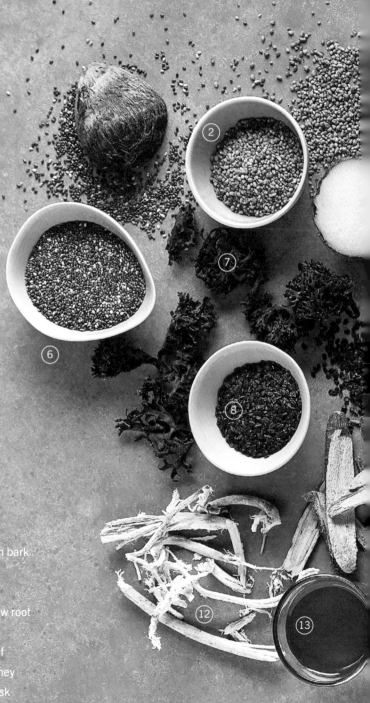

1 + 14 + 18	Licorice root	9	Slippery elm bark
2	Buckwheat	10	Irish moss
3	Jerusalem artichoke	11	Aloe vera
4	Shatavari root	12	Marshmallow root
5	Basil seeds	13	Olive oil
6	Chia seeds	15	Plantain leaf
7	Dulse	16	Manuka honey
8	Chan seeds	17	Psyllium husk

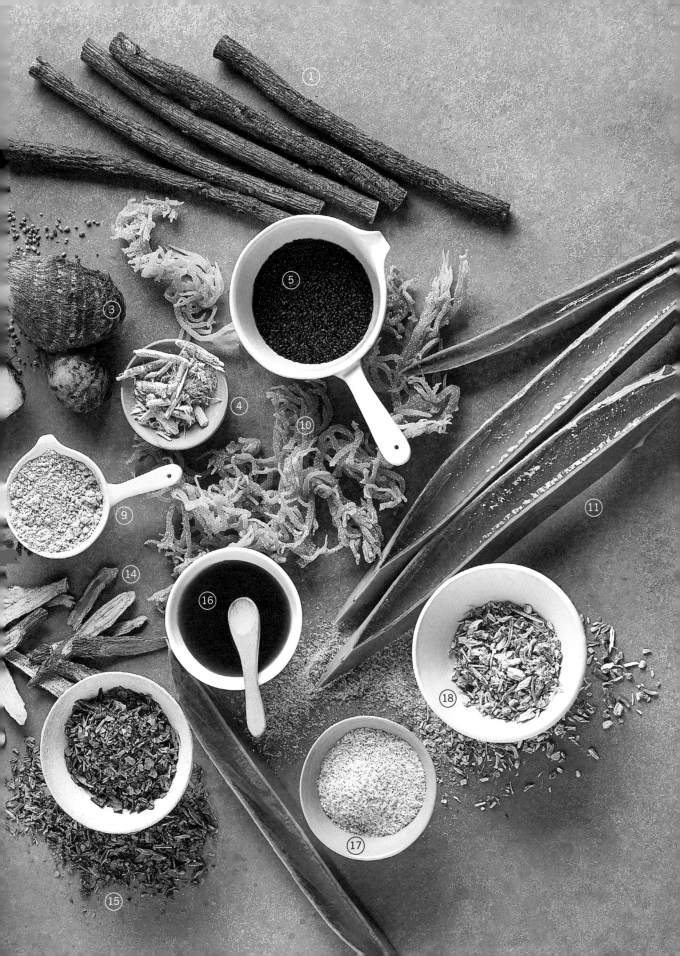

Getting Started

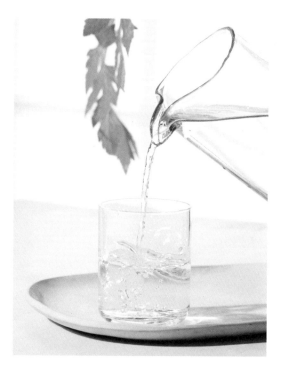

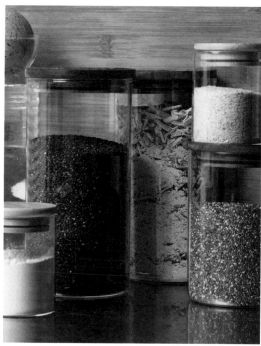

Good Water Source

The first consideration when it comes to hydrating with demulcents is always having a clean, pure source of water. A portable water-purifying pitcher or a faucet-mounted filter is an inexpensive way to keep impurities out of your water. Undercounter filters are more of an investment but work well to remove even more contaminants. There are great portable water bottles with UV filtration to ensure you'll have pure water with you anytime.

Kitchen Setup

Keep your collection of demulcents and supplements—such as powders, seeds, and teas—in a convenient place, near your water source. Store them in airtight containers or sealed bags and keep them in a cool, dry, dark place. Aloe (whether gel, water, or leaf) should always be kept in the fridge.

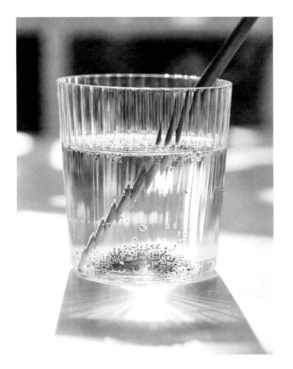

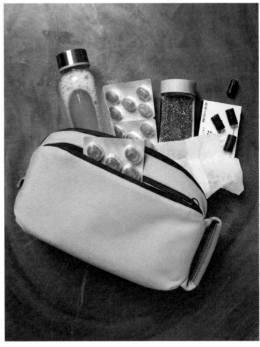

Mixing

It's important to mix demulcents properly so that you don't end up with something chunky, gloopy, or gritty. Basil and chia seeds are best mixed with a fork—stir frequently to avoid a solid chunk forming. A simple handheld milk frother works well with demulcent powders to ensure a smooth, easy-to-drink beverage.

On the Go

Living an active, dynamic life generates a lot of metabolic heat. The farther we go and the more energy we exert—traveling, putting in extended work hours (especially on the computer), attending long meetings, and working out—the more fluids our bodies require to replenish. I recommend carrying a little stash of demulcent powder or balls, chia seeds, slippery elm lozenges, or real licorice candy wherever you go for extra hydrating power when you need it. You can pack them in your suitcase, backpack, workout bag, or water bottle for fast access.

How to Saturate Your Day

Demulcents can be somewhat filling and are best consumed on an empty stomach and in between meals for maximum functional benefits. Soaking demulcent herbs in room-temperature water is all that's needed to extract the mucilage or gel. As a rule, the longer demulcents sit in water, the thicker and more viscous they become. If they become too viscous, simply add more water to thin out.

Whenever possible, drink or eat demulcents. The viscous consistency of demulcents in the mouth has the unique effect of stimulating a nerve reflex that generates moisture throughout the body's mucous membranes. For convenience, though, tablets and/or lozenges will work fine and provide certain benefits, especially in the GI and respiratory tracts.

Lighter demulcents like aloe vera and chia seeds make for refreshing and rehydrating morning beverages, while more-fibrous demulcents like psyllium husk, slippery elm, and marshmallow—rich in viscous, water-soluble polysaccharides—are often taken in the afternoon or evening. Most have an unremarkable, neutral flavor (sort of like white rice) that's agreeable enough on its own. You can enhance the taste by combining them with culinary spices like cinnamon, ginger, nutmeg, or vanilla. This lightly kindles agni and helps the body better digest the soluble fibers.

Morning Rehydration

We all need to rehydrate upon waking. Hydrating first thing in the morning stimulates the production of new red blood cells essential for increasing oxygenation and energizing the body. Morning hydration also catalyzes the production of digestive enzymes, increases metabolism, flushes out toxins and wastes, and stimulates elimination. Drinking a demulcent preparation first thing in the morning amplifies the power of water, setting you up for long-lasting hydration all day.

Daytime Maintenance

Embrace a "slow drip" method of enhanced hydration by using demulcents in various forms throughout the day. These beverages aren't meant to replace drinking water; rather, they add depth to your normal hydration strategy.

Nighttime Restorative

Use demulcents to supply the moisture needed to carry out critical detoxification functions during sleep, rejuvenate the hardworking digestive system, nourish the microbiome, and encourage healthy elimination in the morning. Create a regular habit of drinking a demulcent-rich fiber blend of some sort in the evening, about two hours after your last major meal.

AIR TRAVEL: DEMULCENTS TO THE RESCUE

The dehydrating effects of air travel make us more susceptible to jet lag, fatigue, and opportunistic pathogens. Drinking a lot of water while you're flying can be inconvenient and insufficient on its own. Using demulcents on the flight more effectively replenishes your body's moisture so that you arrive at your destination fresher and more hydrated.

SAMPLE DAILY MENUS

MINIMUM DAILY DOSE

At least two demulcent beverages of your choice: one first
thing in the morning on an empty stomach and one sometime
in the evening, at least two hours after your last meal.

MENU 1

Upon waking:
Chia-Aloe-Lime Rehydrator (page 193)

Throughout the day:
Marshmallow root powder in your water bottle

Post-workout:
Irish Moss–Cacao Nib Elixir (page 188)

After dinner:
Linden tea

Before bed:
Prebiotic fiber drink

MENU 2

Upon waking:
Water with manuka honey and lemon

At breakfast:
Mango–Basil Seed Pudding (page 194)

Throughout the day:
Aloe vera gel in a water bottle

After dinner:
Real black licorice candy

Demulcent Powder Blend

MORNING REHYDRATION • DAYTIME MAINTENANCE • NIGHTTIME RESTORATIVE

See page 189 for a recipe for a synergistic blend of several key demulcent powders. It's combined with a small amount of fennel and orange peel to improve flavor and digestibility.

Demulcent Water

MORNING REHYDRATION • DAYTIME MAINTENANCE

Put approximately 1 teaspoon marshmallow or shatavari powder or Demulcent Powder Blend (page 189) into 2 cups (480 ml) room-temperature or warm water. Stir well or use a mini immersion blender to mix. Adjust the ratio of demulcent to water for your preferred consistency.

Hydration-Enhanced Water

MORNING REHYDRATION • DAYTIME MAINTENANCE • NIGHTTIME RESTORATIVE

To form a less-concentrated version of the demulcent water above, add small amounts of a demulcent powder (such as slippery elm bark, marshmallow root, shatavari root), the Demulcent Powder Blend on page 189, or chia or basil seeds to your normal daily water intake for a simple hydration boost. Use approximately 1 teaspoon powder or seeds per 3 cups (720 ml) water. This preparation should be light enough to sip throughout the day; it's just a bit more viscous than tap or filtered water.

Chia or Basil Seed–Infused Water

MORNING REHYDRATION • DAYTIME MAINTENANCE

Put approximately 1 teaspoon chia or basil seeds into 2 cups (480 ml) room-temperature or warm water. Let sit for 3 to 5 minutes, stirring periodically. (Note that basil seeds become viscous faster than chia seeds.) Add a squeeze of lemon and enjoy.

Aloe Vera Drinks

MORNING REHYDRATION • DAYTIME MAINTENANCE • NIGHTTIME RESTORATIVE

The healing gel contained in aloe vera leaves is an excellent addition to water and a deeply hydrating base for all sorts of beverages, tonics, and elixirs. You can find fresh aloe vera leaves in the produce section of most grocery stores or even grow it yourself under the right conditions. See page 193 for a step-by-step illustrated guide to cutting and extracting the gel from an aloe leaf. Once the gel is extracted, mince it and add to water, smoothies, green drinks, and other beverages (such as the Chia-Aloe-Lime Rehydrator, below) to enhance hydration and demulcency.

Chia-Aloe-Lime Rehydrator

MORNING REHYDRATION • DAYTIME MAINTENANCE

This delicious, rehydrating elixir (page 193) is easy to prepare, especially when you have a batch of fresh aloe vera gel in the fridge (more on this on page 193). It's an ideal drink first thing in the morning, after a workout, or anytime.

Teas and Infusions

MORNING REHYDRATION • DAYTIME MAINTENANCE • NIGHTTIME RESTORATIVE

Many demulcent herbs are available in tea bags or cut and sifted for infusions. Herbs in tea bags are finely cut so the demulcent properties extract very efficiently. Hot water isn't necessary to extract demulcent constituents, but it works fine—and many people simply prefer a hot tea. Some herbs to consider for these preparations include plantain leaf, which has a unique flavor and combines anti-inflammatory and demulcent properties; linden, a famed after-meal European tea of choice that adds calming aromatic constituents to its demulcent actions; licorice, another European favorite that is both sweet and soothing; and sobacha, a nutty-flavored and highly nutritious Japanese tea made from roasted buckwheat.

Cold Infusions

MORNING REHYDRATION • DAYTIME MAINTENANCE • NIGHTTIME RESTORATIVE

Make a cold infusion by placing a couple teaspoons of cut-and-sifted demulcent herbs or seeds (marshmallow root, slippery elm bark, licorice root, chia seeds, or basil seeds) into a quart (1 L) canning jar, filling it with water, and leaving it sealed in the fridge for a few hours or overnight. Strain off the solids; you'll be left with a viscous, demulcent-rich liquid that can be consumed on its own or added to tap or filtered water to enhance the water's hydrating power.

Irish Moss Gel

MORNING REHYDRATION • DAYTIME MAINTENANCE • NIGHTTIME RESTORATIVE

Made from whole unprocessed dried Irish moss, this unique preparation (see page 188) will keep for a week in the fridge and is perfect for adding demulcency to smoothies, shakes, and other beverages.

Irish Moss–Cacao Nib Elixir

MORNING REHYDRATION • DAYTIME MAINTENANCE

This exceptionally delicious smoothie (page 188) is velvety and nourishing. It's packed with vitamins, minerals, and hydrating compounds and makes a replenishing accompaniment to a hike or a beach day.

Demulcent Hydration Balls

DAYTIME MAINTENANCE • NIGHTTIME RESTORATIVE

Eat your demulcents with these tasty treats (page 189) made by blending powdered demulcents with a small amount of honey and water. You can prepare a week's worth of demulcents in only minutes, and they're highly portable.

Mango–Basil Seed Pudding

MORNING REHYDRATION • DAYTIME MAINTENANCE

This delicious pudding (page 194) combines basil seeds with soothing aloe for an excellent breakfast food or a nourishing snack. It's hydrating, high in fiber and nutrients, and great for digestion.

Chia/Basil Seed Pudding

MORNING REHYDRATION • DAYTIME
MAINTENANCE

This very simple preparation combines chia and/
or basil seeds with a plant-based milk for a quick
and nourishing meal. A good beginning ratio is
3 tablespoons seeds to 1 cup (240 ml) liquid;
adjust to your desired consistency. Add a natural
sweetener to taste and embellish the simple base
with fresh berries, nuts, and/or granola. Super Berry
Power Powder Blend (page 158) is a great flavor-
enhancing addition. Make ahead of time and store in
the fridge as an overnight oats alternative.

Prebiotic Fiber Blends

MORNING REHYDRATION • NIGHTTIME
RESTORATIVE

You can purchase pre-made prebiotic fiber drinks
(see Resources, page 352) or make your own (see
page 194). Drink these first thing in the morning on
an empty stomach to encourage healthy elimination,
or at least 2 hours after dinner to help maintain
hydration while you sleep. Either way, they will
nourish the microbiome.

Real Black Licorice Candy

DAYTIME MAINTENANCE • NIGHTTIME
RESTORATIVE

Licorice is an often overlooked, beneficial source of
demulcency. Real black licorice candy is a simple
and delicious delivery mechanism for demulcent
effects (for more on licorice, see page 77).

Supplements and Lozenges

DAYTIME MAINTENANCE • NIGHTTIME
RESTORATIVE

Many demulcent herbs (such as slippery elm bark,
licorice root, marshmallow root, shatavari root,
and Irish moss) can be taken as capsules and
tablets, either alone or combined in formulations
for convenience. Emptying the capsules or chewing
the tablets a bit will increase their effectiveness.
Keeping a package of slippery elm or licorice
lozenges with you is another way to get a small
amount of demulcency throughout the day.

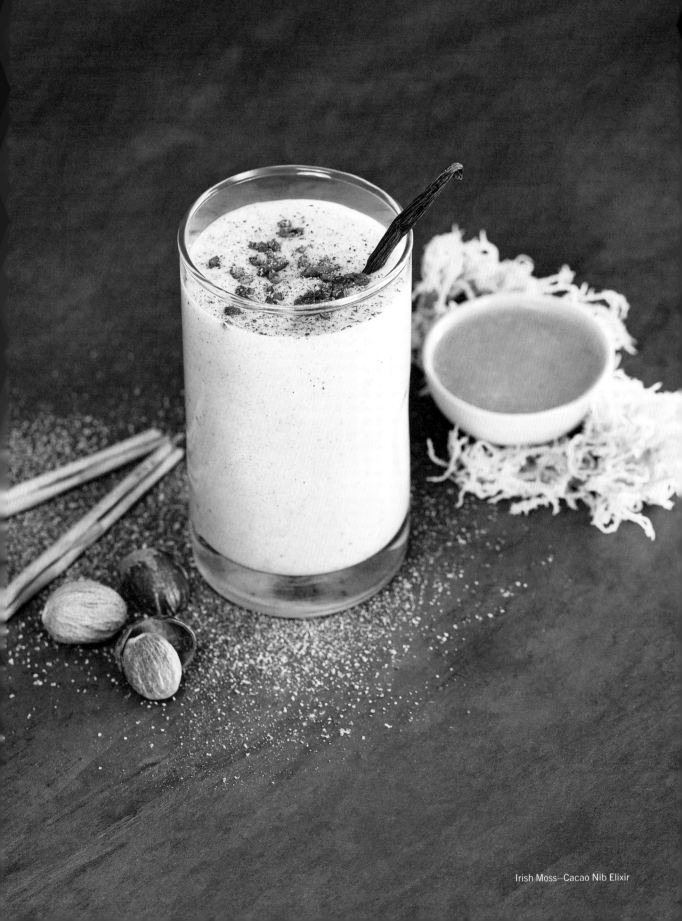

Irish Moss–Cacao Nib Elixir

Morning Demulcent Rituals Around the World

The ritual consumption of a rich demulcent in the morning is something found in many healthy cultures. When you want to go the extra mile to hydrate and lubricate your system, I recommend giving one of these a try. Do it as regularly as you like, or just try one for a week or two to see the benefits.

- **Olive oil.** In a number of Mediterranean countries, it's a well-known traditional health practice to consume a little extra-virgin olive oil first thing in the morning. Though it technically contains no mucilage, olive oil has demulcent properties that emolliate, soothe, and lubricate the GI tract, stimulate digestive secretions, nourish the microbiome, mildly activate liver detoxification, and encourage morning elimination. In addition to its moistening qualities, olive oil contains flavonoids, fatty acids, a plethora of antioxidants, and essential micronutrients. Make your own morning olive oil elixir by taking 1 to 3 teaspoons extra-virgin olive oil first thing in the morning, on an empty stomach, immediately followed by a 12- to 16-ounce (360 to 480 ml) glass of warm water with lemon or the morning demulcent drink of your choice. Wait approximately 30 minutes to an hour before eating your first meal.

- **Ghee.** Some of the Ayurvedic doctors I studied with in India recommended taking a teaspoon of ghee (clarified butter) with a small pinch of trikatu, a classic Ayurvedic spice blend, first thing in the morning. Aside from being moistening, this ritual is particularly beneficial to support gentle cleansing and detoxification. Ghee is revered for its ability to remove toxins and stimulate the liver. The effect is gentle and won't imbalance any constitution, so it works both daily and periodically.

- **Cod liver oil.** In Iceland, it's traditional to have a couple spoonfuls of strong-tasting cod liver oil in the morning, often chased down with a small glass of juice.

- **Manuka honey.** New Zealand's famous medicinal elixir and number one export is the honey derived from the flowers of the native manuka bush (*Leptospermum scoparium*). All parts of manuka—the bark, leaves, and flowers—contain powerful medicinal compounds. New Zealand's indigenous Māori use manuka honey extensively in their traditional medicine as a cure-all.

  All honey has emolliating properties that soothe and moisten the GI tract, but manuka stands out among them for its unparalleled antimicrobial, anti-inflammatory, and antiseptic constituents; it also has a relatively moderate glycemic index compared to other natural sweeteners. Many New Zealanders begin each day with a teaspoon of manuka honey melted into 1 cup (240 ml) hot water with a squeeze of lemon. This morning demulcent elixir revitalizes the GI tract and neutralizes opportunistic microbes at the same time.

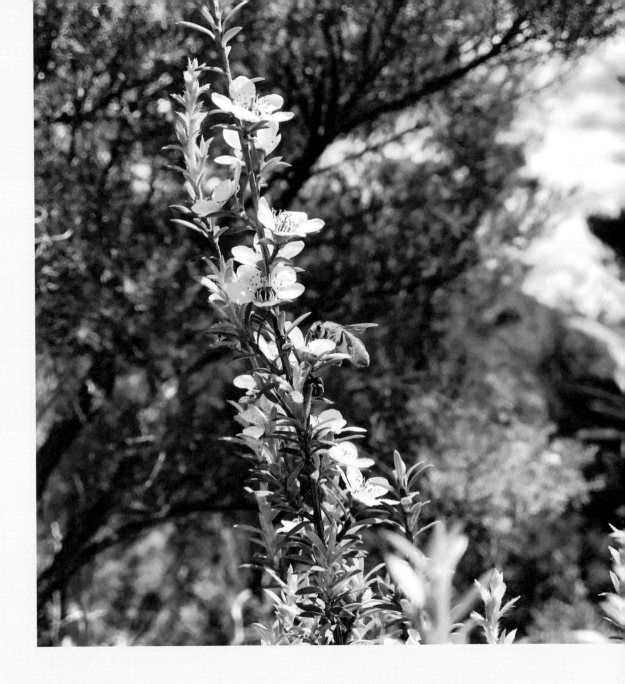

Note: New Zealand maintains high standards for measuring the quality of its manuka honey. Look for the UMF (Unique Manuka Factor) number on the label. This is a quantifiable measurement of the constituents that give manuka its antimicrobial and antioxidant properties. The higher the UMF, the stronger the medicinal effects of the honey. A UMF of 10 or above is generally considered to be

A manuka bush in bloom in Abel Tasman National Park, New Zealand

medicinal grade. Another measurement used in New Zealand is MG, which calibrates manuka's antimicrobial potency; anything above 265 is equivalent to 10 UMF. Both measurements will point you to the good stuff.

Irish Moss Gel

Rinse **1 cup (80 g) dried Irish moss** in a strainer under cold water to remove any sand or impurities. Combine the Irish moss with **½ cup (120 ml) water** and **1 teaspoon fresh lemon juice** in a bowl. Let soak for 3 to 4 hours. After soaking, blend the contents of the bowl with an immersion blender or a high-speed blender. Add small amounts of water as needed to ensure the gel is thick but not too sticky. Transfer the finished gel to a well-sealed glass container; it can be stored in the fridge for up to a week.

On its own, Irish moss has a rather bland and unremarkable flavor that blends well with other beverages. It dissolves instantly and turns any drink into a deeply hydrating and nutrient-dense elixir. Just stir **1 to 2 teaspoons gel** into approximately **2 cups (480 ml) liquid**, adjusted for your preferred consistency.

Irish Moss–Cacao Nib Elixir

Using an immersion blender, combine in a bowl **1 cup (240 ml) water, ½ cup (120 ml) coconut cream, 2 tablespoons Irish moss gel** (above), **1 tablespoon natural sweetener of your choice, 1 or 2 teaspoons cacao nibs, ½ teaspoon cinnamon powder, ½ teaspoon vanilla extract**, and **a pinch of nutmeg**. Process until smooth and chill in the fridge for 30 minutes before serving. Garnish with **more cacao nibs** and **cinnamon powder**.

Demulcent Powder Blend

Mix **1½ cups (312 g) marshmallow root powder**; **½ cup (40 g) each slippery elm bark powder, shatavari root powder, and licorice root powder**; and **2 tablespoons each fennel powder and orange peel powder** in a large bowl. Transfer the blend to an airtight container. If properly stored in a cool, dark, dry place, the blend will last for up to a month. Dry powders lose potency if stored improperly. Makes approximately 3½ cups (450 g).

Demulcent Hydration Balls

Put **½ cup (40 g) of your favorite powdered demulcent** in a bowl. (I recommend slippery elm, marshmallow, shatavari, or Demulcent Powder Blend, above, because of their high mucilage content and fibrous texture). Add **1 or 2 teaspoons manuka or other honey of your choice**, slightly warming the honey if it's not pourable so that it doesn't glob up when mixing. Slowly incorporate the powder and honey with a fork or flexible spatula, then **add water in teaspoon increments** while constantly stirring to thin out the mixture. Keep adding water until you reach a dough-like consistency that is moist enough to remain intact but not overly sticky. Form the dough into one large ball (which you can later break into bize-size pieces) or form several gumball-size balls. Add a little more demulcent powder to the bowl and roll the ball (or balls) in it to coat.

   Put the ball(s) in a resealable container and store for up to 1 week in the fridge. Chew or let a ball or piece dissolve in your mouth. You can also dissolve the balls in water or other beverages to make instant demulcent drinks (use 1 or 2 gumball-size demulcent balls per 2 cups/480 ml liquid).

Note: Feel free to add a small pinch of cinnamon, ginger, orange peel, or other culinary spices to the mix to enhance the flavor.

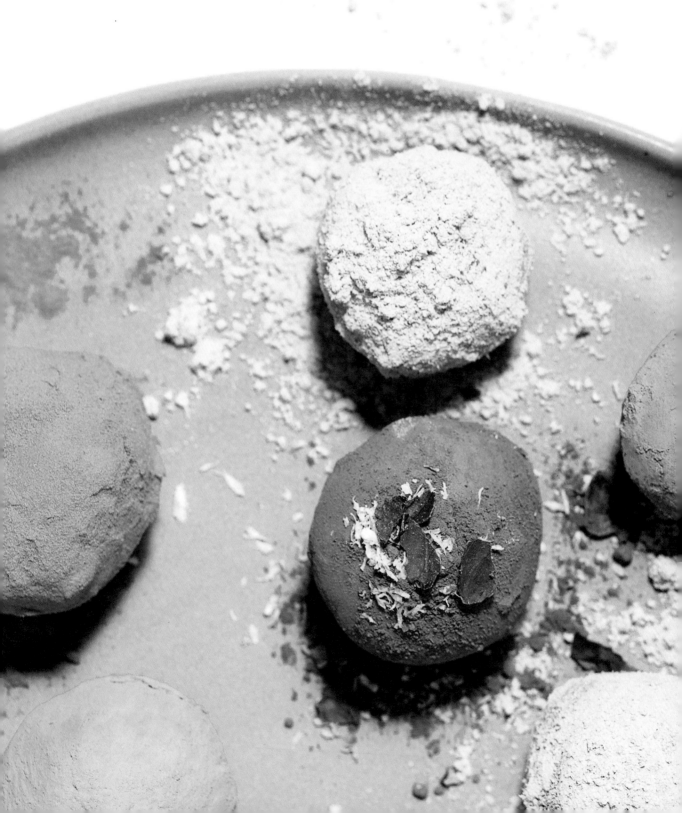

Turmeric Balls (page 123), Nutritive Green Power Balls (page 163), Demulcent Hydration Balls (page 189), and Cacao Adaptogenic Energy Balls (page 255)

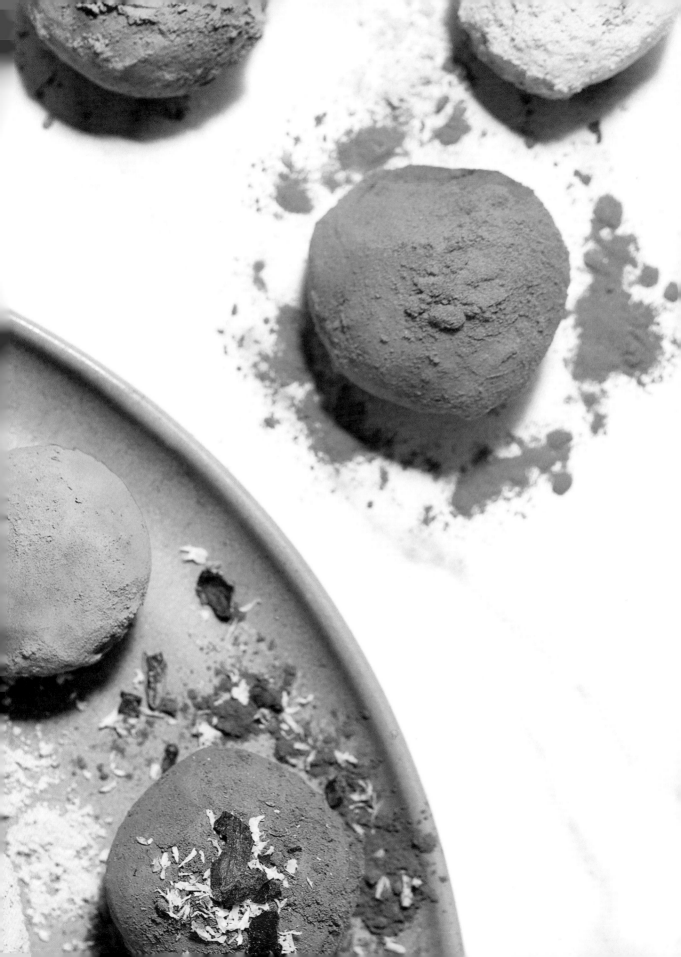

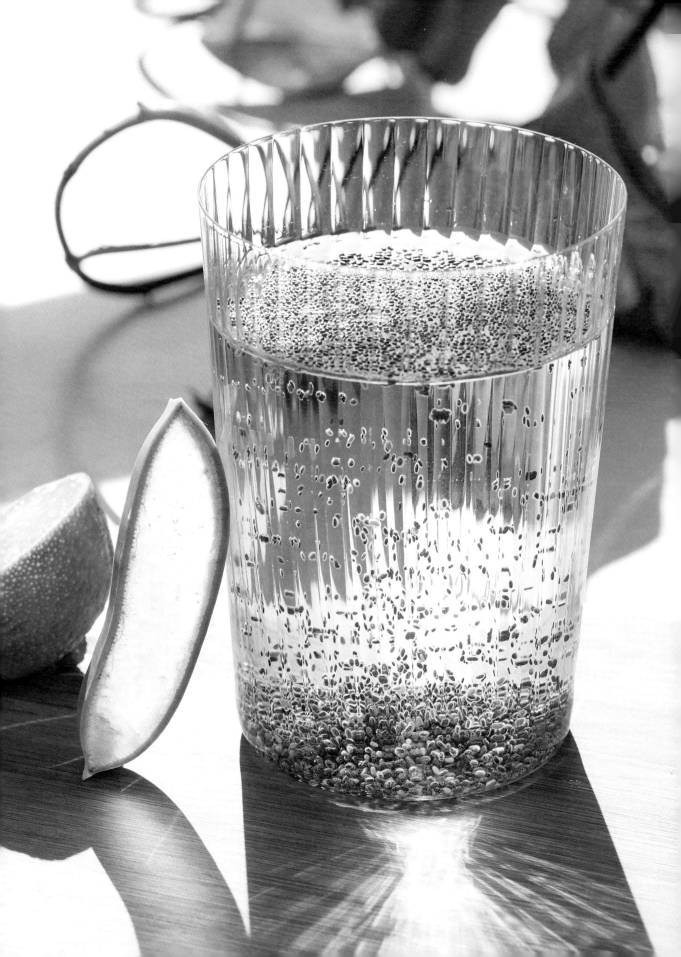

Chia-Aloe-Lime Rehydrator

Add **1 heaping teaspoon chia seeds** to **2 cups (480 ml) water**. Add **2 tablespoons chopped aloe vera gel** (see below), **a squeeze of fresh lime juice**, and **a natural sweetener of your choice** to taste. Let the beverage sit for a few minutes, stirring occasionally, until it becomes visibly viscous.

HARVESTING FRESH ALOE

You can find food-grade aloe vera gel (distinct from the topical or cosmetic preparations) in grocery or health food stores, but the most potent gel comes directly from fresh leaves. To harvest:

1) Slice the spiked sides off lengthwise in very thin slivers.

2) Slice a small sliver off across the leaf at the wider end to reveal the clear gel inside.

3) Insert a paring knife beneath the top of the leaf where the clear gel begins. Remove and discard the top.

4) Slice along the bottom edge of the clear gel to separate it from the outer leaf.

5) Cut the gel into small cubes and store them in an airtight container in the fridge, where they will keep for up to 10 days.

The gel can be blended into a hydrating elixir, smoothie, or beverage (like the Chia-Aloe-Lime Rehydrator, see above), or it can be applied directly to the skin to soothe irritations or as an impromptu moisturizer.

Mango–Basil Seed Pudding

Combine **½ to ¾ cup (120 to 180 ml) cashew or macadamia milk**, **3 tablespoons basil seeds**, **1 teaspoon natural sweetener of your choice (or to taste)**, **½ teaspoon vanilla extract**, and **a pinch of sea salt** in a bowl. Whisk together and let soak for 15 to 30 minutes, stirring occasionally, until the mixture thickens. Meanwhile, puree **½ cup (85 g) fresh mango chunks** and **1 to 2 tablespoons aloe vera gel** (see page 193) in a blender or food processor. Once the basil seed pudding has thickened, fill one tall glass or two small glasses with alternating layers of pudding and mango-aloe puree. Top with **crumbled macadamia nuts**, **coconut flakes**, and/or **cacao nibs**, plus **a few pieces of chopped mango**, and garnish with **a slice of aloe and/or mango or a sprig of spearmint**. Leftovers can be covered and stored in the fridge for 4 or 5 days. Makes 1 to 2 servings.

Prebiotic Fiber Blend

Mix **1 ounce (30 g) psyllium husk powder**; **½ ounce (15 g) chia seed powder**; **¼ ounce (7 g) each slippery elm bark powder, marshmallow root powder, and shatavari root powder**; and **⅛ ounce (4 g) licorice root powder** in a large bowl. Add **1⁄16 ounce (2 g) cinnamon powder** (or another culinary spice) to enhance the flavor and support digestion. Transfer the blend to an airtight container. If properly stored in a cool, dark, dry place, the blend will last for up to a month. Dry powders lose potency if stored improperly.

Note: To make your prebiotic fiber drink, vigorously stir 1 to 2 tablespoons powder into 1½ cups (360 ml) room-temperature water and drink quickly on an empty stomach. You may wish to follow with another glass of water to help with assimilation.

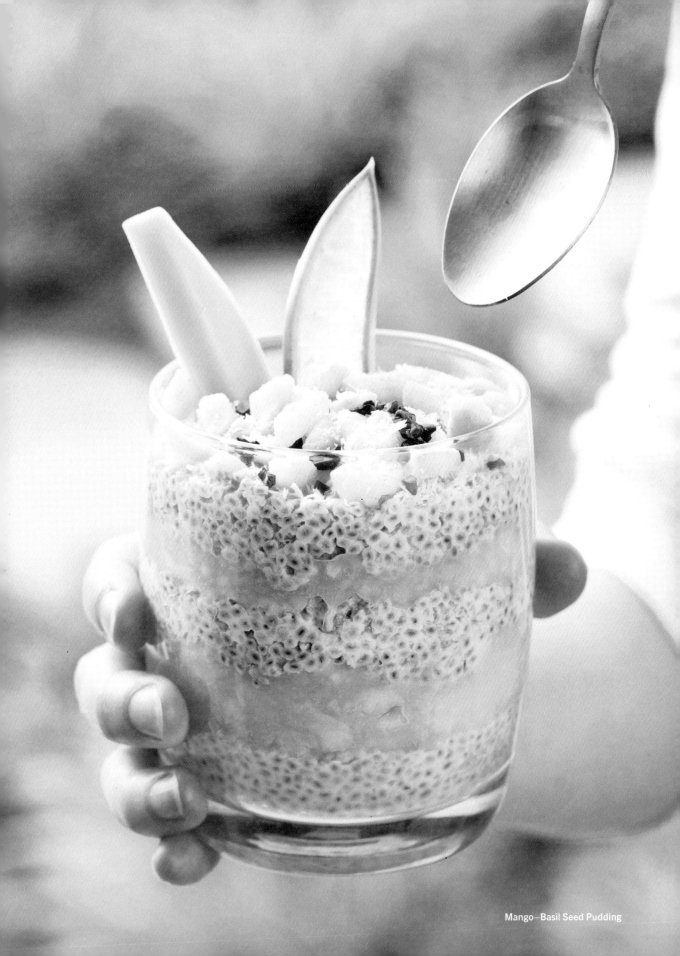

Mango–Basil Seed Pudding

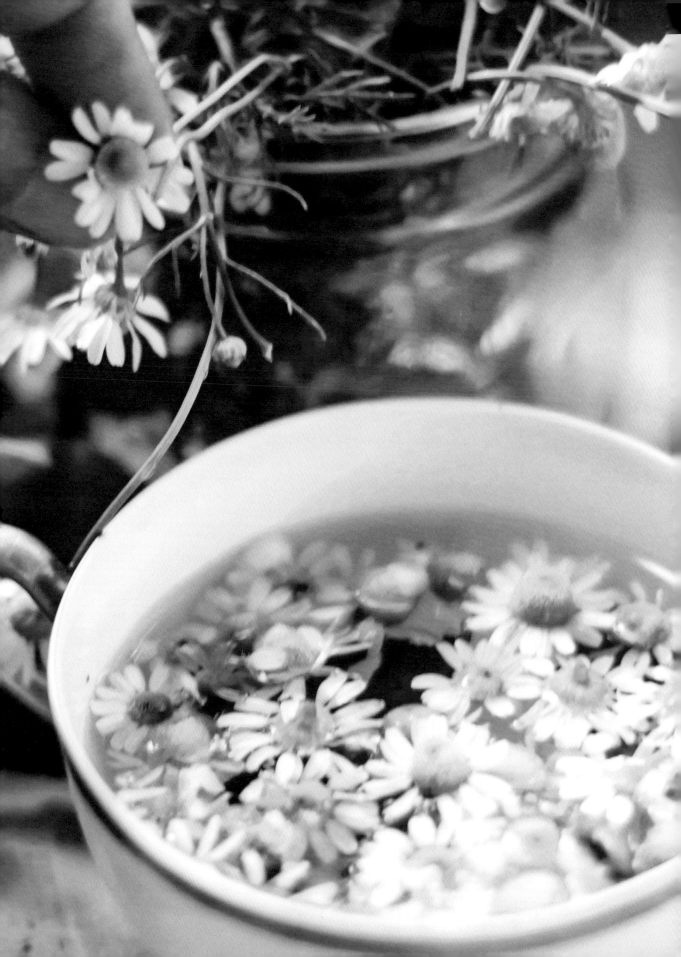

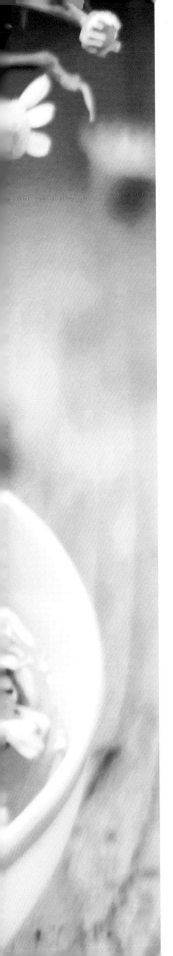

step # 4 | Nervines

THE FOCUS OF THIS STEP IS TO ESTABLISH A RELAXED MIND and body, elevate the mood, and encourage deep restorative sleep by utilizing nervine calmatives, fragrant relaxants, and floral oils. Keeping a balanced nervous system and relaxed state of mind ensures the free-flowing transmission of nerve signals throughout the body. Nervines encourage nerve flow while relaxing tension, thus improving energy and clarity, calming anxiety, relaxing muscle tension, and reducing insomnia. Incorporating them into our daily routine helps us establish a place of calm and inner poise amid the constant demands and stimulation of modern life.

WHAT TO EXPECT

- Improved digestion and an overall more relaxed gut and diaphragm area

- Eased muscular tension, particularly in the neck, shoulders, jaw, and head

- Improved clarity and focus

- More restorative sleep

- More consistently deep breathing

- An uplifted mood, with less anxiety and irritability

- Improved circulation and less frequent cold hands and feet

Plants & Other Ingredients You'll Be Using

Nervines come in a wide range of forms and preparations with varying potency and effects, so you can use them throughout the day for different purposes. Over time, you'll develop your own relationship with these plants and get a feel for how the various preparations work best in your daily routine. *Note:* Essential oils will be covered in depth on the following pages.

Fragrant Relaxants

Fragrant relaxants contain a rich assortment of aromatic oils that gently relax the body and mind. Plants like chamomile, lavender, lemon balm, linden, and spearmint calm the enteric nerves lining the gut and increase vagal nerve tone. Relaxing the densely packed nerves in the gut is essential for good digestion and effectively unravels tension throughout the entire body. These herbs can be used both fresh and dried to make hot and cold infusions, teas, and aromatic waters to drink after meals or sip on throughout the day.

Nervine Calmatives

Soothing the nervous system at a deeper level, nervine calmatives are stronger in their sedative effects, making them especially helpful for promoting sleep and reducing insomnia. They can be used during the day in lower dosages, and they can serve as long-term rejuvenators to restore a chronically overstimulated and exhausted nervous system. These plants can also provide quick relief from acute anxiety. Nervine calmatives are not as flavorful as fragrant relaxants, so they're most often taken in tincture, tablet, or capsule form. Common plants in this group include skullcap, valerian root, hops, passionflower, kava, CBD, and California poppy.

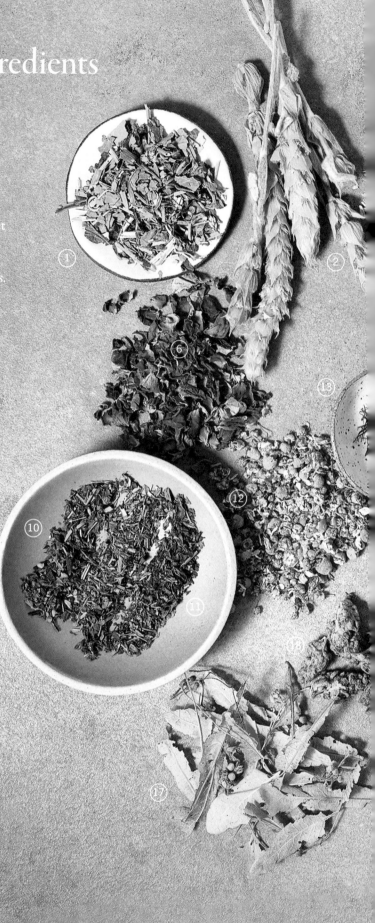

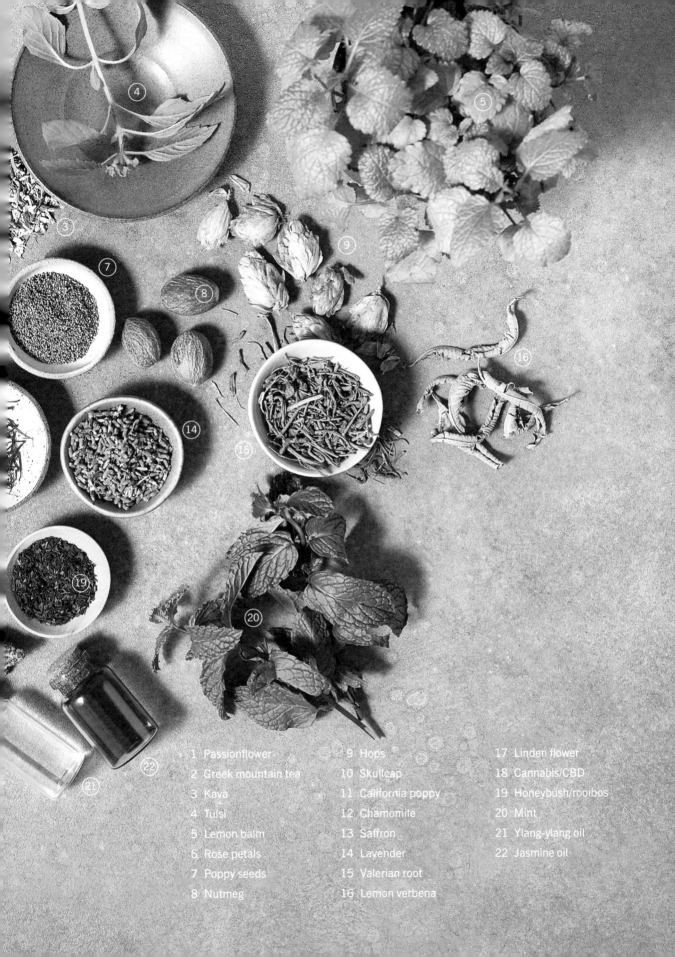

1 Passionflower

2 Greek mountain tea

3 Kava

4 Tulsi

5 Lemon balm

6 Rose petals

7 Poppy seeds

8 Nutmeg

9 Hops

10 Skullcap

11 California poppy

12 Chamomile

13 Saffron

14 Lavender

15 Valerian root

16 Lemon verbena

17 Linden flower

18 Cannabis/CBD

19 Honeybush/rooibos

20 Mint

21 Ylang-ylang oil

22 Jasmine oil

Essential Oils

Essential oils are the fragrant and highly concentrated molecules contained within the flowers, fruits, stems, leaves, and roots of approximately 10 percent of all plants. Many of the plants in this book derive some of their medicinal benefits from their essential oil content. The power of fragrance is subtle but substantial. The sense of smell is directly linked to the limbic system, an area of our brain involved with the production of neurotransmitters that influence mood, cognition, and emotion. Inhalation of essential oils activates the olfactory receptors, which in turn catalyze a range of physiological functions related to overall nervous system health.

Along with helping plants communicate with their environment, essential oils are also part of their immune response; they serve to neutralize harmful pathogens. These antimicrobial and antiseptic actions benefit our immune systems in similar ways: The oils purify respiratory passages when inhaled and neutralize airborne pathogens when diffused into the atmosphere. We can access the benefits of essential oils not just by inhaling them but also by applying them topically or ingesting them in the form of culinary spices, or drinking infusions and teas made from the plants that contain the oils. (An important note: One should never ingest essential oils directly, as they are far too potent and potentially damaging to the gut.)

Below are some of the most vital and useful essential oils for your plant-powered lifestyle.

- **Lavender.** Emblematic of southern France, lavender is the world's top-selling essential oil, and for good reason. Lavender oil is a virtual panacea with a gentle nature. It is a soothing relaxant for the nervous system, with cooling, anti-inflammatory actions for both mind and body that enhance concentration and improve sleep quality. In addition, lavender oil is beneficial when applied topically as a remedy for burns and skin irritations.

- **Helichrysum.** The best oil for skin regeneration and wound healing—including soft tissue injury, bruises, and scar tissue repair—helichrysum (from the *Helichrysum italicum* plant) has potent anti-inflammatory, blood-vitalizing, and antimicrobial actions, which are highly beneficial for skin beautification. Its fresh fragrance is reminiscent of the Mediterranean seaside where it originates.

- **Jatamansi.** A fragrant root from the Himalayas related to valerian, and with a similarly pungent aroma, jatamansi has relaxing and hypnotic qualities beneficial for improving sleep, encouraging pleasant dreams, and easing tension and chronic overstimulation of the sympathetic nervous system.

- **Frankincense.** Frankincense oil is derived from a tree resin native to the deserts of North Africa. Both the oil and the resin have a relaxing, mood-elevating fragrance and are used for ceremonial and ritual purposes all over the world. In addition, when applied topically, frankincense has significant anti-inflammatory, antimicrobial, and blood-vitalizing actions that are beneficial for the skin and soft tissue.

- **Respiratory oils.** Eucalyptus, rosemary, lemon myrtle, and evergreen tree oils (such as spruce, pine, and fir) are excellent for atmospheric purification and reducing airborne pathogens. These oils improve breathing and respiratory immunity, reduce symptoms of colds and flus, clear sinus congestion, and increase mental clarity.

- **Ceremonial oils.** Palo santo, sandalwood, agarwood, mastic, copal, and cedar are used extensively to shift consciousness, improve cognition, calm the nervous system, and elevate mood.

- **Citrus oils.** The bright, fragrant oils of lemon, lime, orange, grapefruit, mandarin, clementine, and neroli have potent antidepressant effects. They are especially uplifting and energizing and beneficial for clearing the mind and improving concentration.

- **Floral oils.** Sultry floral oils—including rose, jasmine, ylang-ylang, clary sage, rose geranium, blue lotus, champa, and vanilla—induce euphoric states, ease tension, increase libido, and improve sleep.

Rose oil distillation in Bulgaria

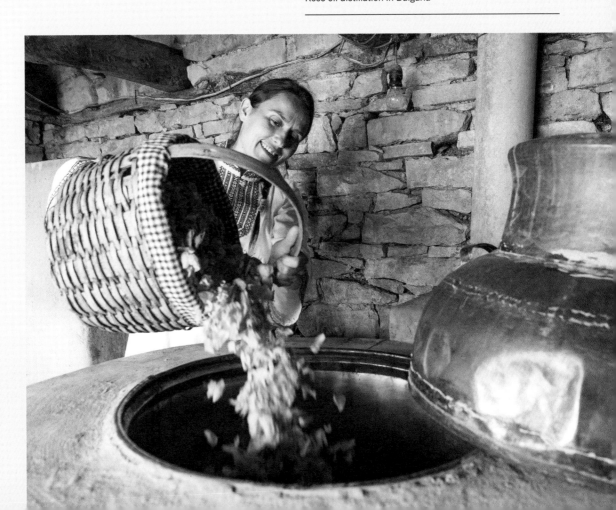

Buying & Administering Essential Oils

The key considerations when buying essential oils are quality and sustainability. It's important to determine the origin and purity of the essential oils you're using, as adulteration and contamination are common problems within the industry. As with many industrial agricultural products, essential oils can be contaminated with pesticides or chemical residues. Adulteration of essential oils with synthetic compounds or substitute oils is unfortunately also something to be aware of. In terms of sustainability, it takes a large volume of plant material to get a small amount of essential oil (for example, 250 pounds/113 kg of lavender flowers yields approximately 1 pound/455 g of lavender oil). To sustain healthy plant populations, especially those harvested in the wild, it's imperative to purchase your essential oils from reputable, responsible producers that ensure the oils are coming from sustainable sources and projects. See suggested sources on page 353.

Once you are assured of an oil's quality, focus on its safe application and administration. Essential oils are powerful, concentrated compounds that need to be used in a thoughtful and safe way. Cinnamon, clove, and thyme, for example, can be irritating if applied directly to the skin. Other oils, such as lemon, orange, and other citruses, are phototoxic and should not be applied to skin that is exposed to direct sunlight. On the other end of the spectrum, oils such as lavender and chamomile are relatively safe and gentle, less likely to cause adverse reactions with direct skin contact, and therefore more versatile. In general, do not ingest essential oils, and dilute them with carrier oils like argan or almond oil to guard against potential skin irritation. What follows are two of the easiest and most effective ways to interact with essential oils; see page 214 for more.

- **Diffusion.** Diffusion uses heat or vibration to liberate aromatic molecules directly into the air we breathe, purifying the atmosphere, calming the nervous system, elevating mood, and creating subtle shifts in consciousness. There are four main types of diffusers: nebulizing, evaporative, ultrasonic, and electric. An ultrasonic or humidifying diffuser uses a base of water to evaporate the oils into a fine mist that permeates the space. This does not use heat, which preserves the beneficial constituents of the oil. How much oil to use in your diffuser will vary based on the size of the water tank, the potency of the particular oil you're using, and your desired effect. For a small diffuser, I recommend starting with five drops of oil. For larger diffusers, I use between ten and fifteen drops. The advantage of using a diffuser is that you get a great effect with minimal effort. Some diffusers can run for six hours straight without needing to be refilled or restarted. If done consistently, this deceptively simple technique can make a significant improvement in one's health and state of mind.

- **Direct palm inhalation.** Gentle oils like floral relaxants and eucalyptus and other respiratory oils work well for direct palm inhalation (very strong oils like cinnamon, oregano, thyme, and other spice oils shouldn't be used in this way). Place two or three drops of essential oil on your palms, rub them together, and cup your hands over your nose and mouth (avoiding the eyes). Inhale slowly and deeply for several breaths. Bring mindfulness to the process: Pay close attention to how you feel before, during, and after the inhalations. Notice the subtle shifts that occur in your state of mind and body and how long they last.

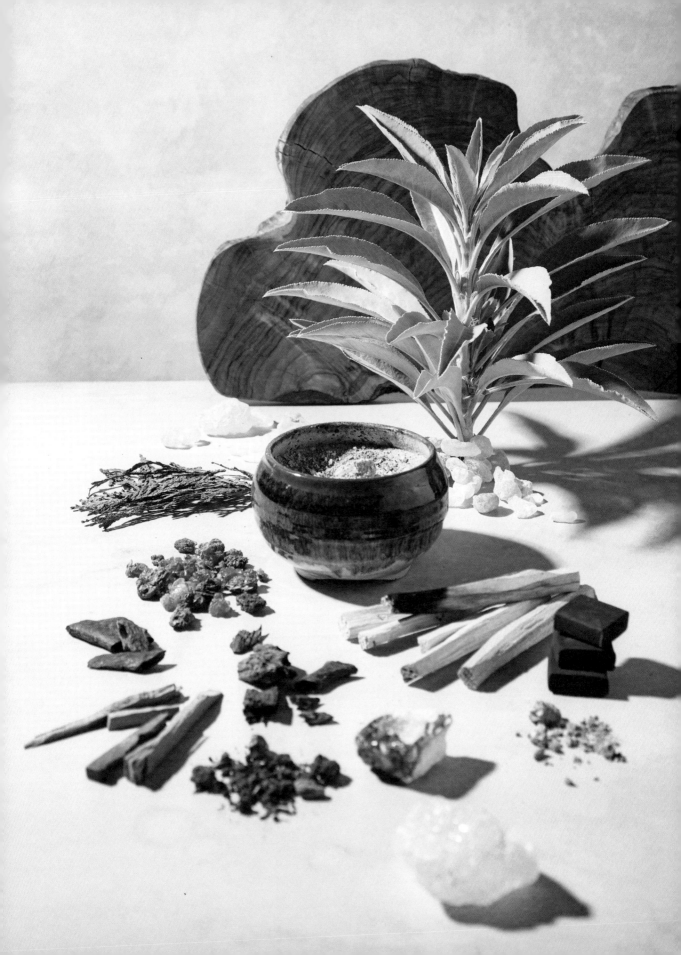

Getting Started

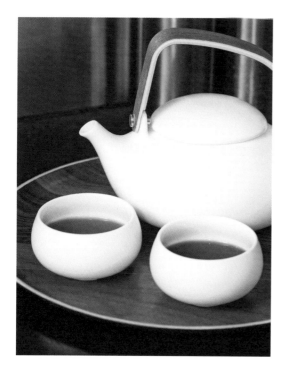

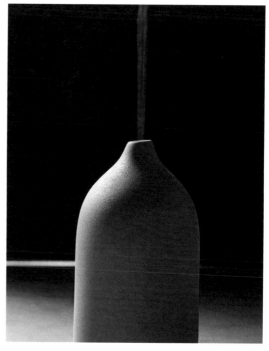

Tea Station

The simplest way to consume fragrant relaxants is in teas or infusions. Creating a dedicated tea-making zone in your house or workplace makes it easy and enjoyable to develop a daily drinking ritual. Gather a varied collection of your favorite loose herbs and bagged teas. Your tea station might include a teakettle, a French press, a teapot with a removable infuser basket, tea infusers (baskets, balls, or canisters), self-fill tea bags, teacups or mugs, a glass pitcher for cold infusions, natural sweeteners (honey, agave, monk fruit blend, or the sweetener of your choice), and fresh lemons or a small bottle of lemon juice. Storing herbs in glass containers adds a nice aesthetic touch; just be sure to keep containers away from direct sunlight to maintain their potency. Small metal containers with airtight lids also work well.

Diffusers

Having essential oil diffusers around the house and workspace is a simple way to generate an atmosphere of mood-elevating good vibes wherever we are. Choose different oils to diffuse depending on your desired effect. Rosemary, citrus, and melissa oil, for example, have an uplifting quality that encourages a clear, focused, and creative state of mind and thus are good options for a work area. Diffusing lavender or clary sage in the evening while reading or watching TV creates a calm ambience that encourages your nervous system to unwind from the stimulation of the day. Rose, jasmine, or ylang-ylang in the bedroom creates a sultry atmosphere that puts mind and body at ease and promotes good dreams as you drift off to sleep.

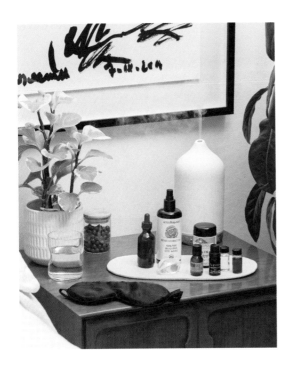

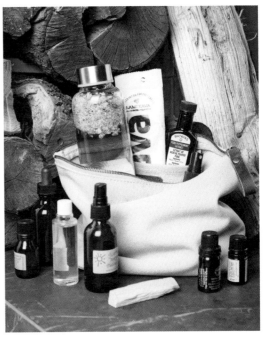

Bedside Table

Keep nervine tinctures, tablets, capsules, or CBD oil in or on the bedside table to create a sustainable sleep-optimizing routine. Tablets and capsules need to be digested for their effects to be felt, so take them approximately half an hour before sleep, as you wind down for the evening. Nervine tinctures such as skullcap, passionflower, valerian root, or hops are absorbed quickly, providing fast-acting relaxation to quiet the mind and initiate sleep. Their immediate effects also make them especially helpful to put you back to sleep if you awaken in the night. Keep oils like lavender, ylang-ylang, jasmine, jatamansi, and rose in the bedroom as well. A few drops of oil dispersed through a diffuser, sprinkled on your pillow, or mindfully inhaled in the palms helps you slip peacefully into sleep.

On the Go

Use nervines to create a little force field of calm wherever you are. Carry a small bottle of floral essential oil (such as rose, neroli, lavender, geranium, mandarin, or lemon) as you travel. Anoint your neck with a drop or two or do direct palm inhalations (see page 202) to quickly restore a feeling of ease and flow. Fill an insulated thermos with hot, fragrant, relaxant tea to sip throughout the day. Or simply drop a handful of fresh-cut herbs like lemon balm, mint, or tulsi into a water bottle. Nervine tinctures made with lavender, chamomile, skullcap, or passionflower travel well and work quickly to calm the nervous system; keep a small bottle in your backpack or purse. Kava or CBD oil capsules and/or gummies help alleviate anxiety, ease muscle tension, and diminish jet lag.

How to Saturate Your Day

The sympathetic nervous system is more active during the daytime when we're action oriented and amped up. It can be difficult to sufficiently circulate the energy we generate, which, according to TCM, leads to qi stagnation, tension, and anxiety. Using nervines throughout the day keeps us from accumulating too much tension that would otherwise interfere with our ability to unwind and sleep when the time comes. In the evening, nervines encourage a naturally occurring progressive relaxation, ultimately easing us into deep and restful sleep.

Daytime Qi Regulation

The best times to reach for nervines during the day are after meals, during intensive work sessions or meetings, or any time you're feeling overstimulated. Focus on fragrant relaxants and essential oils for daytime use. You can brew tea, drink a cold infusion, or take a supplement to ease tension in the gut, uplift the mind, and encourage feelings of ease and flow.

Evening Unwind

At the end of a workday, we naturally look to shift gears into evening relaxation-and-renewal mode. Incorporate nervines thirty minutes to one hour after the evening meal. For restorative sleep, continue using nervines into the evening and/or at bedtime with the pulse-dosing method (see page 216).

Instant Chill

Certain herbs in the nervine category can quickly alleviate anxiety and tension when we need to relax and shift the state of our nervous system relatively immediately. You might do a few direct palm inhalations of rose oil, drink a cup of kava or take a dose of CBD oil. Nervines can shift us out of fight-or-flight mode, to help our bodies better navigate the stress response. They provide fast relief for an anxious mind, soothe tense muscles, improve circulation, relieve pain, and speed healing in many common conditions, such as headaches, menstrual cramps, sports injuries, muscle tension, and TMJ syndrome.

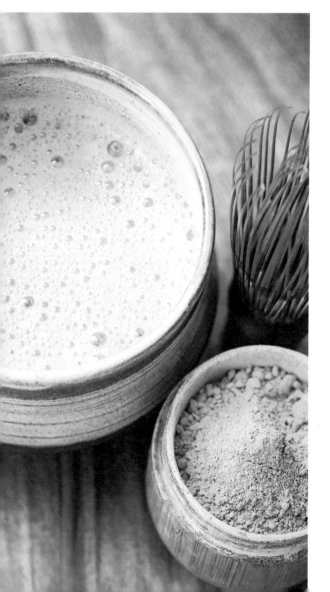

Matcha Latte (page 220)

SAMPLE DAILY MENUS

MINIMUM DAILY DOSE

Drink a strong cup or two of a fragrant relaxant tea of your choice twice a day, preferably after lunch and in the evening after dinner to wind down. Use mood-elevating essential oils in a diffuser as you work, and take direct palm inhalations of your favorite calming oil in the evening before bed.

MENU 1

In the morning:
Lemon balm tea after breakfast and a direct palm inhalation of rosemary oil for a few minutes before work

After lunch:
Greek Mountain Tea (page 218) and a diffusion of grapefruit oil

In the evening:
Lavender tea

Before bed:
Nutmeg-Saffron Deep Sleep Elixir (page 224) and an application of jasmine oil

MENU 2

In the morning:
Peppermint extract after breakfast (see page 210) and rose geranium oil in a diffuser at work

In the afternoon:
Honeybush Latte (page 218) and a direct palm inhalation of neroli oil

After dinner:
Chamomile tea and a diffusion of ylang-ylang oil

Before bed:
Pulse dosing of skullcap tincture

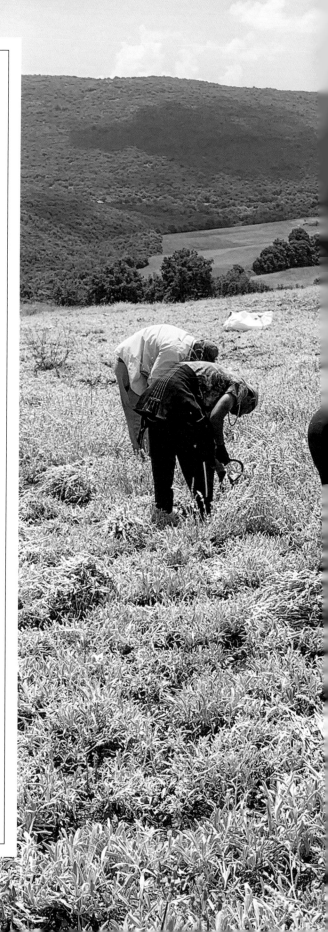

TSAI TOU VOUNOU: THE IKARIAN ELIXIR OF LONGEVITY

On a sourcing trip to Greece, my wife and I took a side journey to the island of Ikaria, one of the original Blue Zones famous for having uncommonly high numbers of people living lives of enviable health and happiness well into their nineties and beyond. Many factors are involved in the longevity experienced by Ikarians, including the regular consumption of a wide variety of wild medicinal herbs gathered throughout the island. Among the most treasured of these is Greek mountain tea, aka ironwort—*tsai tou vounou* in Greek, meaning "tea of the mountain," or simply "mountain tea," as it's called here—made from the flowers and leaves of small perennial plants with silvery leaves and bright clusters of yellow flowers in the *Sideritis* genus. As a member of the mint family, mountain tea has a delicious flavor reminiscent of mint and sage that makes a highly aromatic tea widely consumed for its flavor and health benefits (see its profile on page 320). On the island of Ikaria, sharing a pot of mountain tea is a daily ritual not to be missed.

During the visit, I made a point of drinking as much tea as I could, especially to warm up after harvesting plants in the mountains. When my hosts sat down to drink mountain tea, it was a vehicle for stepping out of time, chatting, laughing, and enjoying each other and the moment. Mountain tea relaxes tension in the gut and diaphragm, deepens the breathing, increases circulation, and makes the body feel at ease. Drinking it several times a day helped get me into the relaxed rhythm of the Ikarians.

Whenever I sip mountain tea at home now, it reminds me of the Ikarian way of life, and what the ease-and-flow herbs are all about: creating healthy rituals on our own or with others to calm down, lighten up, take a minute, and let go of concerns and agendas. Make your own cup of tea with fragrant relaxants and allow the moment to find you.

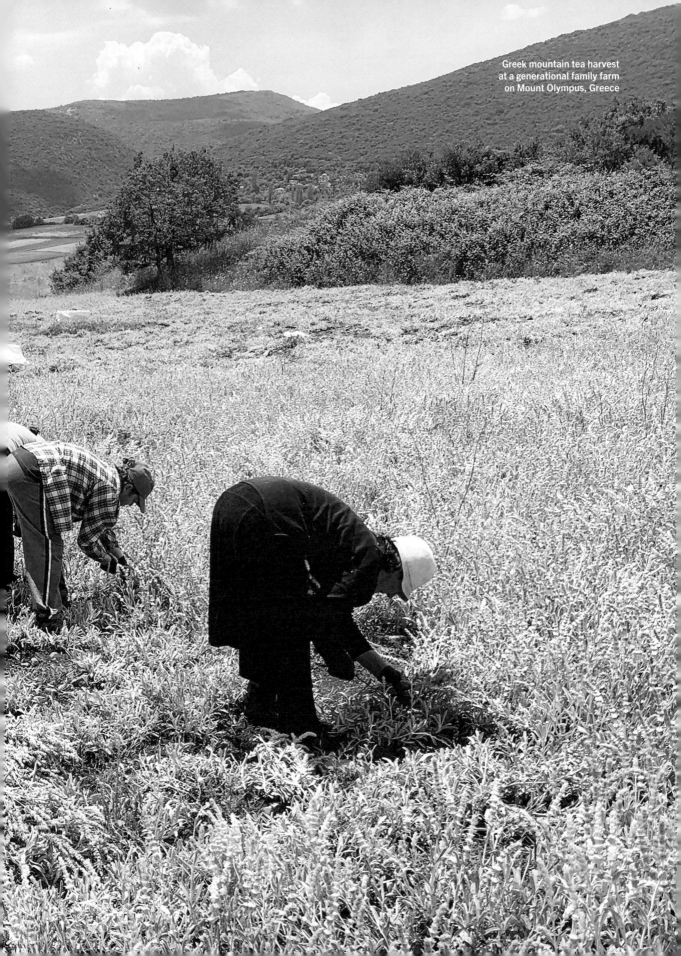

Greek mountain tea harvest
at a generational family farm
on Mount Olympus, Greece

step 4 | Options

Teas and Infusions

DAYTIME QI REGULATION • EVENING UNWIND •
INSTANT CHILL

Infusions and teas are effective and enjoyable ways to regularly incorporate fragrant relaxants into our lifestyle. A good time to do this is after major meals, but it's fine to drink them any time of day or night. The herbs in this category are for the most part interchangeable, but each one does have a slightly different effect based on its specific constituents. (See page 94 for more on teas and infusions, and the plant profiles beginning on page 300 for specific actions of individual fragrant relaxants.)

Greek Mountain Tea

DAYTIME QI REGULATION • EVENING UNWIND

This tea (page 218) is an apothecary in one plant. It's deliciously aromatic, full of phytonutrients, immune enhancing, and calming to frazzled nerves. In Greek culture, mountain tea is an essential part of daily life (for more on this, see page 208).

Aromatic Herb-Infused Water

DAYTIME QI REGULATION • EVENING UNWIND

Aromatic waters infused with fragrant relaxants fulfill the same function as teas or infusions, just in a slightly more dilute and refreshing form. They are a great option during the warmer months when you're not as inclined to drink hot tea and want something a bit more refreshing.

Peppermint Elixir

DAYTIME QI REGULATION • EVENING UNWIND

Peppermint extract is made from macerating peppermint leaves in alcohol—similar to the way vanilla extract is made. To make a quick and easy peppermint elixir, dilute ¼ to ½ teaspoon peppermint extract in 1 to 1½ cups (240 to 360 ml) water. This refreshing drink is excellent after meals to help settle digestion—reducing any excess gas or bloating and the sluggishness you may feel after a big meal. For a more concentrated, fast-acting version, use less water and drink it like a shot. You can also add ¼ teaspoon extract to a shot of bitters. Peppermint extract is available online and in grocery stores in the cooking and spices section (see the Resources section on page 352 for recommended sources).

Lattes
DAYTIME QI REGULATION • EVENING UNWIND

Herbal tea lattes, like Lavender Flower Latte (page 221), Chamomile Latte (page 221), Cacao Rose CBD Bliss Latte (page 221), and Honeybush Latte (page 218), are great after meals or as a relaxing evening beverage.

Matcha Latte
DAYTIME QI REGULATION

Treasured in Japan for its ability to enhance energy without causing jitters, matcha has been a portal into elevated states of mind for millennia. Drinking this frothy green beverage increases oxygenation to the brain, sharpens focus, brightens the mood, and gets the synapses firing. Packed with antioxidants and other constituents that increase overall health, this is a great tonic to drink daily to increase vitality and reclaim our attention. See page 220 for the recipe.

Kava Koolada
DAYTIME QI REGULATION • EVENING UNWIND • INSTANT CHILL

This tropical refresher (page 224) transports you to the beaches of the South Pacific. Juicy pineapple and creamy coconut are the perfect flavor combination to accentuate kava's "instant chill" effect. For more on kava, see page 226.

Blue Poppy-Seed Sleep Elixir
EVENING UNWIND

Poppy is commonly consumed in the Ayurvedic tradition for its relaxing qualities. Culinary poppy seeds are rich in fiber, essential fats, vitamins, and minerals—including magnesium, a vital mineral for improving sleep quality. See page 224 for a delicious beverage incorporating poppy seeds with vanilla and cardamom.

Nutmeg-Saffron Deep Sleep Elixir
EVENING UNWIND

This delicious, soothing elixir (page 224) is an Ayurvedic favorite combining two all-star herbs, nutmeg and saffron, for promoting deep calm and relaxation. This is a reliable sleep elixir—drink about an hour before sleep.

CBD (Cannabidiol)
DAYTIME QI REGULATION • EVENING UNWIND • INSTANT CHILL

CBD comes in a wide variety of forms and preparations (see page 309). CBD preparations usually begin to work in about 30 minutes, and the effects tend to last for at least 3 to 4 hours. Dosages vary depending upon the individual and preparation, but research suggests a guideline for an effective starting dose for most people is somewhere around 10 milligrams. A good general guideline: Start low and work up to determine the right dosage for you.

Cacao Rose
CBD Bliss Latte

DAYTIME QI REGULATION • EVENING UNWIND •
INSTANT CHILL

As the name suggests, this recipe (page 221) is
deeply relaxing and delicious. The combination
of cacao and CBD is a match made in heaven—
excellent for unwinding, elevating the mood, and
getting good vibes going.

Essential Oils

DAYTIME QI REGULATION • EVENING UNWIND •
INSTANT CHILL

Diffusing essential oils promotes a calm, balanced
atmosphere around the house, workplace,
classroom, or wherever you happen to be—and
it's often the easiest way to integrate herbs from
this category into your daily routine. Direct palm
inhalations of essential oils can also be used
intermittently throughout the day as a quick-and-
easy way to calm the mind, improve your mood,
and rebalance the nervous system. See more on
essential oils on page 200.

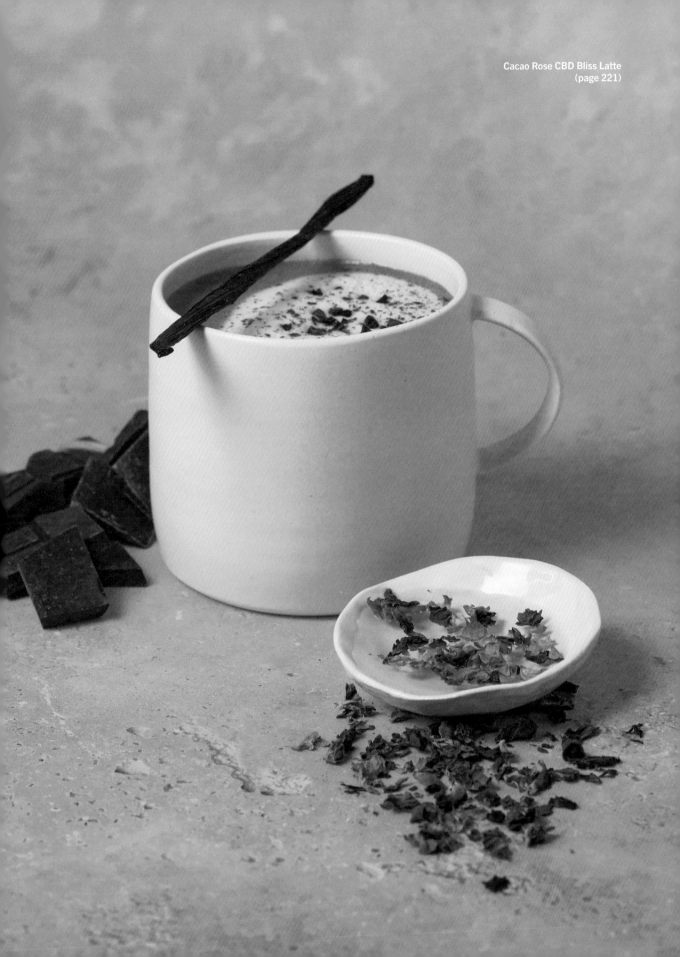

Cacao Rose CBD Bliss Latte
(page 221)

Rituals for Shifting Gears

Think of these rituals as aromatic baths of a sort, cleansing you of the concerns and unfinished business of the day, clearing the mind, and renewing your intentions.

Allow the experience and sensations of inhaling the fragrance to anchor your attention into the present moment, letting go of thoughts and resting in the body. Linking our intention to shift into a more relaxed and balanced state of mind with inhalation of fragrances reinforces the development of new neural networks, making their effects stronger and more immediate over time. Essential oils and/or aromatic resins and woods that work well for the first two rituals are frankincense, palo santo, sandalwood, copal, lavender, rose, or any centering and uplifting scent of your choice.

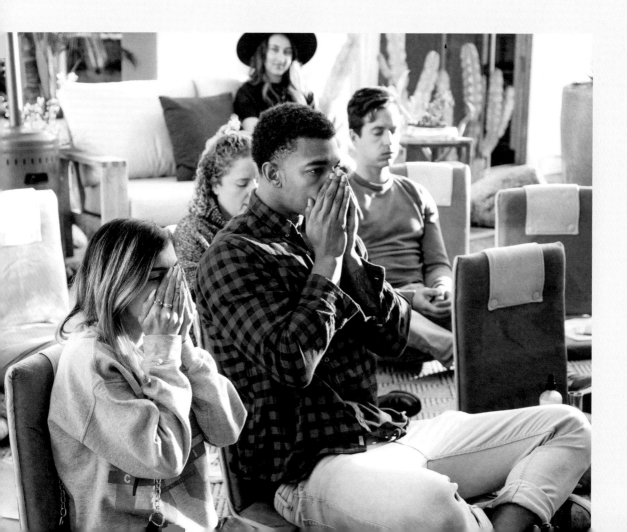

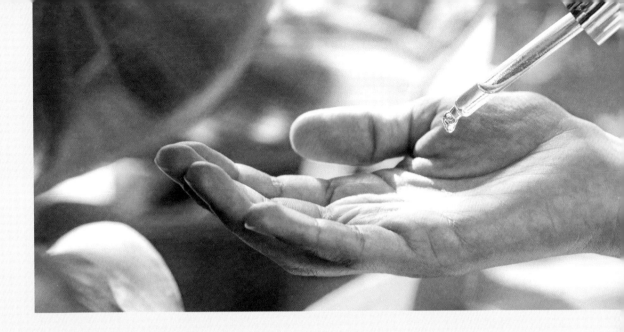

Palm Inhalations

Place a few drops of essential oil in the center of your palm and rub them between your hands. Cup your hands around your nose and mouth (avoiding the eyes) and take five slow, deep inhalations. Repeat for at least three or four cycles. Take care not to get the oil directly in your mouth or eyes. For more on direct palm inhalation, see page 202.

Burning Resins

Make sure you're doing this ritual outside or in a room with plenty of ventilation. Set up a ceramic bowl with Japanese charcoal bricks placed in fine volcanic ash on which to burn the resin or aromatic wood of your choice. Hold one charcoal brick to a flame using small wooden or metal tongs until it sustains an orange glow along one side. When it is sufficiently ignited, nest it into the ash so that it has a stable base. Then use the tongs to place a small piece of resin or wood onto the burning part of the charcoal. It should begin to smoke immediately. You can add more resin or wood as the smoke dies down. Spend ten minutes allowing the smoke to swirl around you while you gently breathe in the aromatic vapors from the air.

Note: Don't breathe in the smoke directly; the aromatic compounds will diffuse through the air sufficiently that you can experience their effects without getting smoked out.

Abhyanga Massage

Our skin contains many sensitive nerve endings, making it an excellent place to directly access and calm the nervous system. Ayurveda considers the unctuous, moistening, and heavy qualities of oil combined with aromatic calming herbs and massage to be the perfect antidote to a hyperactive nervous system. The powerful practice of self-massage, called *abhyanga*, delivers the calming, antispasmodic, muscle-relaxing effects of nervines directly into the body. Abhyanga is best done with warm oil in the morning after bathing or in the evening before bed. You can easily find oils for abhyanga online or in health food shops, or make your own by adding some of your favorite soothing essential oils (floral oils like lavender, ylang-ylang, rose, and jasmine are good options) to a carrier oil like sesame, coconut, or jojoba. (Carrier oils dilute the potency of essential oils, which can be strong and irritating to the skin if applied directly.)

Pulse Dosing for Sleep

Persistent sleep challenges are one of the most prevalent health issues I see in my practice and one of the first things I aim to correct because it's simply impossible to be healthy without getting good sleep.

Over the years, I developed a method called pulse dosing to progressively ease body tension and wind down mental activity from the stimulation of the day. The method uses nervines taken in small amounts at regular intervals throughout the evening to gradually relax the nervous system and shift the body's internal chemistry. It's a natural complement to any wind-down routine and a subtle retraining process that teaches the nervous system how to relax. It is far more effective than trying to knock ourselves out with a single dose of a sleep supplement at bedtime.

Picture a completely still pond where the water is flat. If you drop a pebble into the pond, a ripple will form and shift the state of the water momentarily, but the water will quickly return to its previous state. If you drop pebbles in continuously at regular intervals, eventually the ripples will remain and the state of the water will have a new vibration. Pulse dosing has this same effect on our bodies. To shift the state of our nervous system, we have to apply the nervines like pebbles in the pond, gradually altering our internal chemistry and nerve flow until a relaxed and easeful state is established. Herbs often have a reputation for being too subtle to affect seriously entrenched or challenging sleep or nervous system issues. Pulse dosing is a method that allows you to access the true effectiveness of these plants to create deep relaxation and sleep.

This method specifically employs tinctures for their rapid absorption and immediate effects. Some of the recommended plants to use in this way include skullcap, California poppy, passionflower, valerian root, or hops, alone or in combination. While it is possible to overdo anything (and nervines are no exception), in my experience it's more common to underdo it and not get the proper results. The nervines suggested (above) have a high degree of safety, and waking up slightly groggy is usually the only side effect of taking too much. The most important thing is to find the herb that works best for you and feels right for your system. Refer to the plant profiles (page 300) for guidance on the specific actions of the individual nervine calmatives.

Pulse dosing with nervines works best for short-term stints to shift the body back to a normal sleep pattern. Eventually the body can achieve this state even without the use of the tinctures. The more mindful or present you are to the subtle shifts in the way you feel with each subsequent dose, the more you'll establish a new reference point for what normal and progressive evening relaxation feels like. The difference when using nervines, as opposed to alcohol or sedative pharmaceuticals, is that you feel relaxed without numbing yourself into a loss of connection to mind and body. *Note:* Generally, combining nervine tinctures or nervines with sedative pharmaceuticals or alcohol amplifies their effects, is contraindicated, and is something I don't recommend. Stick to the basic parameters presented below, and you're unlikely to overdo it.

1) Two to three hours before your anticipated bedtime, as you begin to wind down, take a dropperful or two of tincture (approximately ½ teaspoon), either alone or with a small amount of water. Pay attention to the subtle shifts in the way this makes you feel.

2) Twenty to thirty minutes later, take another dose of the same amount and repeat this dosing method at the same time intervals until bedtime.

3) If your day has been particularly stressful and you feel amped up, experiment with a slightly higher dosing regimen. For example, take a double dose before turning out the light and hitting the pillow.

As you practice this method, calibrate the amounts of tincture you take to the level of calming and relaxation you need. Over time, you'll get a feel for what doses of calming nervine tinctures are right for you.

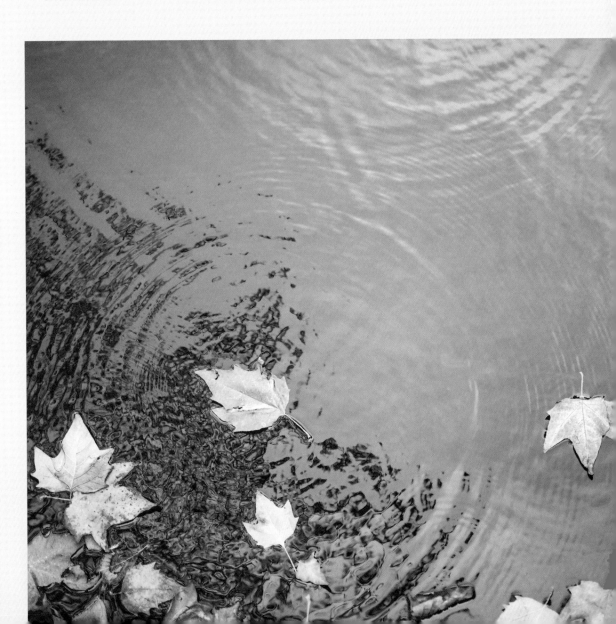

Each recipe makes one serving unless stated otherwise.

Greek Mountain Tea

Briefly simmering mountain tea is the best way to extract maximum flavor and benefits. Note that mountain tea is most often found in whole uncut form (as stems, leaves, and flowers). Start off by putting **a small handful of Greek mountain tea** (maybe 4 or 5 stems to start) in **1½ cups (360 ml) water**. Lightly simmer in a covered pan for 3 to 5 minutes. Turn off the heat and let steep for 2 to 3 minutes. Strain into a mug, then add **honey or a natural sweetener of your choice** and **a squeeze of lemon** like the Greeks do—this really takes the beverage up a notch.

Notes: To make a stronger tea, add more plant material and/or let steep for an additional 5 minutes. You can experiment with adding other herbs like a sprig of rosemary, a cinnamon stick, or any other culinary spice you like when simmering. You can also chill the strained tea in the fridge for a few hours and serve over ice.

Honeybush Latte

Heat **1 cup (240 ml) water** and pour it over **2 honeybush tea bags or 2 teaspoons loose honeybush** in a mug. Steep, covered, for 5 to 7 minutes, then remove the tea bags or strain the herbs into another cup. Add **½ teaspoon vanilla extract** and **1 teaspoon honey or a natural sweetener of your choice**. In a separate bowl, froth **½ cup (120 ml) oat milk**. Slowly add the frothed milk to the tea and sprinkle **a pinch of cinnamon powder** on top before serving.

Note: For an iced latte, use half to two-thirds the amount of liquid. Chill the mixture, pour over ice cubes, top with the milk frothed on the cold setting, and garnish with the cinnamon.

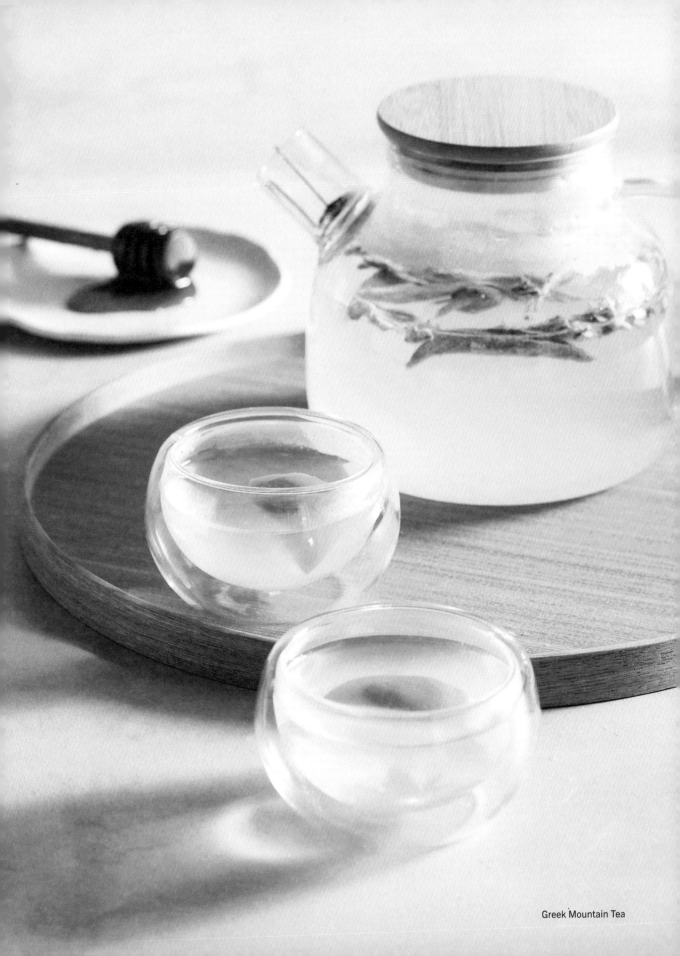

Greek Mountain Tea

Matcha Latte

Heat water in a kettle to just under the boiling point. Carefully spoon out (or use a chashaku to ladle) **1 to 2 teaspoons matcha powder** into a traditional matcha bowl (or another bowl or mug). Slowly pour approximately ¾ cup **(180 ml) water** from the kettle into the bowl and whisk with a traditional bamboo matcha whisk (or an electric version) until frothy bubbles show up. Use quick, light, back-and-forth movements (not circular), with the whisk just barely touching the bottom of the bowl. In a separate bowl, froth **¼ cup (60 ml) oat milk or plant-based milk of your choice**. Pour the matcha mixture into a mug and top with the frothed milk. If you like, add **a natural sweetener of your choice to taste**.

Note: For an iced latte, use half to two-thirds the amount of water. Chill the mixture, pour over ice cubes, and top with the milk frothed on the cold setting.

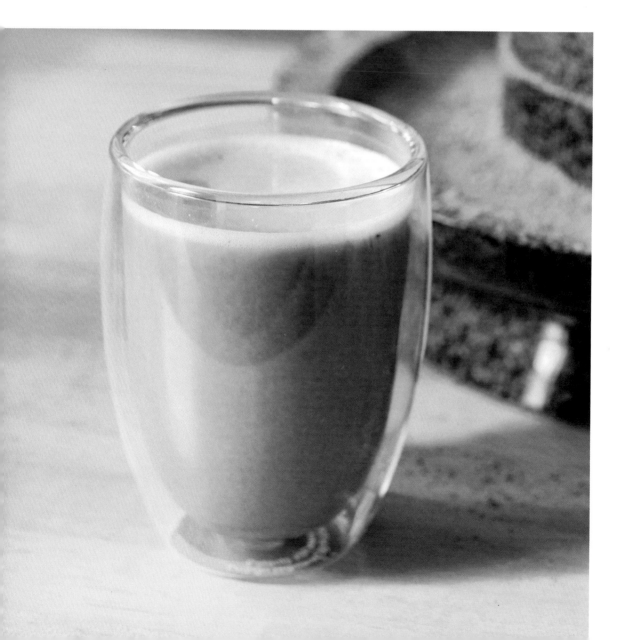

Lavender Flower Latte

Combine **1 tablespoon dried lavender flowers** and **½ teaspoon butterfly pea flowers** in a small bowl and spoon into a self-fill tea bag or a removable infuser basket in a mug. Fill the mug with **1 cup (240 ml) hot water**, cover, and steep the tea for 5 minutes. In a separate bowl, froth **½ cup (120 ml) plant-based milk of your choice**. Remove the tea bag or infuser. Add **1 teaspoon honey or a natural sweetener of your choice** and top with the frothed milk.

Note: For an iced latte, use half to two-thirds the amount of liquid. Chill the mixture, pour over ice cubes, and top with the milk frothed on the cold setting.

Chamomile Latte

Heat **1 cup (240 ml) water** and pour it over **4 chamomile tea bags or 2 tablespoons loose chamomile flowers** in a mug. Steep, covered, for 10 minutes, then remove the tea bags or strain the herbs into another cup and stir in **1 tablespoon honey or a natural sweetener of your choice** until dissolved. Add **⅛ teaspoon vanilla extract**. In a separate bowl, froth **½ cup (120 ml) oat milk or plant-based milk of your choice**. Slowly add the frothed milk to the tea and sprinkle **a pinch of cinnamon powder** on top before serving.

Note: For an iced latte, use half to two-thirds the amount of liquid. Chill the mixture, pour over ice cubes, top with the milk frothed on the cold setting, and garnish with the cinnamon.

Cacao Rose CBD Bliss Latte

Place **1 cup (240 ml) water** and **½ to 1 ounce (15 to 30 g) unsweetened or semisweet cacao chunks** in a saucepan. Gently warm over low heat, stirring occasionally, until the cacao starts to melt, 2 to 3 minutes. Turn off the heat and let cool for a few minutes. Add **1 teaspoon vanilla extract, 1 teaspoon cinnamon powder, 1 teaspoon food-grade rose hydrosol, 10 to 20 mg CBD oil**, and **1 tablespoon natural sweetener of your choice** or to taste. Mix thoroughly with an immersion blender or whisk until frothy bubbles appear. In a separate bowl, froth **⅓ cup (80 ml) oat milk**. Pour the cacao mixture into a glass or mug and top with the frothed oat milk. Sprinkle **finely chopped dried rose petals** on top before serving.

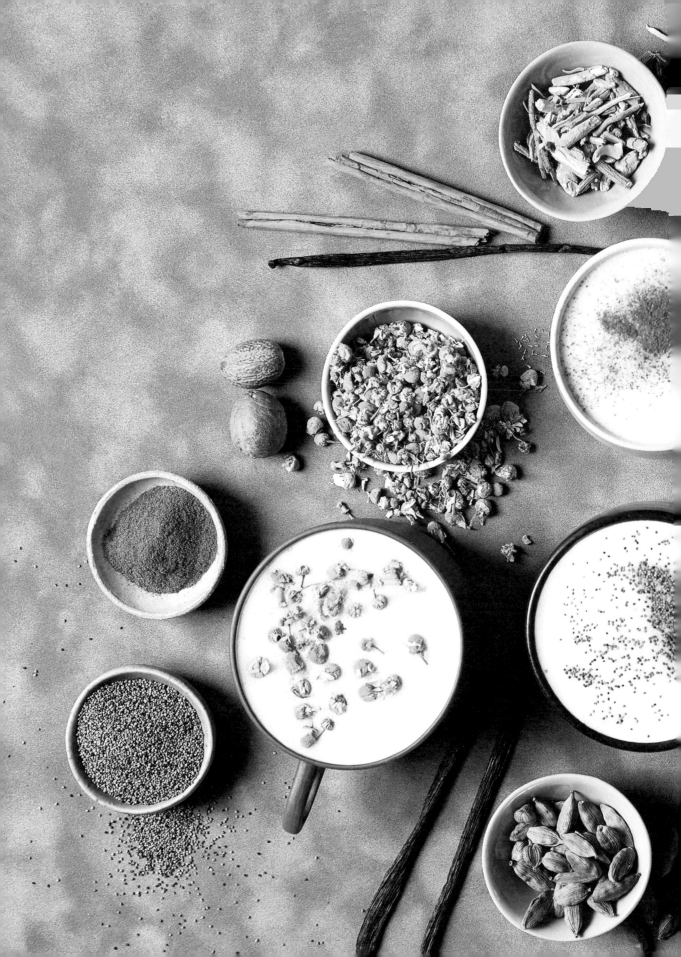

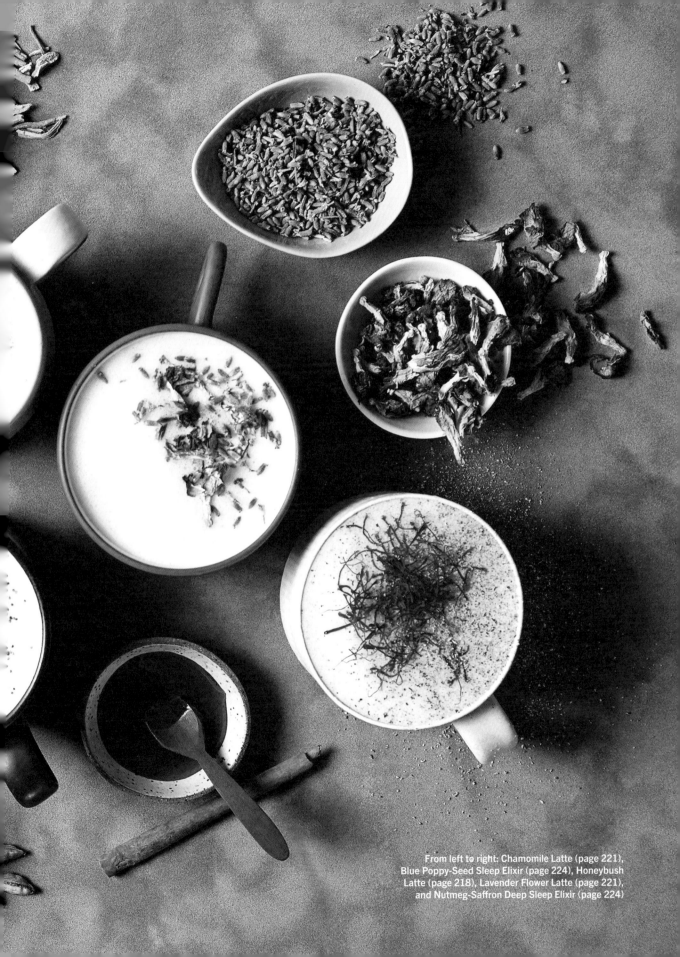

From left to right: Chamomile Latte (page 221),
Blue Poppy-Seed Sleep Elixir (page 224), Honeybush
Latte (page 218), Lavender Flower Latte (page 221),
and Nutmeg-Saffron Deep Sleep Elixir (page 224)

Kava Koolada

Using a blender, thoroughly combine **1 cup (240 ml) pineapple juice, ½ cup (120 ml) plant-based milk, ¼ cup (60 ml) coconut cream, 1 to 3 teaspoons kava powder** (see Note), **1 teaspoon maple syrup or a natural sweetener of your choice** (if desired), and **2 or 3 ice cubes.** Add more ice cubes before serving, if you'd like.

Note: The dosage of kava depends on the effects you're after and the type of kava you're using—some kava varieties are inherently stronger than others (for more on this, see page 230). Adjust the recipe based on the strength of the effect you are looking for.

Blue Poppy-Seed Sleep Elixir

Soak **1 tablespoon culinary poppy seeds** in warm water for 15 minutes to soften. Strain. Add the seeds to **¾ to 1 cup (180 to 240 ml) oat milk** in a saucepan and simmer over low heat for 5 minutes. Turn off the heat and add **⅛ teaspoon vanilla extract or a pinch of vanilla powder, a pinch of cardamom powder,** and **1 teaspoon honey or a natural sweetener of your choice,** if you'd like. Pour into a cup, including the seeds, and drink a half hour before bedtime.

Notes: This recipe uses the culinary poppy seeds you get at grocery stores, *not* the unwashed variety from the internet that contains opiates. If you don't like the sensation of drinking the seeds, you can give the elixir a quick whiz in a blender to break up the seeds before pouring the beverage into a cup.

Nutmeg-Saffron Deep Sleep Elixir

Grate a whole nutmeg with a small hand grater to get **¼ to ½ teaspoon nutmeg powder.** Warm **¾ to 1 cup (180 to 240 ml) oat milk** in a saucepan or use a milk frother to heat. Pour the heated milk into a cup and add the nutmeg, **⅛ teaspoon vanilla extract or a pinch of vanilla powder,** and **1 teaspoon honey or a natural sweetener of your choice,** if desired. Blend thoroughly. Sprinkle **2 or 3 saffron stamens** on top.

Note: This recipe calls for using a whole nutmeg because the powder is most potent when freshly grated.

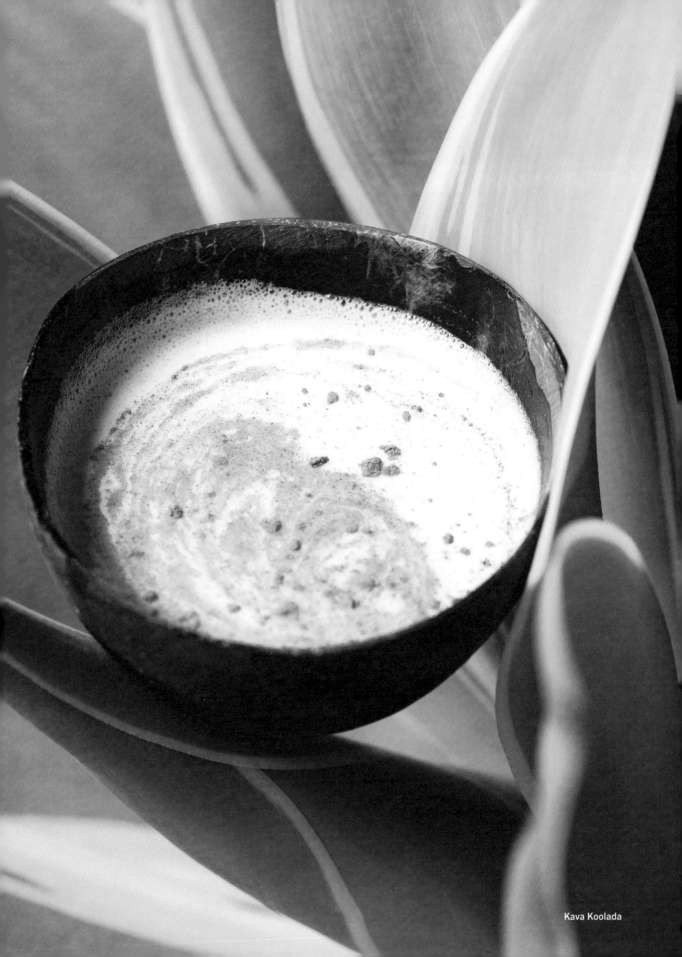

Kava Koolada

Kava: Get Happy

For centuries, people throughout the South Pacific have consumed a magical brew made from the dried roots of kava to promote feelings of peace and tranquility. A tall jungle shrub related to black pepper, kava (*Piper methysticum*) has great cultural and spiritual significance throughout this region, where drinking kava is an integral part of everyday life. It's consumed in both formal and informal settings: to welcome foreign dignitaries, to help facilitate delicate negotiations and settle disputes among villages, or simply to relax at the end of a workday and have fun with friends.

The active constituents in kava, kavalactones, are responsible for its relaxing effects and the distinctive numbing or tingling sensation felt in the mouth when drinking it (this sensation is temporary and recedes after a few minutes). Kava simultaneously relaxes the body while leaving the mind feeling clear, increasing one's calmness and contentment without dullness or lethargy. It can be mildly relaxing to downright euphoric depending on how much is consumed and can be used to promote deep and restful sleep. In recent decades, kava has found its way to the West and gained some well-deserved attention for its anxiety-reducing, mood-elevating, and sleep-enhancing effects.

In places where kava is regularly consumed, it plays a role somewhat similar to alcohol in our modern culture. But in contrast to alcohol, kava doesn't cause intoxication or the loss of control over the mind and emotions—there are no barroom brawls during a kava ceremony. In fact, kava is often referred to as the "drink of peace" because it facilitates communication and goodwill. Lastly, kava is far easier than alcohol for the body to metabolize, so it can be consumed in moderate amounts without concern for toxicity or even a hangover.

A few years ago, my wife and I went on a surfing honeymoon adventure in Fiji with a side mission of diving deep into kava culture. Officially designated as the national drink of Fiji, kava is a source of pride and identity for the country and one of the reasons for Fiji's reputation as the happiest place on earth. Visitors are offered kava the moment they land, both in the spirit of welcome and to help them downshift to the relaxed pace locals call "Fiji time" (and no doubt because it's amusing to see how foreigners react to their first drink). Kava is the perfect elixir to sync up with the easygoing vibes of the warm Fijian people, the swaying palms, aqua-blue water, green mountains flowing into the sea, and the sounds of gently lapping waves on white sandy beaches.

In Fiji, kava is called *yaqona* or, more often, *grog* by the locals, and when participating in a kava ceremony, the legendary friendliness and enthusiasm for life of the Fijian people is on full display. On this plantventure, we were lucky enough to experience several ceremonies in settings throughout the islands. One particularly

A mature kava plant in Fiji

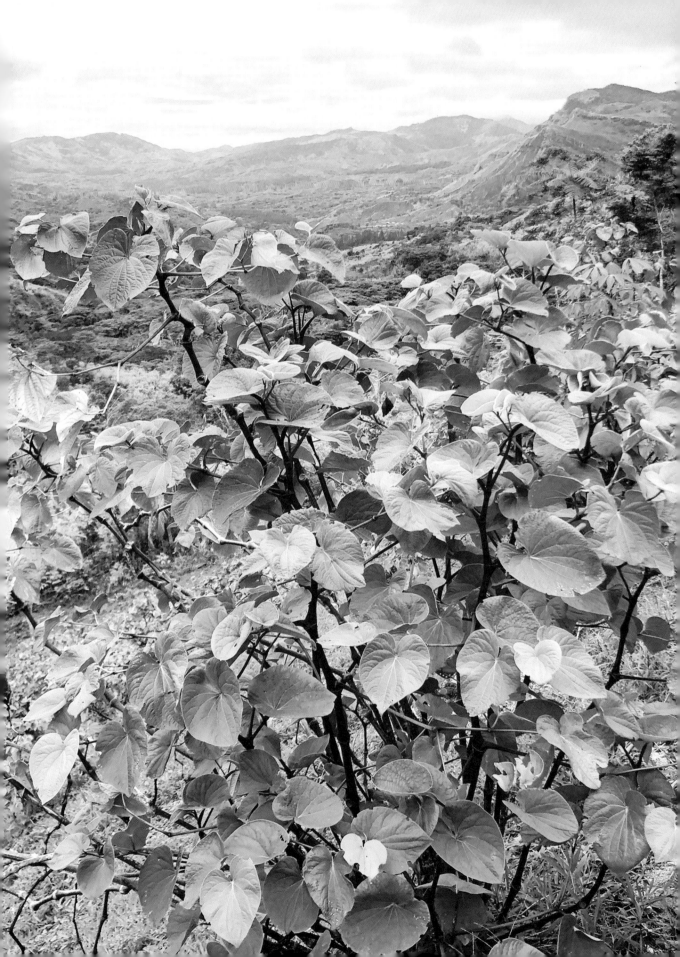

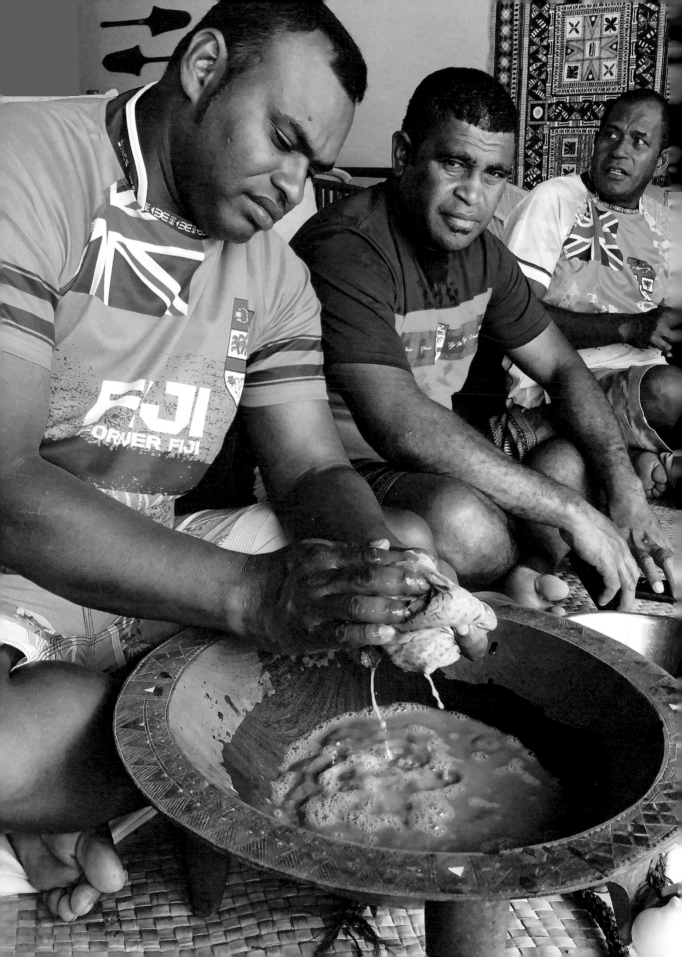

memorable ceremony happened while we were visiting farmers in a village deep in the mountains to secure a source of kava for Goldthread.

After offering a bundle of kava roots to the village chief, a customary gift and gesture of respect in Fiji, we were invited to drink kava with him and his family. No matter the setting, drinking kava involves a certain protocol and etiquette. About twenty of us were seated on woven mats on the floor of the chief's hut. The kava ceremony commenced with the chief sharing stories about the joys of drinking kava, how it enhances one's health, and its importance to Fijian culture. Several teenage boys took turns dunking powdered kava roots wrapped in T-shirts in water and then straining the fragrant, muddy-colored liquid into a tanoa (a traditional wooden bowl). The kava was plunged, kneaded, and squeezed for ten to fifteen minutes to ensure extraction of the active constituents. In Fiji, kava is traditionally consumed from halved coconut shells, and guests are always served first as a sign of respect and hospitality. As is the custom, we clapped once before downing the entire cup in one continuous gulp and then three more times afterward while exclaiming *"Bula!"* (the Fijian word for "cheers!" and "love of life"). This ritual, repeated by each participant, served to accentuate the increasingly jovial atmosphere. As the coconut cups were passed and the kava continued to flow, the physical-relaxation and mood-elevating effects started to take hold, and a palpable sense of effervescent cheer filled the hut. Laughter and easy-flowing talk were punctuated by the occasional story, joke, or song as a natural feeling of ease and connectedness took hold among us. The evening ended with smiles and hugs as we stepped into the cool night air, under a sky filled with stars. My mind felt calm and refreshed, and my body was relaxed and grounded, as I reflected on the experience.

Feelings of social isolation are increasingly understood to be a real and pervasive form of chronic stress, on par with smoking tobacco in terms of their negative impact on health. In a communal culture like Fiji's, drinking kava with others is a natural way to bring people together. Its effects help decrease feelings of social anxiety and increase communication and self-expression.

Opposite and below: Fijians preparing for a traditional kava ceremony

---

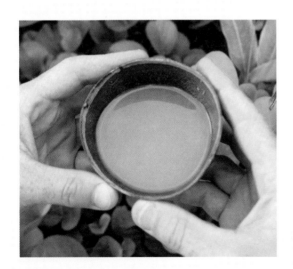

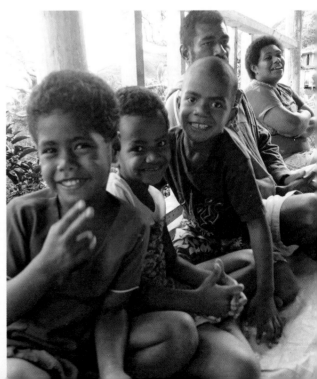

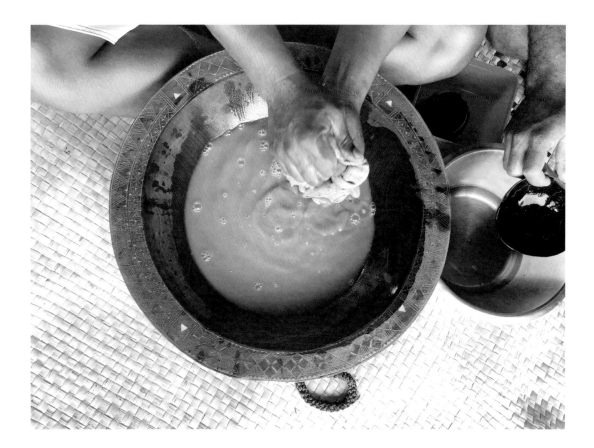

Traditional Kava Preparation Method

There are many options when it comes to using kava. Throughout the South Pacific, hundreds of different cultivars of kava have been developed, each with its own active constituents and slightly different effects. Those with mood-elevating, somewhat energizing, and euphoric effects are considered better for drinking during the daytime. Others are heavier and best served in the evening to relax the nerves and enhance restorative sleep. Still others are somewhere in between.

When it comes to buying kava, quality matters. Look for sellers who offer what is called "noble" varieties of kava (versus "tudei" varieties). Noble is easier to metabolize and best for regular consumption, while tudei-grade kava is more medicinal in its action and constituent profile and historically was not cultivated for everyday drinking purposes. See the Resources section (page 352) for recommended suppliers; their websites offer good information on which strains of kava to purchase for the specific effects you're going for, from sleep or relaxation to mental clarity.

Note: Kava has a unique, earthy flavor and is somewhat of an acquired taste. Feel free to add a little fruit juice or cool it down in the fridge to make it more enjoyable. Or see the Kava Koolada recipe (page 224) for a slightly less traditional but definitely more delicious version.

The following is the traditional kava preparation method, a process that has remained alive and well in the South Pacific for some three thousand years.

Because it typically takes fifteen to thirty minutes to feel the full effects of kava, pace yourself before drinking another cup to get a sense of how it is affecting you. You'll tend to feel groggy if you overdo it, so let your body tell you when you've had too much. Over time, you'll be able to gauge the right amount for you.

1) Measure out the powdered kava root. Serving sizes vary somewhat depending on a variety of factors (such as one's individual constitution and the specific type of kava used), but 2 to 3 tablespoons powder per 1¼ to 1½ cups (300 to 360 ml) water is a good baseline for an individual serving size. (It's typical for several cups to be consumed during a single session, so make enough for multiple servings for each person joining you.)

2) Add the kava powder to a muslin strainer bag and knot the top. Place the bag in a medium to large bowl and pour in room-temperature water; let sit for 5 minutes.

3) Now the fun part: With clean hands, begin mixing, churning, kneading, and squeezing all the liquid from the kava bag before dunking it in again. Dunk and knead and swish and swirl and dunk and knead again. You'll notice the water start to turn a muddy color, and fragrance will begin wafting from the bowl. Do this for about 10 minutes to extract all the kavalactones and make a potent brew.

4) Remove the strainer bag and give it one final squeeze to coax all remaining liquid out.

5) The kava is now ready to drink! Use a small cup or ladle to scoop the kava from the bowl and into individual 8-ounce (240 ml) cups, remembering to always serve guests first.

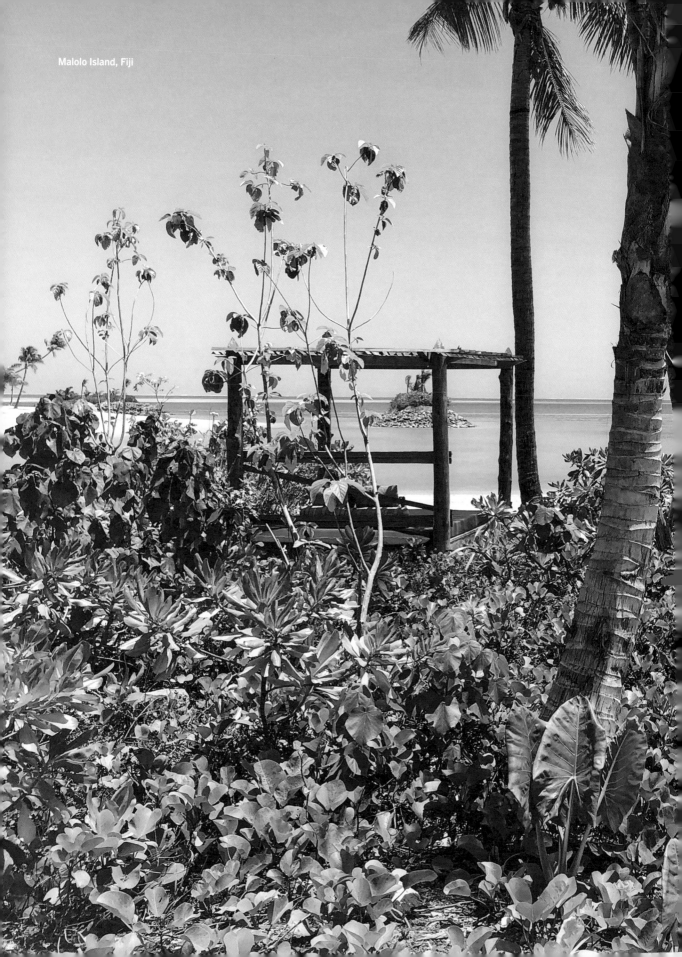

Malolo Island, Fiji

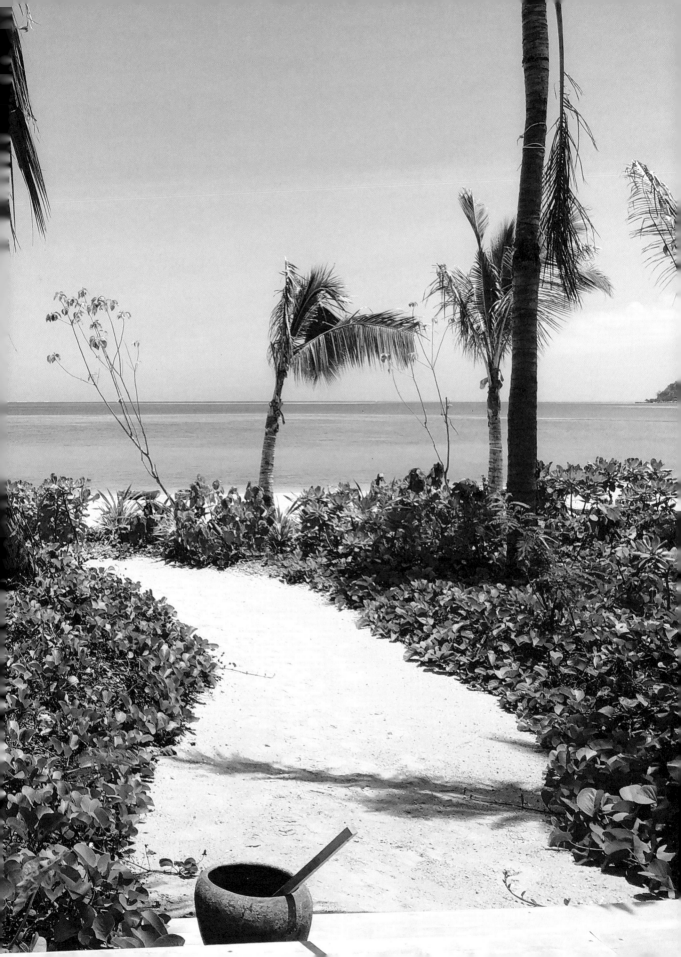

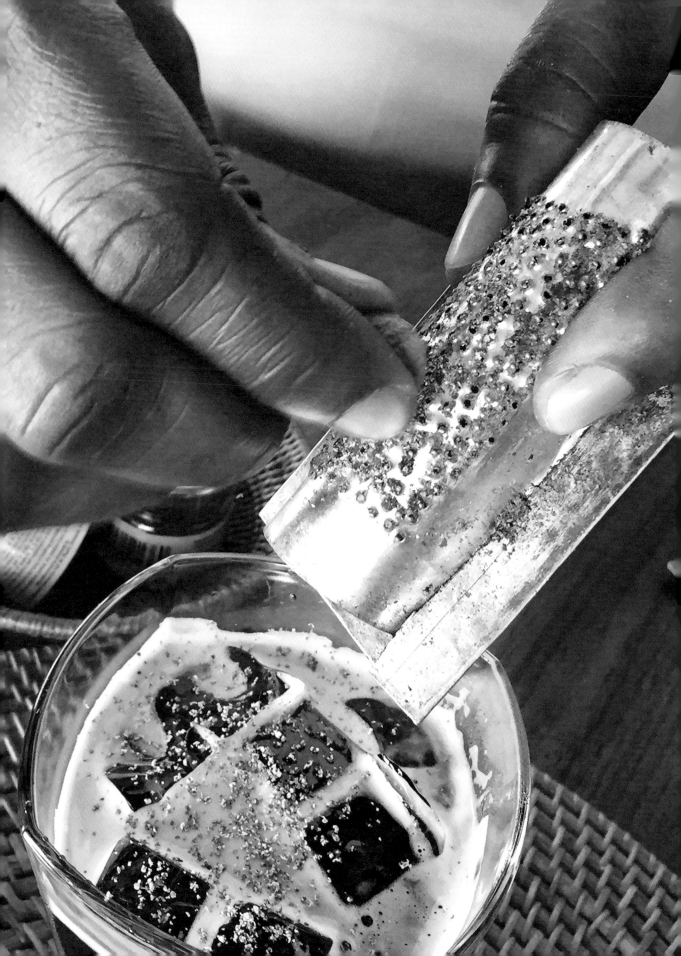

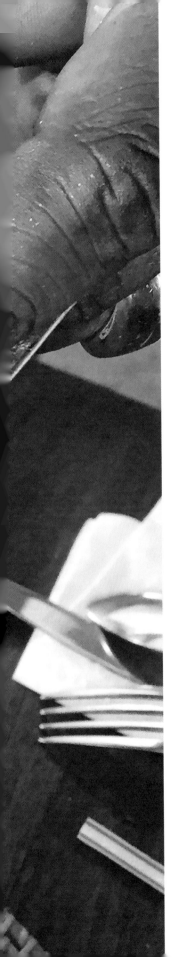

Adaptogens

THE FOCUS OF THIS STEP IS BUILDING ENERGY, ENDURANCE, and deep immunity with adaptogenic tonics and medicinal mushrooms. Adaptogens help to restore hormonal balance, reduce the toll of physical and mental stress, and increase the inner resources needed to navigate the constant change and challenges of daily life. Incorporating a variety of these plants into our daily routine fuels our ability to achieve greatness and sets a solid foundation for longevity.

WHAT TO EXPECT

- Less-frequent bouts of illness

- Faster recovery from physical exertion

- More energy and endurance, both mental and physical

- Deeper and more restorative sleep

- Enhanced libido

- Less jet lag when traveling

- More resilience and better function during demanding transitions like starting a new job, having a child, moving houses, or writing a book

- Greater emotional stability and a higher quality of attention

Plants & Other Ingredients You'll Be Using

The benefits from adaptogens occur gradually and build until a critical mass is reached and you begin experiencing noticeably higher levels of functioning. A number of adaptogens *do* have perceptible, fast-acting effects, however, depending on preparation and dosage. Tulsi leaf, for example, can immediately affect our state of alertness, attention, and overall cognitive function. Ginseng root, rhodiola, and cordyceps taken in sufficient quantities will produce noticeable improvements in energy and physical performance. In this step, you'll be using adaptogens in both ways: taking certain ones at effective doses to boost energy and endurance in the short-term, and consuming others in smaller daily increments as part of a long-term strategy to build physical and mental resilience.

Some adaptogens have overlapping benefits and indications with other nutritive categories. Goji berries, schisandra, amla berries, and maca root, for example, could easily find themselves in the nutritive category. This protocol includes medicinal mushrooms among the adaptogens. Some, such as shiitake, maitake, and turkey tail, are not technically classified as adaptogens but function similarly to a traditional adaptogen, thanks to their powerful, long-term immune-enhancing effects. Cordyceps and reishi, however, are true adaptogens.

All adaptogens offer benefits such as increasing resistance to physical and mental stress and enhancing energy, endurance, fertility, libido, cognitive, and immune functions. They each also have their own specific strengths and ideal applications. For in-depth information on individual adaptogens, see the plant profiles beginning on page 300. They can be used alone or combined into synergistic blends for a broader range of effects.

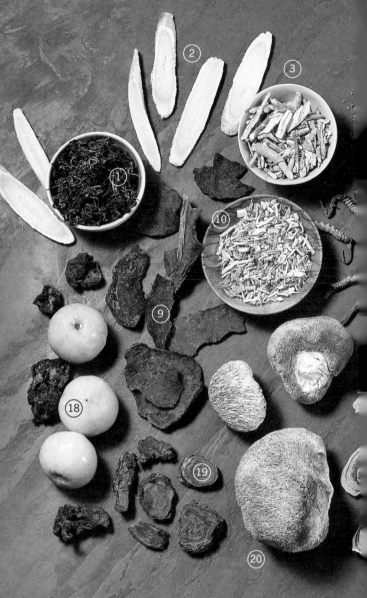

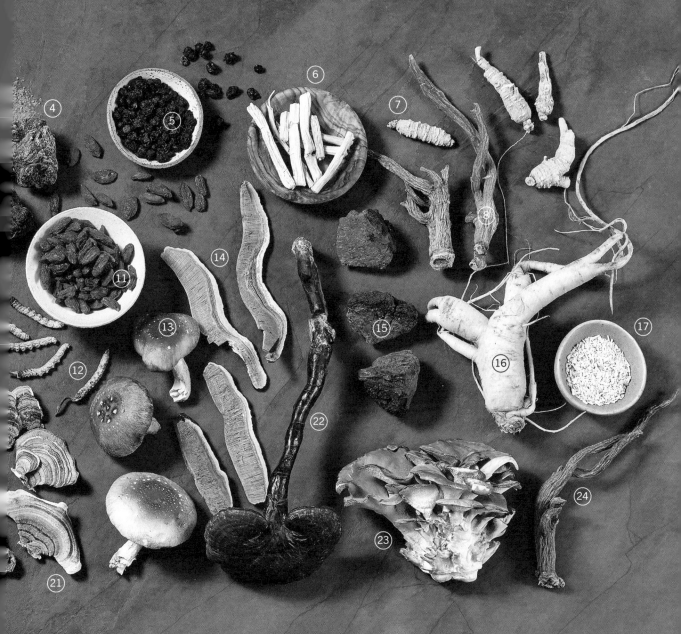

1 Gymnostema

2 Astragalus root

3 Ashwagandha root

4 Maca root

5 Schisandra berries

6 Shatavari root

7 + 16 + 17 American
   ginseng root

8 + 24 Korean red
   ginseng root

9 He shou wu

10 Eleuthero

11 Goji berries

12 Cordyceps

13 Shiitake

14 + 22 Reishi

15 Chaga

18 Amla berries

19 Rhodiola root

20 Lion's mane

21 Turkey tail

23 Maitake

Getting Started

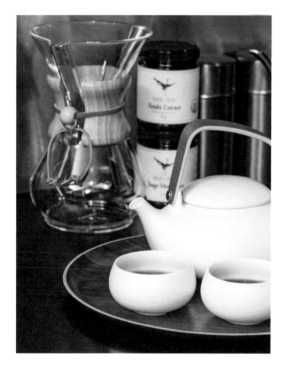

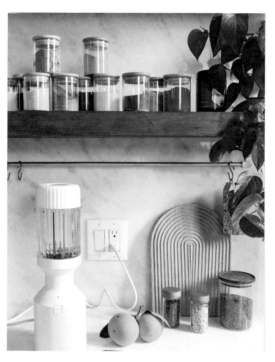

Supercharger Station

Collect adaptogenic powders and powdered extracts—including medicinal mushrooms (cordyceps, reishi, chaga, and maitake) and shatavari—to put into your morning coffee, tea, cacao, or chai, and keep them near the coffeemaker or kettle.

Smoothie Setup

Adaptogens are vital ingredients for the serious smoothie maker. Powders and extracts such as maca, ashwagandha, schisandra, shatavari, goji, and he shou wu should be kept in airtight jars or bags, in a cool, dry spot easily accessible to where you make smoothies and elixirs.

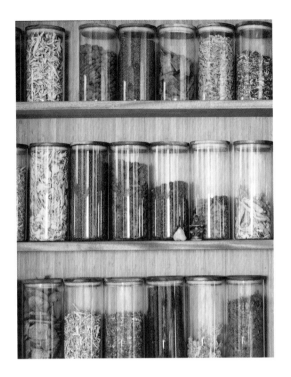

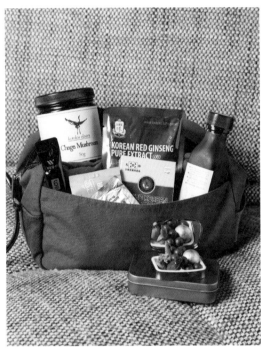

Adaptogenic Kitchen

Adaptogens are often included in meals. Keep a supply—including goji and schisandra berries, ginseng and astragalus roots, and some whole medicinal mushrooms like shiitake, chaga, and maitake—for adding to your food and for making decoctions. The kitchen is also a good place for a jar of chyawanprash (see page 246) and any adaptogen supplements you're using.

On the Go

Most of us are constantly moving from one activity to another, so having a portable source of adaptogens helps with maintaining consistent usage; supplements work well for this purpose. Tablets, capsules, and tinctures are widely available and effective options to have on hand when traveling or busy. Medicinal mushroom powdered extracts come ready to use in single-serve packets, or you can easily construct your own blends from bulk sources. Pack ginseng liquid pouches in your workout bag for an energizing pre- or post-workout tonic. Decoctions and infusions are on-the-go options as well.

How to Saturate Your Day

You'll find many opportunities and occasions to integrate adaptogens into your routine. Adaptogens can be combined with food in recipes, eaten between meals, or added to all types of flavorful elixirs, tonics, and infusions to drink from morning to night.

Morning Liftoff

A morning energy drink is a perfect place to incorporate adaptogens. They set the tone for balanced energy throughout the day. Many of the options listed on the following pages can be used at this time, so feel free to experiment and choose your favorites.

Mind-Body Workouts

Activities that involve physical exertion are a natural time to include adaptogens. These plant materials enhance performance when consumed before physical activity and are helpful in replenishing the system afterward. Adaptogens are equally valuable to support *mental* exertion.

Evening Replenisher

The grounding and nourishing actions of adaptogens make them supportive to winding down in the evening. Adaptogens help shift our endocrine system into a state of rest, rejuvenation, and deep replenishment, allowing us to sleep more soundly. Nighttime is a good opportunity to turn to standouts such as reishi, ashwagandha root, and shatavari root.

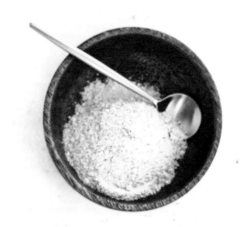

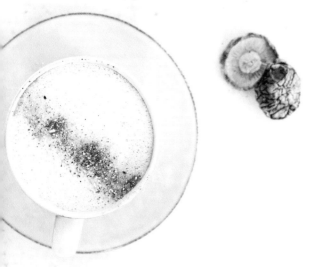

Adaptogenic mushroom latte

SAMPLE DAILY MENUS

MINIMUM DAILY DOSE

Integrate two servings of adaptogens per day. The easiest
option is usually to add one serving to your morning drink.
For your second, choose from the options in this step based
on your lifestyle. If you find yourself frequently hitting
only the minimum amount, make sure to be consistent—
adaptogens often need to build up in the system to gain
momentum, and that requires consistent use.

MENU 1

In the morning:
Reishi powdered extract added to
coffee or tea

In the afternoon:
Pouch of ginseng extract

Post-workout:
Peanut Butter–Maca–Goji Berry
Smoothie (page 250)

At dinner:
Adaptogen-infused Wei Qi Soup (page 255)
and a post-meal mug of tulsi tea
with lemon and honey

MENU 2

In the morning:
Chaga Chai Latte (page 249)

In the afternoon:
Cordyceps powdered
extract in water

Post-workout:
Schisandra Berry–Rose Energizing
Lemonade (page 253)

In the evening:
Ashwagandha Deep Rest Replenisher
(page 253)

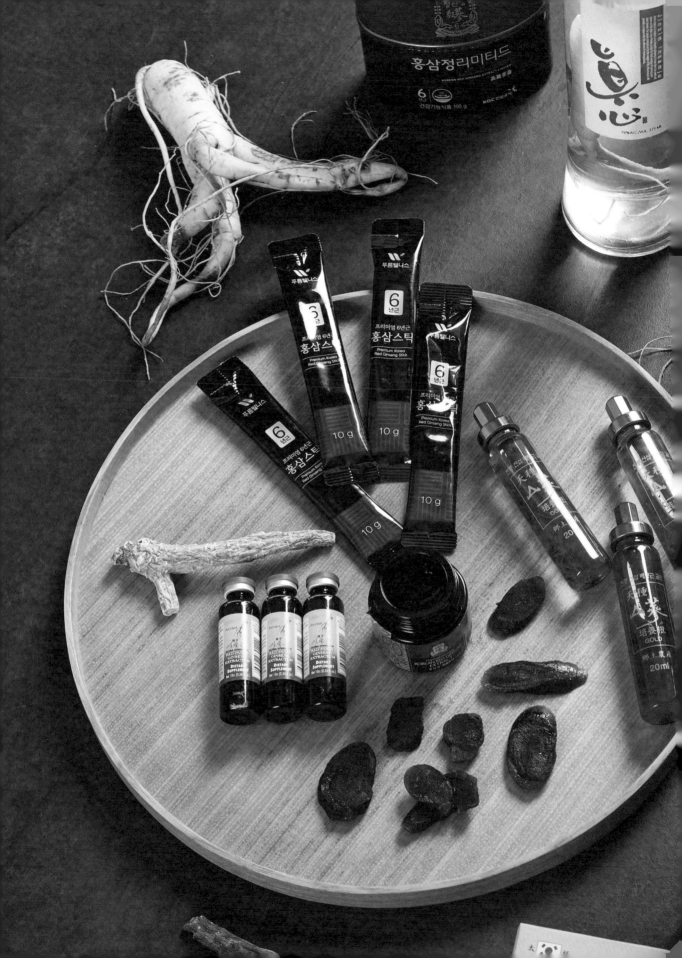

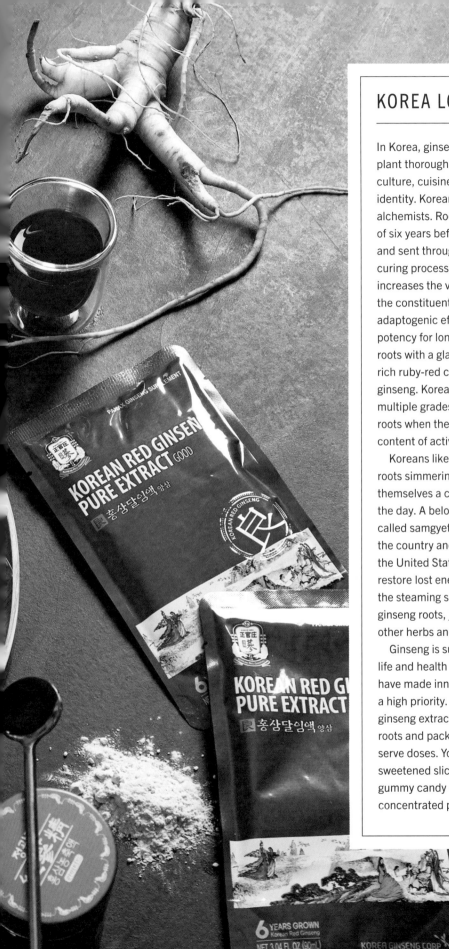

KOREA LOVES GINSENG

In Korea, ginseng is a treasured medicinal plant thoroughly woven into the nation's culture, cuisine, folklore, and national identity. Koreans are true ginseng alchemists. Roots are grown for a minimum of six years before being harvested, dried, and sent through a slow steaming and curing process that concentrates and increases the variety of ginsenosides, the constituents that give ginseng its adaptogenic effects, and preserves their potency for long periods. The result is roots with a glass-like consistency and a rich ruby-red color—hence the name red ginseng. Korean ginseng is available in multiple grades based upon the age of the roots when they were harvested and their content of active compounds.

Koreans like to keep a pot of ginseng roots simmering on the stove and pour themselves a cup several times throughout the day. A beloved, nourishing chicken soup called samgyetang is served throughout the country and in Korean communities in the United States. Traditionally eaten to restore lost energy and boost immunity, the steaming soup contains fresh and dried ginseng roots, jujube dates, and a variety of other herbs and spices.

Ginseng is such an integral part of daily life and health optimization that Koreans have made innovating portable preparations a high priority. Look for the popular liquid ginseng extracts made from pre-decocted roots and packaged in pouches for single-serve doses. You can also find honey-sweetened sliced roots with the texture of gummy candy or choose from a variety of concentrated pastes, capsules, and tablets.

Morning Adaptogenic Coffee

MORNING LIFTOFF • MIND-BODY WORKOUTS

Several adaptogens, including reishi, chaga, cordyceps, and maitake, have the perfect flavor profile for blending into coffee.

Cacao-Reishi-Cordyceps Latte

MORNING LIFTOFF • MIND-BODY WORKOUTS

This delicious tonic (page 249) combines the mood-elevating, cardioprotective, energizing effects of cacao with the adaptogenic immune-enhancing powers of medicinal mushrooms in what is sure to become a healthy obsession. You can drink it hot, cold, or blended with ice.

Chaga Chai Latte

MORNING LIFTOFF • MIND-BODY WORKOUTS

This simple elixir (page 249) is an easy way to get some immune-enhancing chaga mushrooms in a warm, tasty beverage. The earthy, nutty flavor of chaga blends well with pungent chai spices.

Powerful Powders

MORNING LIFTOFF • MIND-BODY WORKOUTS

Many adaptogens (such as ashwagandha root, he shou wu, cordyceps, reishi, chaga, maitake, shatavari root, schisandra berry, astragalus root, maca root, and ginseng root) are available as powders and powdered extracts, making them easy to add to your daily routine. Dosages vary depending on the type of adaptogen you're using and the concentration of the extract (see page 259 for more). A simple guideline: Blend 1 teaspoon to 1 tablespoon powder, or ¼ to ½ teaspoon powdered extract, into 1 to 1½ cups (240 to 360 ml) liquid per serving. Drink twice a day.

Adaptogenic Decoctions

MORNING LIFTOFF • MIND-BODY WORKOUTS • EVENING REPLENISHER

Most adaptogens—like ginseng, ashwagandha, astragalus, and medicinal mushrooms—are tough and woody in their whole form and require simmering to extract the active constituents. A process known as decoction (see page 94) also works well to create flavorful medicinal broths made with ginseng, astragalus, and medicinal mushrooms (see the recipe for Wei Qi Soup on page 255).

Adaptogenic Infusions

MORNING LIFTOFF • MIND-BODY WORKOUTS •
EVENING REPLENISHER

You can achieve a strong extraction from whole dried herbs without simmering by using a long or overnight infusion. The cut size of the plant material (and time) determines the level of active constituents you will be able to extract. The finer the plant is cut, the more surface area is exposed to water, and the more efficient the extraction. For a long or overnight infusion, look for herbs that have already been cut and sifted, and simply pour hot water over them to steep (see more on page 94). Ginseng, ashwagandha, and astragalus root, and medicinal mushrooms will all work well prepared in this way. Tulsi and gymnostema are two of the rare adaptogens derived from leafy material, and they easily lend themselves to a simple infusion method or even a strong tea.

Ginseng-Ginger Lemon Tonic

MORNING LIFTOFF • MIND-BODY WORKOUTS

This fresh and flavorful tonic (page 250) offers an invigorating lift. It's great over ice or heated up on chilly days.

Ashwagandha and Shatavari Coconut Replenisher

MORNING LIFTOFF • MIND-BODY WORKOUTS •
EVENING REPLENISHER

Combining two of Ayurveda's most powerful rejuvenating tonics, this delicious drink (page 250) contains an assortment of aromatic spices and essential fats. It's a deeply nourishing and replenishing elixir you can drink anytime.

Peanut Butter–Maca–Goji Berry Smoothie

MORNING LIFTOFF • MIND-BODY WORKOUTS

Maca is prized for its nutritional value, fiber content, and energy-boosting effects. The nourishing smoothie on page 250, with goji and cacao, makes the perfect post-workout replenisher or long-workday revitalizer.

Strawberry Shatavari Smoothie

MORNING LIFTOFF • MIND-BODY WORKOUTS •
EVENING REPLENISHER

Shatavari has been used in Ayurveda for centuries as a women's revitalizing tonic, yet everyone can benefit from this rejuvenating herb. It is a rich source of phytonutrients and unique compounds that increase energy and stamina. There are many ways to incorporate this wonderful herb into our routines; see page 251 for a nourishing, delicious smoothie.

Schisandra Berry–Rose Energizing Lemonade

MORNING LIFTOFF • MIND-BODY WORKOUTS

Schisandra berries are an adaptogen from Asia with a tart, delicious flavor reminiscent of cranberries that makes for a refreshing and restorative beverage. Providing ample electrolytes to replace ones lost during exercise, this schisandra-ade (page 253) is both energizing and rehydrating.

Tulsi Tea

MORNING LIFTOFF • MIND-BODY WORKOUTS •
EVENING REPLENISHER

This miraculous herb is known in India as the "incomparable one" for its strengthening effects. The active constituents in tulsi are found in its leaves and are easy to extract with a simple infusion or strong tea.

Ashwagandha Deep Rest Replenisher

EVENING REPLENISHER

There's nothing better than ashwagandha to nourish and stabilize a short-circuiting nervous system. The tonic on page 253 helps you feel grounded and relaxed so you can sleep more soundly and wake up refreshed and revitalized.

Ginseng Pouches and Honey Sliced Roots

MORNING LIFTOFF • MIND-BODY WORKOUTS

See "Korea Loves Ginseng," page 243, for more on these. Both are portable, convenient, and effective preparations that you can easily find online (see Resources, page 352).

Ginseng Root Paste

MORNING LIFTOFF • MIND-BODY WORKOUTS

Word has it that Mick Jagger keeps his energy up during concerts by drinking Korean red ginseng paste mixed into water. Dissolve ¼ to ½ teaspoon paste in 1 cup (240 ml) hot water. You can find these concentrated pastes online and in Asian food stores (see Resources, page 352).

Maca-Vanilla-Coconut Tonifying Honey

MORNING LIFTOFF • MIND-BODY WORKOUTS

This delicious strengthening honey (page 253) combines maca with healthy-fat coconut butter and a hint of sultry vanilla. Whether you take a spoonful between or after meals or drink it melted in 1 to 1½ cups (240 to 360 ml) warm plant-based milk, this adaptogenic treat provides fast and easy energy replenishment.

Cacao Adaptogenic Energy Balls

MORNING LIFTOFF • MIND-BODY WORKOUTS

These energizing and nourishing snacks (page 255) have lots of protein and healthy fat while serving as the perfect delivery method for a generous dose of adaptogens (including ashwagandha, maca, goji berry, and cordyceps). This combination works well as a spread or spoonable snack, too.

Chyawanprash

MORNING LIFTOFF • MIND-BODY WORKOUTS •
EVENING REPLENISHER

This herbal jam is the premier restorative tonic, immune enhancer, and promoter of longevity in the Ayurvedic tradition. Chyawanprash is a super-nutrient-dense blend containing up to fifty different medicinal plants and aromatic spices, including several key adaptogens such as ashwagandha root, shatavari root, and amla (Indian gooseberry)—the latter an antioxidant powerhouse and the richest known plant source of vitamin C. Eat this by the spoonful or blend a heaping teaspoon or two into 1 cup (240 ml) warm water or plant-based milk for an instant tonic.

Wei Qi Soup

MORNING LIFTOFF • MIND-BODY WORKOUTS • EVENING REPLENISHER

It's a tradition in Asia to combine nourishing adaptogenic tonics and medicinal mushrooms with culinary spices to make healing, immune-boosting medicinal broths. These are great for seasonal changes, during the colder months for increased energy and resilience, or anytime you're feeling depleted. The delicious, savory broth on page 255 can be consumed on its own or used as a base for other soups.

Supplements

MORNING LIFTOFF • MIND-BODY WORKOUTS • EVENING REPLENISHER

Achieving the beneficial effects of adaptogens requires consistency, so including supplements in your routine is a good idea in addition to the other options listed here. Excellent options are available with concentrated or standardized active constituents. Supplements are also useful when you want to emphasize a specific action, such as using a rhodiola extract to enhance cognitive function. See the plant profiles, beginning on page 300, for more on the benefits of individual adaptogens, and what to look for when purchasing them in supplement form.

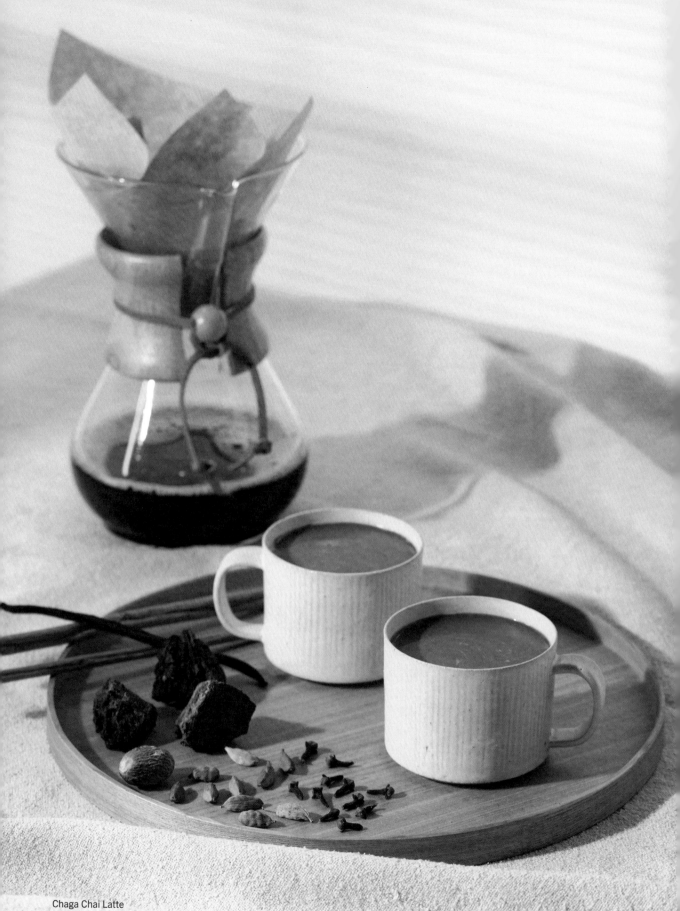

Chaga Chai Latte

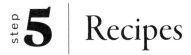

Recipes

Each recipe makes one serving unless stated otherwise.

Cacao-Reishi-Cordyceps Latte

Mix **1 or 2 tablespoons cacao powder** into **1 to 1½ cups (240 to 360 ml) hot water** in a bowl. Add **½ teaspoon cinnamon powder**, **½ teaspoon each reishi and cordyceps powdered extracts**, **¼ teaspoon vanilla extract or powder**, and **⅛ teaspoon allspice powder**. Use a mini immersion blender to mix with **2 to 4 ounces (60 to 120 ml) oat milk**, and sweeten to taste with **a natural sweetener of your choice**.

Note: For an iced latte, use half to two-thirds the amount of liquid. Chill the mixture and oat milk, stir, and pour over ice cubes.

Chaga Chai Latte

Mix **1½ cups (360 ml) plant-based milk of your choice** and **½ cup (120 ml) coconut cream** in a bowl. Using a whisk or an immersion blender, mix in **½ teaspoon chaga powdered extract**, **¼ teaspoon cinnamon powder**, **¼ teaspoon vanilla extract or powder**, **⅛ teaspoon nutmeg powder**, **⅛ teaspoon cardamom powder**, and **a small pinch of clove powder**. Add **a natural sweetener of your choice to taste**.

Notes: You can substitute 1 tablespoon powdered chaga for the extract; pour the liquid through a metal strainer first to remove any grit. You can use a teaspoon or two of premade powdered chai mix instead of the individual spice powders. For an iced latte, use half to two-thirds the amount of liquid. Chill the mixture and pour over ice cubes.

Ginseng-Ginger Lemon Tonic

Put ½ cup (20 to 30 g) **American or Korean dried cut-and-sifted ginseng root** and ½ cup (115 g) **chopped, unpeeled fresh gingerroot** in a saucepan with **4 cups (1 L) water**. Simmer, covered, over low heat for 25 minutes. Remove from the heat and strain. Add ½ cup (120 ml) **fresh lemon juice** and **manuka honey or a natural sweetener of your choice to taste**. Alternatively, place the ginseng and ginger in a 1-quart (1 L) jar, pour in enough **hot water** over the plant material to reach the top of the jar, let stand for 2 hours, then strain and add the lemon juice and honey. The tonic can be stored in the fridge for at least 1 week. Makes 4 servings.

Ashwagandha and Shatavari Coconut Replenisher

This recipe can be made hot or cold. For a hot beverage, place **1½ cups (360 ml) plant-based milk of your choice, ¼ cup (60 ml) coconut cream, 1 teaspoon coconut oil, 1 teaspoon each of ashwagandha root powder and shatavari root powder, ½ teaspoon cinnamon powder, ½ teaspoon vanilla extract or powder, ¼ teaspoon nutmeg powder, ⅛ teaspoon cardamom powder, 2 or 3 saffron threads**, and **1 teaspoon natural sweetener of your choice** in a small saucepan. Cook over low heat for 5 minutes. Use an immersion blender to blend until smooth and creamy. For a cold beverage, combine the milk, cream, oil, powders, and sweetener and mix well with an immersion blender or high-powered blender. Top the drink with **a saffron thread or two**.

Peanut Butter–Maca–Goji Berry Smoothie

Combine **1½ cups (360 ml) plant-based milk, 1 banana (fresh or frozen), 2 tablespoons peanut butter, 1 tablespoon gelatinized maca root powder, 1 tablespoon goji berry powder, 1 tablespoon unsweetened cacao powder, 1 teaspoon coconut oil, ½ teaspoon vanilla extract or powder**, and **½ teaspoon cinnamon powder** in a blender. Process until smooth.

Notes: Feel free to sprinkle some shaved coconut or cacao nibs on top at the end. If the drink is too thick, add a little more milk or water until you reach the desired consistency.

Strawberry Shatavari Smoothie

Combine **1½ cups (360 ml) plant-based milk of your choice,
1 cup (150 g) frozen or fresh strawberries, 2 tablespoons
unsweetened coconut flakes, 2 pitted dates, 2 heaping
teaspoons shatavari root powder, ½ teaspoon cinnamon
powder, ½ teaspoon vanilla extract or powder**, and **2 to
4 saffron threads** in a blender. Process until smooth. Garnish
with **cacao nibs,** if desired.

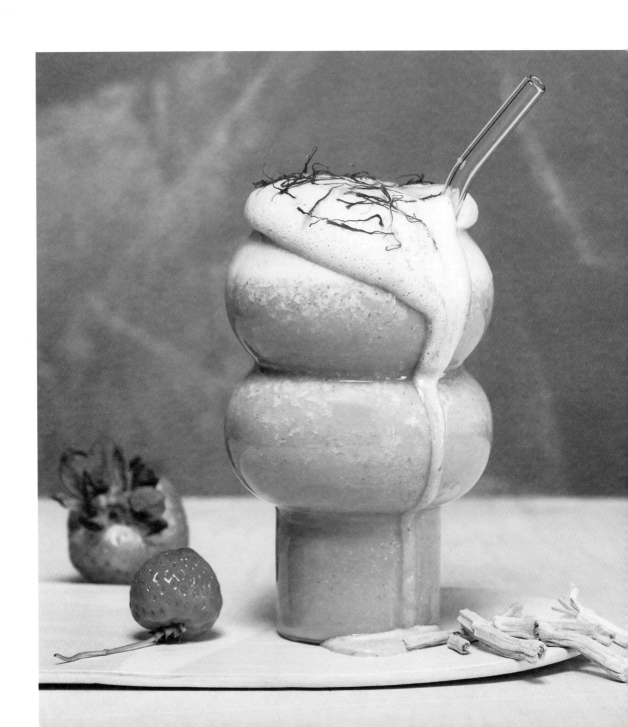

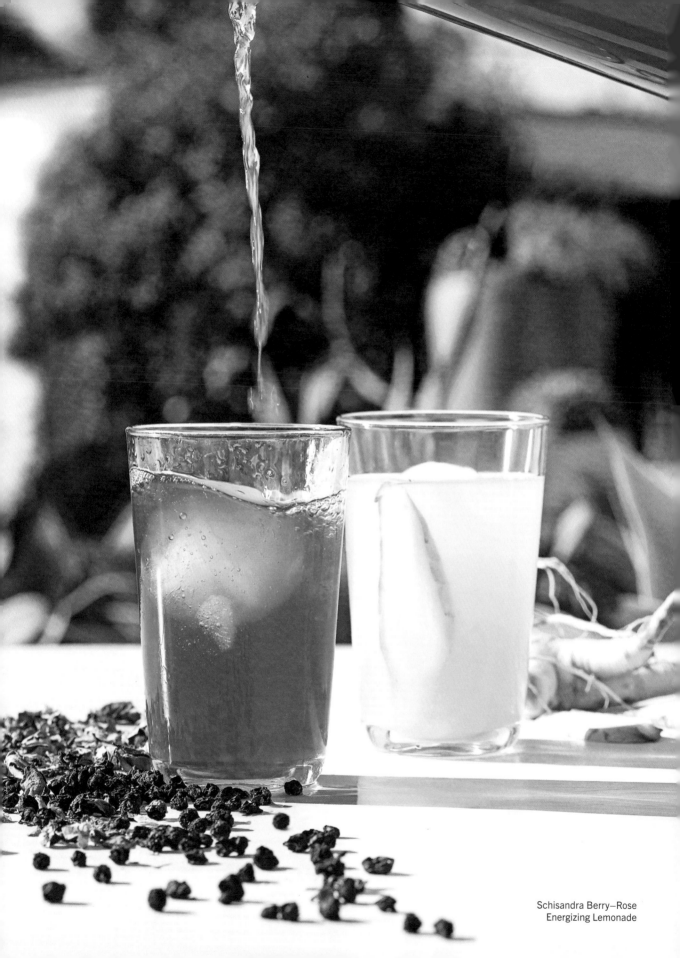

Schisandra Berry–Rose
Energizing Lemonade

Schisandra Berry–Rose Energizing Lemonade

Place **½ to ¾ cup (15 to 20 g) rose petals** and **⅓ cup (30 g) schisandra berries** in a 1-quart (1 L) jar. Pour in enough **hot water** over the plant material to reach the top of the jar. Let stand for 45 minutes to 1 hour. Strain off the plant material and stir in **¼ cup (60 ml) fresh lemon juice** and **honey or a natural sweetener of your choice to taste**. Store in the fridge for up to a week. Makes 4 servings.

Note: For a faster preparation, simmer the ingredients on the stove for 15 minutes. Let cool, then strain.

Ashwagandha Deep Rest Replenisher

Combine **1½ cups (360 ml) oat milk** and **½ cup (120 ml) coconut cream** in a small saucepan. Warm the mixture over medium-low heat for 2 to 3 minutes before stirring in **1 tablespoon coconut oil**, **1 tablespoon honey or a natural sweetener of your choice**, **1 tablespoon ashwagandha root powder**, **1 teaspoon cinnamon powder**, **2 cardamom pods**, **½ teaspoon vanilla extract or powder**, and **¼ teaspoon nutmeg powder** (ideally freshly ground). Simmer for about 10 minutes, stirring occasionally, until the flavors have infused into the milk. Take care not to scald the mixture. Pour through a fine-mesh strainer into cups. Makes 2 tonics.

Maca-Vanilla-Coconut Tonifying Honey

Place **1 cup (240 ml) honey** (pourable kind works best), **⅓ cup (85 g) coconut butter**, **¼ cup (60 g) maca root powder**, and **¼ teaspoon vanilla extract** in a mixing bowl and blend until all the ingredients are completely integrated. (Alternatively, you can blend the ingredients in a food processor—coconut butter takes a minute to blend in properly.) Store in a sealed container in the fridge for 1 to 2 weeks. Makes about 1½ cups (360 ml) honey.

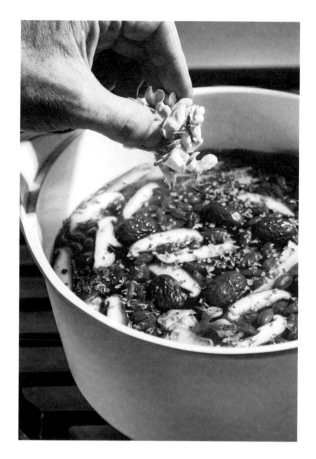
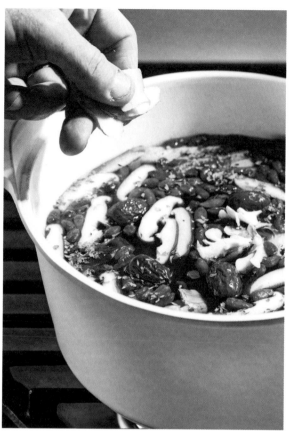
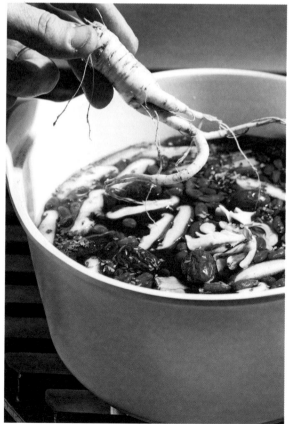

Wei Qi Soup

Cacao Adaptogenic Energy Balls

Place **1 cup (250 g) raw almond butter or a nut butter of your choice, 3 pitted dates, 3 tablespoons melted coconut oil, 2 tablespoons maple syrup, 2 tablespoons cacao powder, 1 tablespoon maca root powder, 1 tablespoon cordyceps powder, 1 tablespoon ashwagandha root powder, 1 tablespoon goji berry powder, ½ teaspoon cinnamon powder, ½ teaspoon vanilla extract or powder**, and a **pinch of salt** in a food processor. Pulse, intermittently pausing and scraping the sides of the bowls, until the ingredients are evenly combined. Mix together small, equal amounts of **coconut flakes, cacao nibs**, and **cacao powder** and spread in a thin layer across a plate. Roll the energy ball mixture into large gumball-size balls, then roll them in the topping mix. Store in an airtight container in the fridge for up to 1 week. Makes 6 to 8 balls; 2 balls constitute a good daily dose of adaptogens.

Note: This same recipe can be used as a spread or spoonable snack by forgoing rolling it into balls.

Wei Qi Soup

Fill a large pot with **12 cups (3 L) water**, then add **1 cup (70 g) chopped fresh shiitake mushrooms or ½ cup (20 g) dried, ½ cup (35 g) chopped fresh maitake mushrooms or ¼ cup (10 g) dried, ½ cup (45 g) goji berries, ¼ cup (60 g) cut and sifted astragalus root (or 2 to 3 tablespoons astragalus root powder), ¼ cup (60 g) cut and sifted ginseng root (or equivalent weight of whole fresh roots)**, and **2 tablespoons cordyceps powder**. Bring to a simmer and cook over low heat, covered, for 45 minutes to 1 hour. Add **4 cloves minced garlic, 2 to 3 tablespoons minced fresh gingerroot, 2 to 3 teaspoons salt (or to taste), 1½ teaspoons onion powder, 1 teaspoon dried oregano, 1 teaspoon dried basil, ½ teaspoon ground black pepper**, and **a pinch of cayenne pepper**. Continue simmering over low heat, covered, for 30 minutes. Remove from the heat, strain into a large bowl, and discard the plant material. Store for 1 week in the fridge or freeze for several months. Makes approximately 9 cups (2 L).

Note: You can consume this medicinal broth on its own, combine it in equal parts with bone broth as a soup base, or use it as a base for soup.

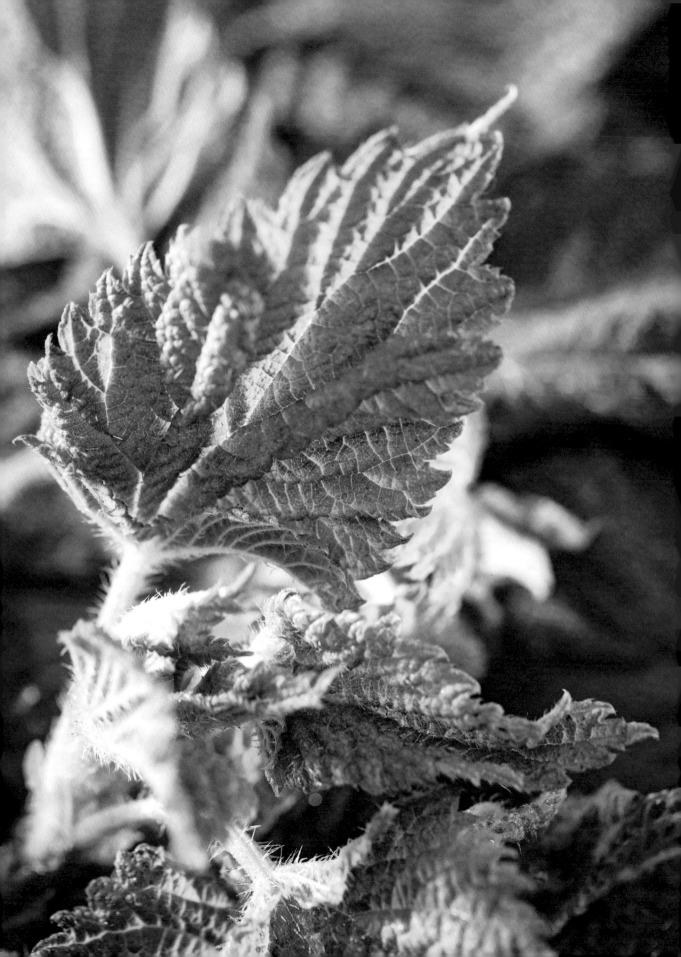

Protocol FAQs

Step 1:
Culinary Herbs, Spices & Bitters

Can I overdo it?

In general, my recommendation is to consume far more of these herbs and spices than you ever have. That said, don't use the hottest spices in excess or activate digestion when there's no food coming (which tends to result in uncomfortable low blood sugar and the feeling of being "hangry"). With the bitter herbs, moderate amounts give you the benefits, so there is no need to consume them in excess.

What if I don't like spicy things?

There are plenty of culinary herbs that are more temperate on the heat scale. See "Some Like It Hot" (page 112) for more on this.

What if I have acid reflux?

Acid reflux is actually the result of weak, rather than too intense, digestive fire—so rejuvenating your agni is very important if you suffer from reflux. That said, the GI tract can be sensitive to heating spices when it's already inflamed and irritated, so it's best to use those that are on the temperate side of the spice scale (like fresh cilantro, fennel, parsley, and coriander) while rectifying the underlying cause of reflux.

Will bitters get me drunk?

Bitter liquors are low in alcohol to begin with (20 to 40 percent), making this post-meal digestif practice sustainable without worrying about excessive alcohol consumption. You don't have to consume a lot to reap the benefits; they are catalyzed just from tasting the bitter flavor, so even a small amount will do the trick. There are bitters supplements and teas for those who prefer to avoid alcohol altogether.

Step 2:
Nutritives

I have a garden with its fair share of weeds, but I wouldn't know purslane from lamb's-quarters. How can I identify wild-growing nutritives?

Check out a copy of the *Peterson Field Guide to Edible Wild Plants* or visit foragers-association .org, which has all kinds of resources. There are also apps for identifying plants on the spot with your phone camera, such as Seek, by iNaturalist (a joint initiative of the National Geographic Society and the California Academy of Sciences) and Wild Edibles Lite. If you're not 100 percent sure of what you're picking, don't do it! And only harvest plants from clean areas not frequented by pets or sprayed with fertilizer or any other chemicals.

I understand stinging nettles can cause a mild sting when your skin touches them. So how do I handle (and cook with) nettles?

When harvesting your nettles, I suggest wearing gardening gloves and a long-sleeved shirt. The formic acid that causes the sting in stinging nettles is destroyed when the leaves are cooked or dried.

Step 3:
Demulcents

What can I do if I don't like a demulcent's consistency?

First off, preparations made with powders (as opposed to loose herbs) have the thickest consistency. Add less powder or more liquid to thin a beverage to your desired viscosity. You can also select lighter demulcents, like linden and plantain leaf, that have a lower mucilage concentration. Adding demulcents to foods with a complementary texture (like yogurt or a smoothie) helps, too.

What if demulcents make me feel full or bloated?

The digestive system and the microbiome need a little time to adjust to the influx of soluble fiber in demulcents. So start slowly, pay attention to how your digestive system feels, and give your body time to adjust. Adding some carminative, agni-enhancing culinary spices (such as cinnamon, ginger, or cardamom) to your demulcents will minimize some of these effects. Using infusions of whole plants where the solids have been strained off (see page 94), as opposed to consuming powder (where you're eating the whole herb), also makes these effects less pronounced.

Can demulcents be used topically?

Yes! Aloe vera has incredible cooling and moisturizing properties and has been shown to speed up healing and regeneration of skin cells. Olive oil is commonly used topically in Mediterranean countries; it is highly antioxidant and reduces free radical damage on skin. In New Zealand, manuka honey is a main ingredient in many skin-care products; it also has antimicrobial properties. Other skin-care products and regimens contain marshmallow and slippery elm.

Can demulcents help with coughs and sore throats?

Yes! In fact, most cough syrups and lozenges contain demulcent herbs, as the soothing, moistening properties of these plants act like a healing balm on sore throats. Demulcents are also a very important category of herb for promoting respiratory health and resolving short-term conditions affecting the lungs and sinuses. The reflex action of demulcents on the mucous membranes helps moisten dry sinuses and bronchioles, loosen and thin out mucus, and improve coughs by aiding expectoration. For more on treating coughs and sore throat, see pages 291 and 292.

Step 4:
Nervines

Can I drink alcohol during this step?

Alcohol is a powerful central nervous system relaxant, so using stronger-acting, more-sedative nervines in conjunction with alcohol will amplify these effects and become overly sedating and unpleasant. That said, a glass of wine with dinner in combination with the lighter forms of relaxants discussed in this step will not be a problem. Nervines can be a healthy alternative to alcohol or other substances in the evenings, if desired.

How do plant-based relaxants stack up to pharmaceuticals?

Plants are gentler in action when compared with pharmaceutical-based sedatives and sleep aids, and that's why they are valuable as a sustainable alternative. Plant-based relaxants are nontoxic, free from side effects, far easier for the body to metabolize, and enhance natural relaxation without disrupting sleep cycles. Unlike many pharmaceutical sedatives, plant-based sleep aids are also non–habit forming.

Can I go about my normal activities while taking these herbs?

Yes, definitely! Most of the nervines here can be used any time of the day and during any kinds of activities without any interference in normal functioning. Generally speaking, only the stronger nervine calmatives could be considered sedative. Nervines do not dull or numb our senses, and they allow us to maintain clear thinking and presence of mind. It's best to keep doses moderate or light on some of the stronger nervines (like skullcap, California poppy, hops, kava, and CBD) if you're planning to drive or need to maintain a degree of alertness.

Are these safe for kids?

They are both safe and recommended for kids. Generally speaking, because kids are smaller and their systems more responsive than adults' are, fragrant relaxants and essential oils will be sufficient for the most part. In some cases, small amounts of the more sedative, stronger-acting nervines can be helpful, but they shouldn't be the first option. See page 296 for more on kids and medicinal plants.

Step 5:
Adaptogens

Will adaptogens keep me up at night?

Part of what makes adaptogens so unique is their harmonizing effects. Adaptogenic plants balance a system that is off-kilter from excess stimulation by calming it down—but they also replenish and energize a system that is depleted and exhausted. A good rule of thumb is to use the high-powered, more energizing adaptogens earlier in the day and to emphasize the more relaxing adaptogens later in the day to benefit from their grounding and sleep-enhancing effects.

Can you overdo adaptogens?

Some adaptogens, including ginseng root, rhodiola, and cordyceps, are more stimulating than others. If taken at too high a dosage, these adaptogens may cause restlessness, anxiety, and insomnia in some people. It comes down to the strength of the preparation and the age and constitution of the individual taking it. In general, younger people with more energy will be more likely to experience excessive stimulation from taking adaptogens. Concentrated extracts or supplements can be potent and thus easier to overdo. If you're feeling restless or jittery, simply lower the dose, choose a different adaptogen, or select a different type of preparation, such as a synergistic formula where the overall effects are distributed. See the Resources on page 352 for suggested formulas.

BEGINNING YOUR NEW PLANT-POWERED LIFE

CONGRATULATIONS! YOU'VE FINISHED THE PROTOCOL.
Yet this is just the beginning of your lifelong plantventure. Bringing these new plant-powered habits into your daily life will be easy now that you've experienced their benefits firsthand.

So what does it look like to shift from the protocol into your new routine? During the protocol, the focus was on strengthening one system of the body with one category of plants at a time. Going forward, you'll support all of the body systems, drawing from all of the plant categories. A good starting place is to continue with the Minimum Daily Dose for all five steps simultaneously, making sure you're incorporating plants from each category every day. Enhancing all of the key body systems in small ways will upgrade the entire body in a big way. As your confidence grows and the routine becomes second nature, continue to layer in more of your favorites from each category until your days are fully saturated with plants.

> "Your experience during the protocol will help you personalize a routine that emphasizes your own needs, tastes, goals, and circumstances."

Like all things health and wellness, there is no one-size-fits-all approach here. Your experience during the protocol will help you personalize a routine that emphasizes your own needs, tastes, goals, and circumstances. As your awareness about how your body feels when working optimally increases, you'll naturally gravitate to the things that work best for you and make you feel good. Allow for some ebb and flow with your new plant practices, while always aiming for consistency. And remember you can repeat one (or more) of the steps anytime to refresh your knowledge or reinvigorate a specific system that seems out of balance.

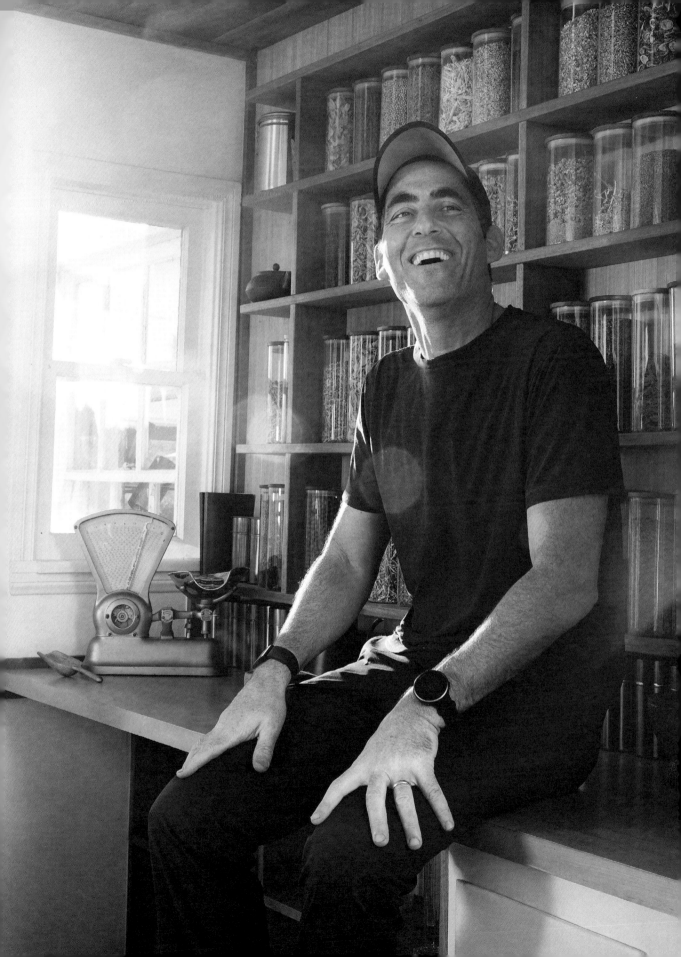

A PLANT-POWERED DAY

Here's what it looks like when the whole protocol comes together. A routine like the following is something to aspire to over time. The increase in energy and vitality you'll experience when fully saturated with plants will blow you away.

Upon waking:
Chia-Aloe-Lime Rehydrator (page 193)

Super Sonic Tonic (opposite)

Before breakfast:
Turmeric shot

At breakfast:
Unsweetened muesli and coconut yogurt mixed with walnuts and Super Berry Power Powder Blend (page 158), and a Super Seed Topper (page 164)

At work:
Peppermint tea

Diffusion of rosemary essential oil

Water bottle with a teaspoon of marshmallow root powder

As a snack:
Nutritive Green Power Balls (page 163)

At lunch:
Seaweed salad with Milk Thistle Detox-Enhancing Dukkah (page 135)

Spicy tuna roll with plenty of ginger and wasabi

Post-meal sip of Swedish bitters

In the afternoon:
Pre-workout ginseng liquid packet

Schisandra Berry–Rose Energizing Lemonade (page 253) during workout

Peanut Butter–Maca–Goji Berry Smoothie (page 250) post-workout

After work:
Frankincense resin ritual for shifting gears (page 215)

At dinner:
Kitchari (page 134) and Horta Vrasta (page 133)

After dinner:
Italian amaro shot

Linden tea

Real licorice candy

Before bed:
Prebiotic fiber drink

Nighttime nervine tincture

Diffusion of lavender oil on the nightstand

Super Sonic Tonic

Unleash a powerful blast of plant-based vitality with a delicious tonic that incorporates a diverse array of medicinal plants from every step of the protocol. This invigorating elixir provides a comprehensive range of benefits, ensuring that you are equipped with the energy and nourishment needed to take on the day with zeal.

Put **2 cups (480 ml) water** and **5 to 7 grams cacao** (discs or chunks) in a saucepan. Gently warm over low heat, stirring occasionally, until the cacao starts to melt, 2 to 3 minutes. Turn off the heat and let cool for a few minutes. **Add 1 teaspoon each cordyceps, ashwagandha, shatavari, and roasted dandelion powders; ½ teaspoon moringa powder; ¼ teaspoon cinnamon powder; and ½ teaspoon vanilla extract.** Mix thoroughly with a mini immersion blender. Top with **¼ to ½ cup (60 to 120 ml) oat milk** and **a natural sweetener of your choice to taste**.

Note: You can substitute cacao powder for the discs or chunks; simply add it to the warmed water along with the other powders.

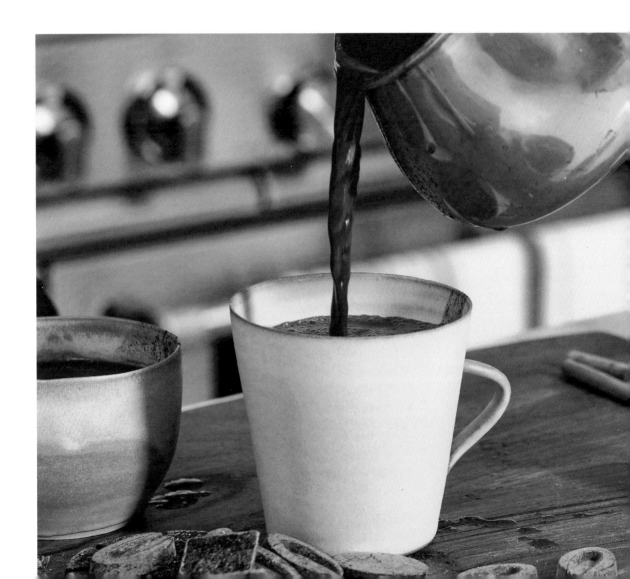

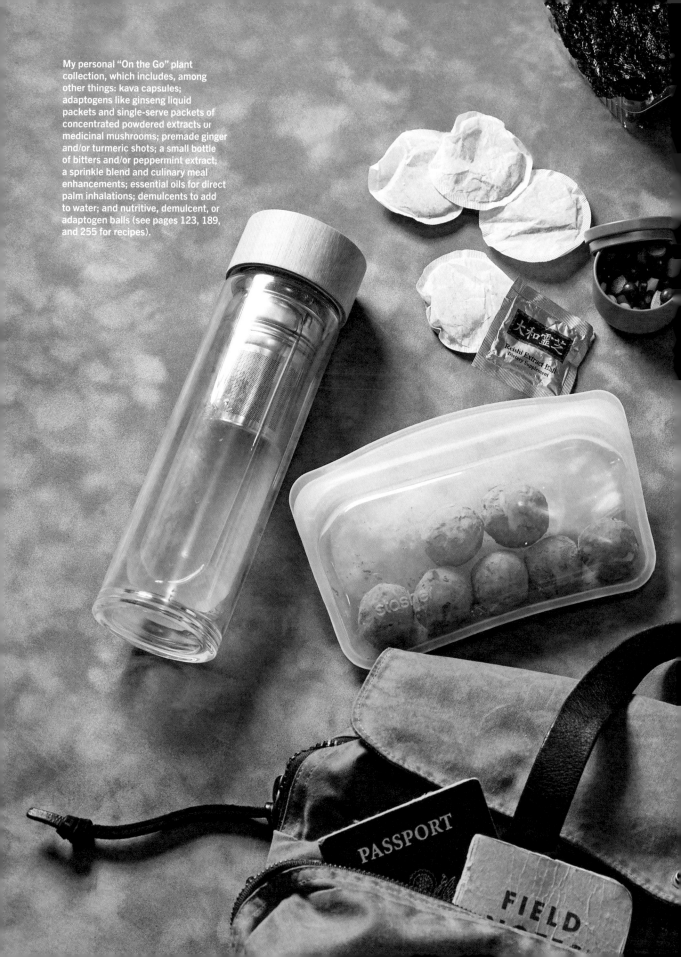

My personal "On the Go" plant collection, which includes, among other things: kava capsules; adaptogens like ginseng liquid packets and single-serve packets of concentrated powdered extracts or medicinal mushrooms; premade ginger and/or turmeric shots; a small bottle of bitters and/or peppermint extract; a sprinkle blend and culinary meal enhancements; essential oils for direct palm inhalations; demulcents to add to water; and nutritive, demulcent, or adaptogen balls (see pages 123, 189, and 255 for recipes).

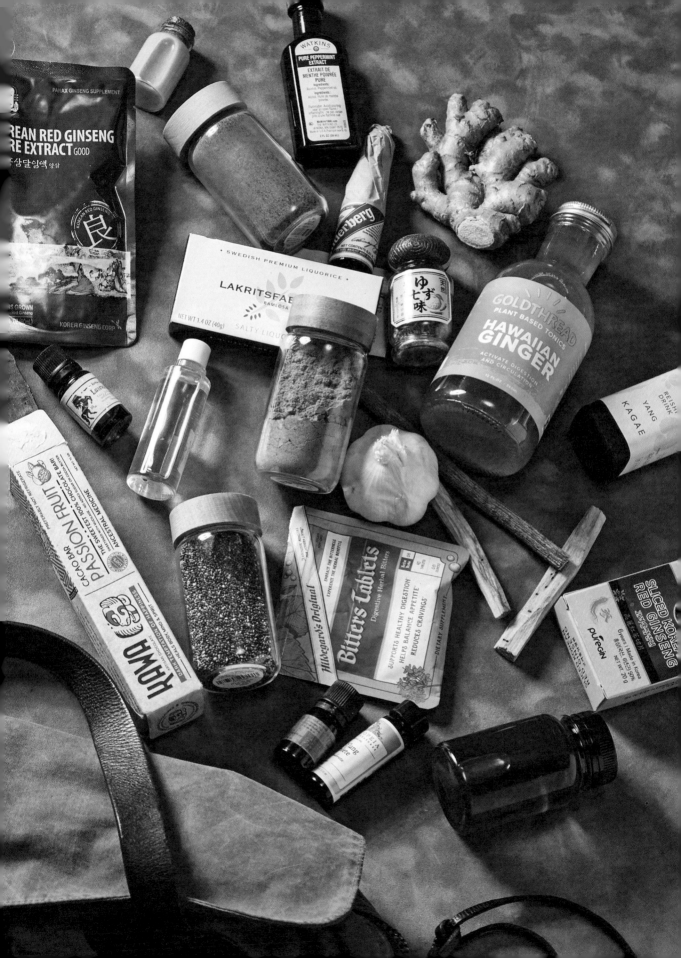

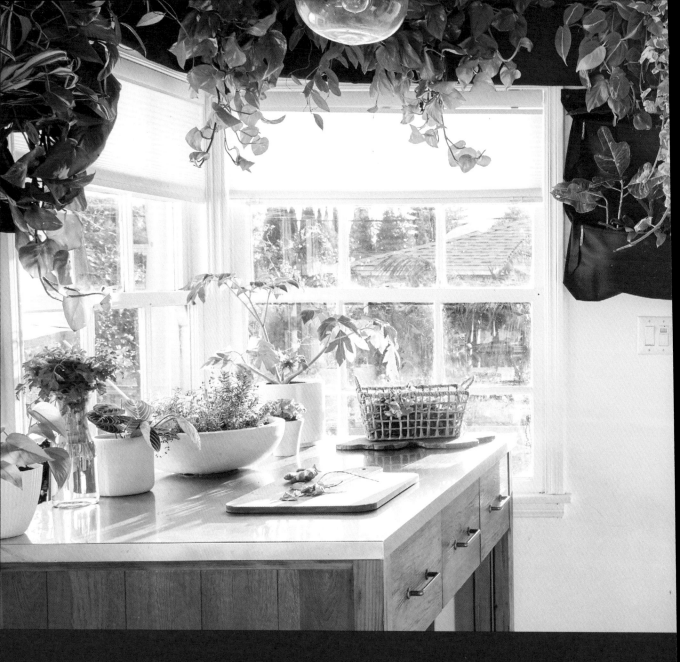

Part III

THE PLANT-POWERED
HOME

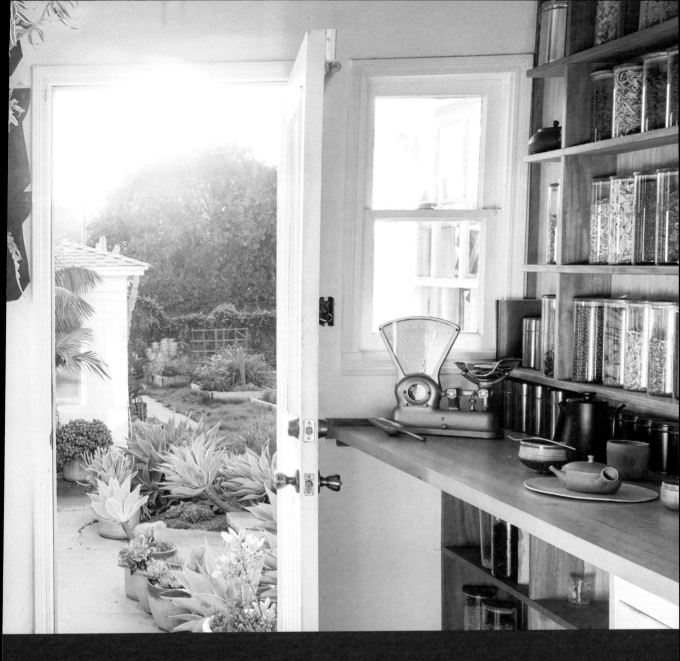

To actualize a lifestyle fully saturated with the health-enhancing power of medicinal plants, create a space that reinforces the new habits you're building. The things we consider essential enough to use on a regular basis are always easily accessible to us. The room-by-room guides on the following pages are designed to illustrate how to create living spaces that reinforce your health and well-being and make the daily consumption of medicinal plants feel almost effortless.

The primary focus of the book so far has been using medicinal plants for prevention and optimization. Since everyone is subject to minor illnesses at times, this section also includes a suggested home apothecary to address common, relatively uncomplicated conditions, using many of the same plants you're now familiar with to complete your plant-powered home setup.

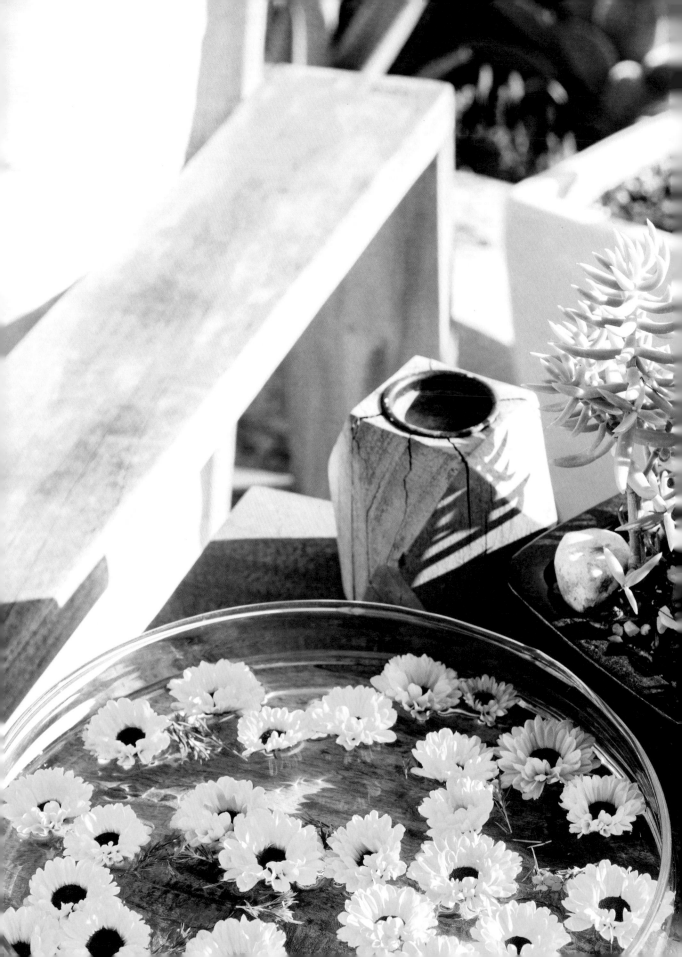

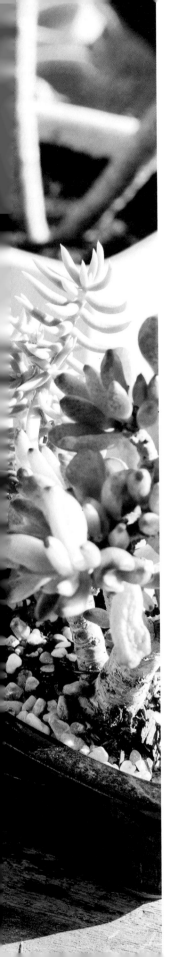

Your Home
On Plants

THE PAGES THAT FOLLOW OFFER INSPIRATION FOR KEEPING your chosen plants and remedies, along with any tools and materials you need to enjoy them, front and center. Seeing them arranged attractively and prominently throughout the home will help renew your intention to use them each and every day.

As you'll see, one room can contain several different "plant moments" without feeling cluttered. Create collections of different kinds of plants to increase the diversity of options and keep things exciting: bitters, aromatic teas, and essential oils, in particular, lend themselves to these sorts of collections.

Enjoy creating a home environment that reinforces your new habits and helps actualize your plant-powered lifestyle.

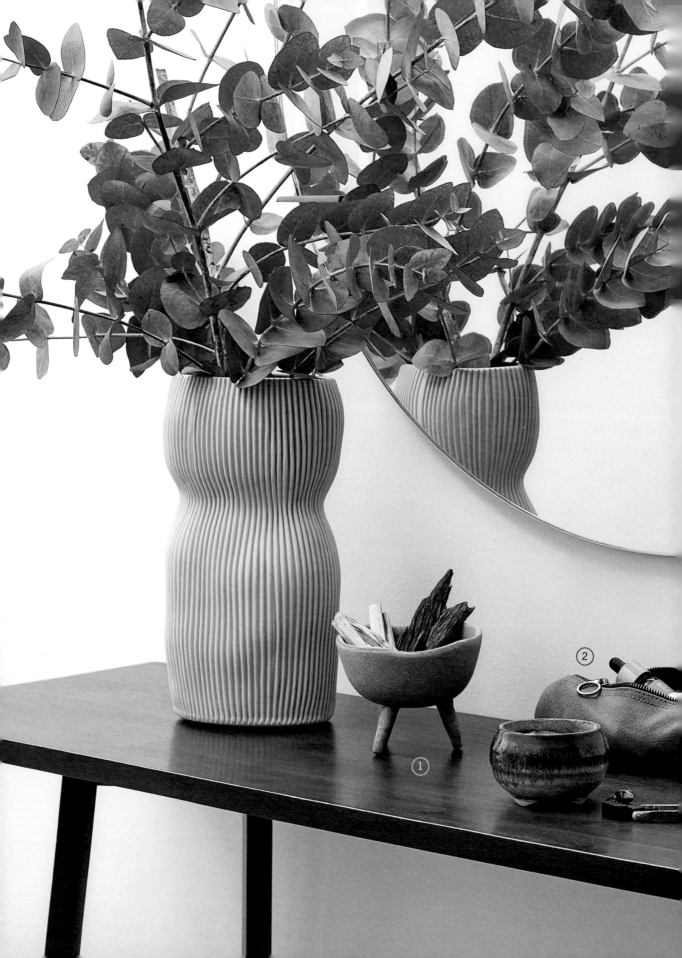

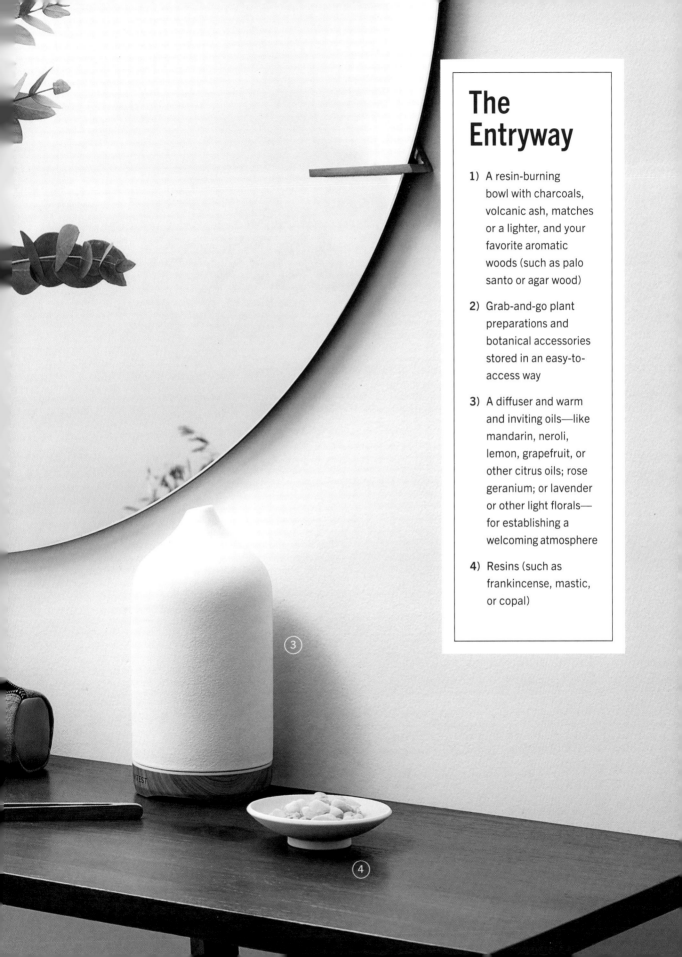

The Entryway

1) A resin-burning bowl with charcoals, volcanic ash, matches or a lighter, and your favorite aromatic woods (such as palo santo or agar wood)

2) Grab-and-go plant preparations and botanical accessories stored in an easy-to-access way

3) A diffuser and warm and inviting oils—like mandarin, neroli, lemon, grapefruit, or other citrus oils; rose geranium; or lavender or other light florals—for establishing a welcoming atmosphere

4) Resins (such as frankincense, mastic, or copal)

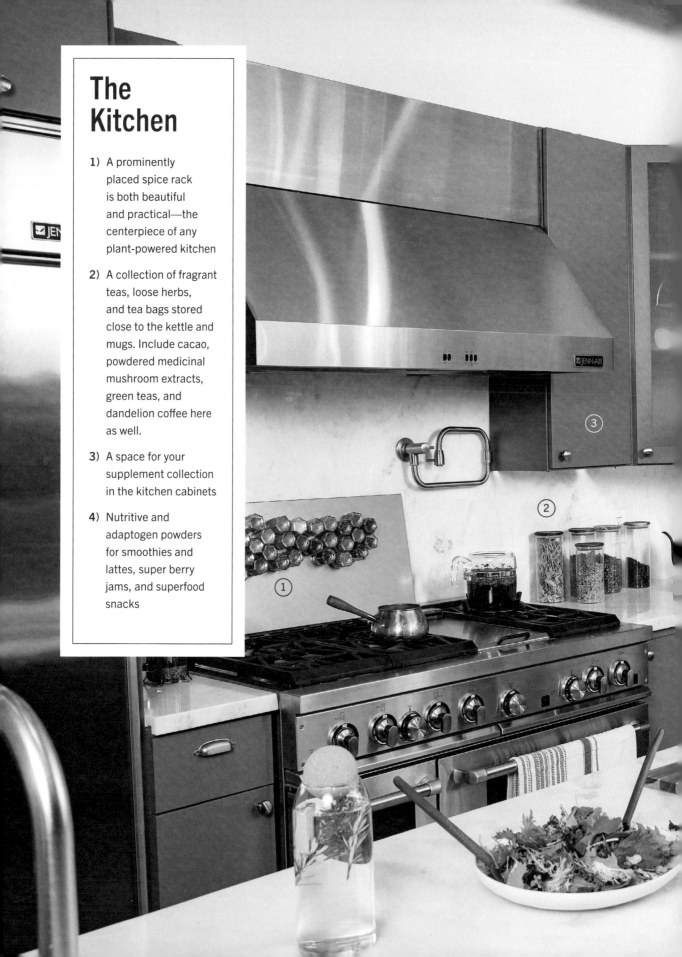

The Kitchen

1) A prominently placed spice rack is both beautiful and practical—the centerpiece of any plant-powered kitchen

2) A collection of fragrant teas, loose herbs, and tea bags stored close to the kettle and mugs. Include cacao, powdered medicinal mushroom extracts, green teas, and dandelion coffee here as well.

3) A space for your supplement collection in the kitchen cabinets

4) Nutritive and adaptogen powders for smoothies and lattes, super berry jams, and superfood snacks

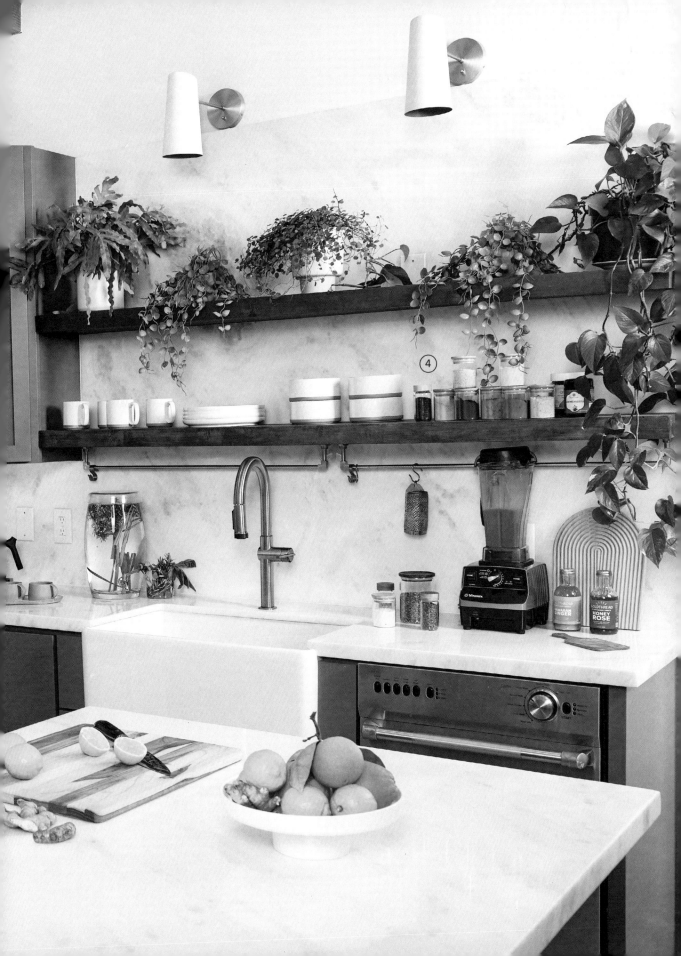

The Refrigerator

1) Fresh culinary herbs

2) Plant-based milks for smoothies and lattes

3) Herbal infusions, plant waters, aloe vera juice and gel, and citrus juice for making elixirs

4) A veggie drawer that includes nutritive roots and bitter greens

5) Delicate powders like matcha and acai

6) A dedicated space for spiced condiments and garnishes (to ensure they don't get lost behind other things and miss their window of freshness)

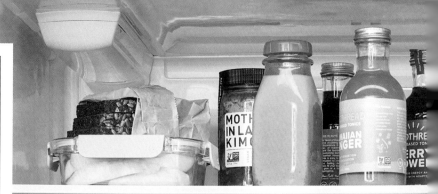

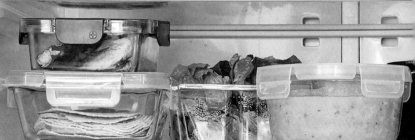

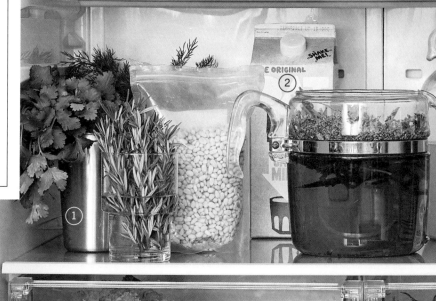

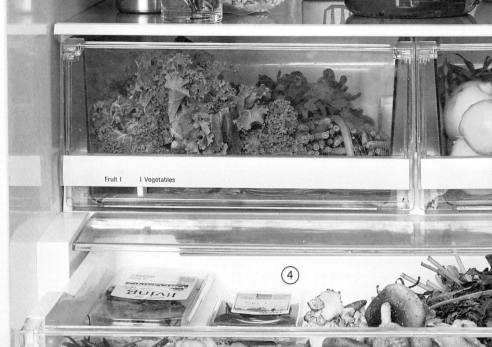

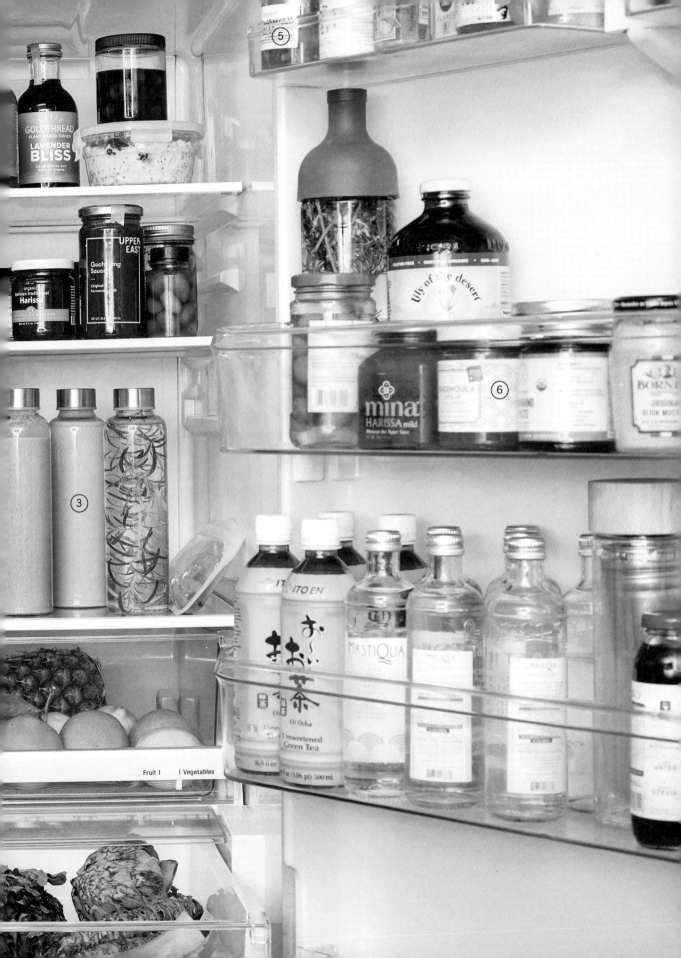

The Dining Room

1) A bitters bar, complete with shot glasses, for an after-meal digestif

2) A tray of various sprinkles and toppers for your meals

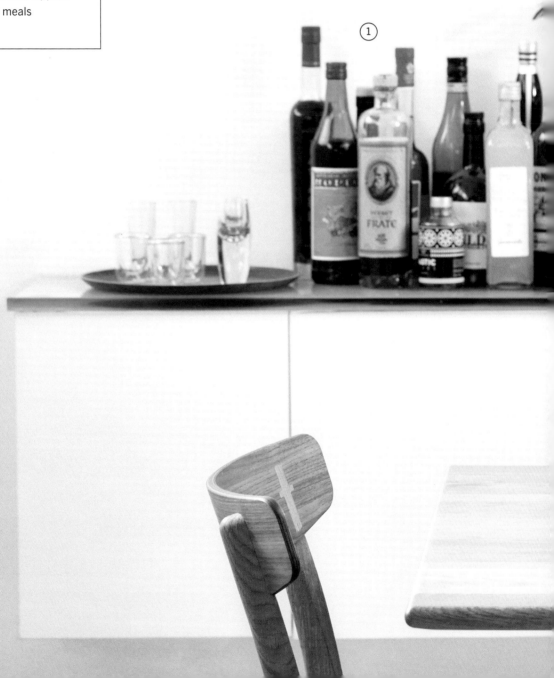

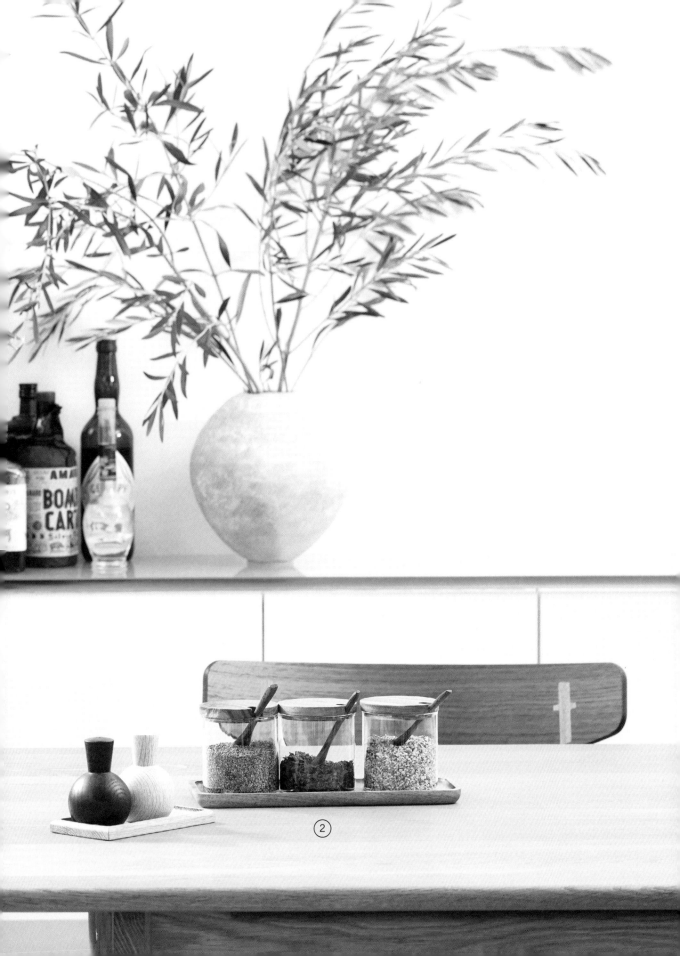

②

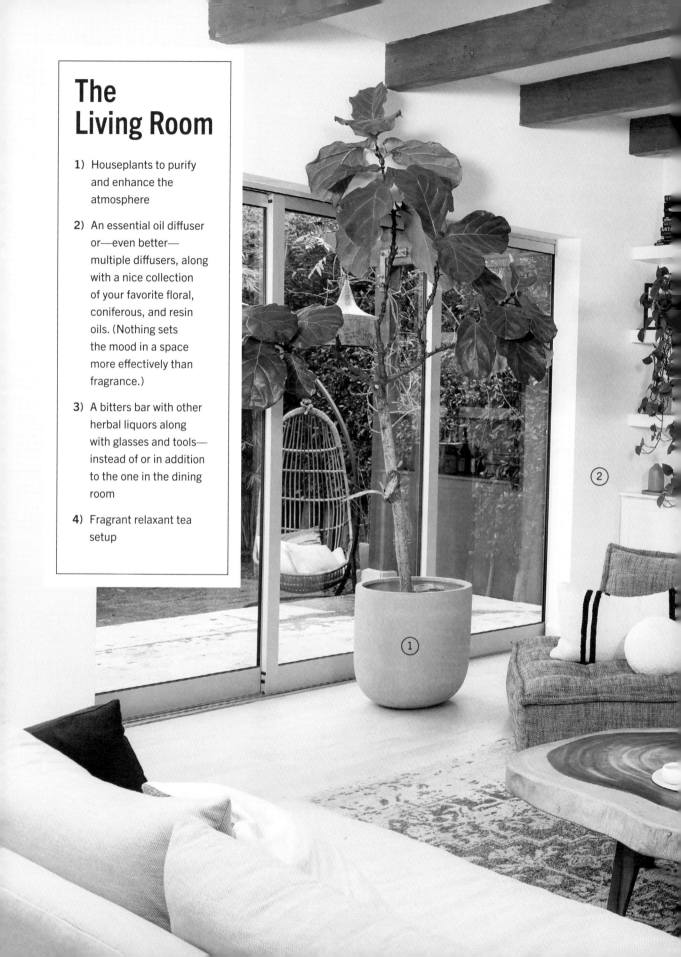

The Living Room

1) Houseplants to purify and enhance the atmosphere

2) An essential oil diffuser or—even better—multiple diffusers, along with a nice collection of your favorite floral, coniferous, and resin oils. (Nothing sets the mood in a space more effectively than fragrance.)

3) A bitters bar with other herbal liquors along with glasses and tools—instead of or in addition to the one in the dining room

4) Fragrant relaxant tea setup

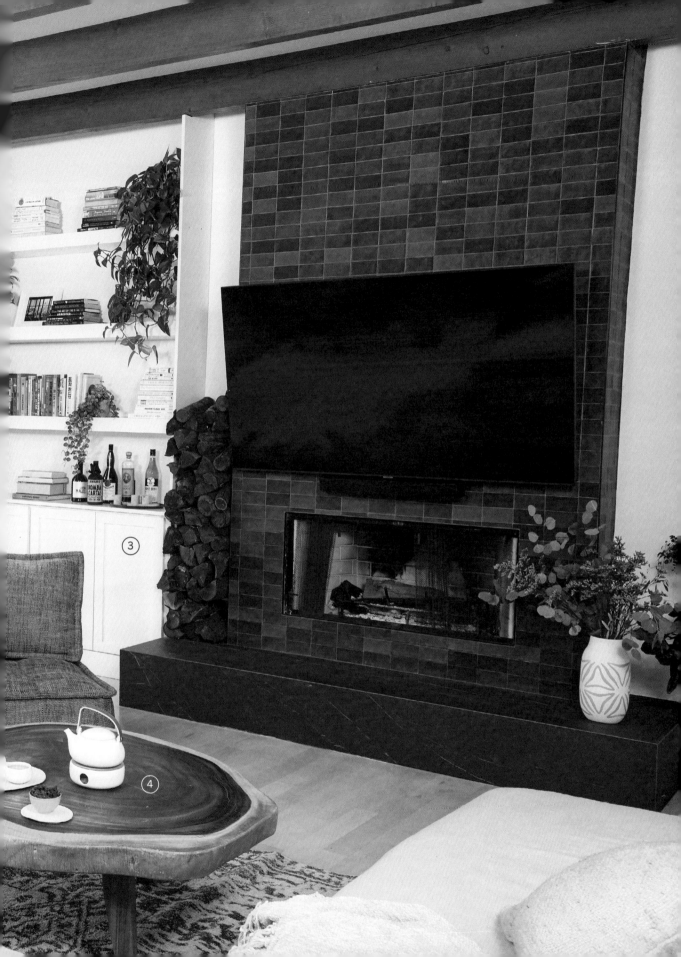

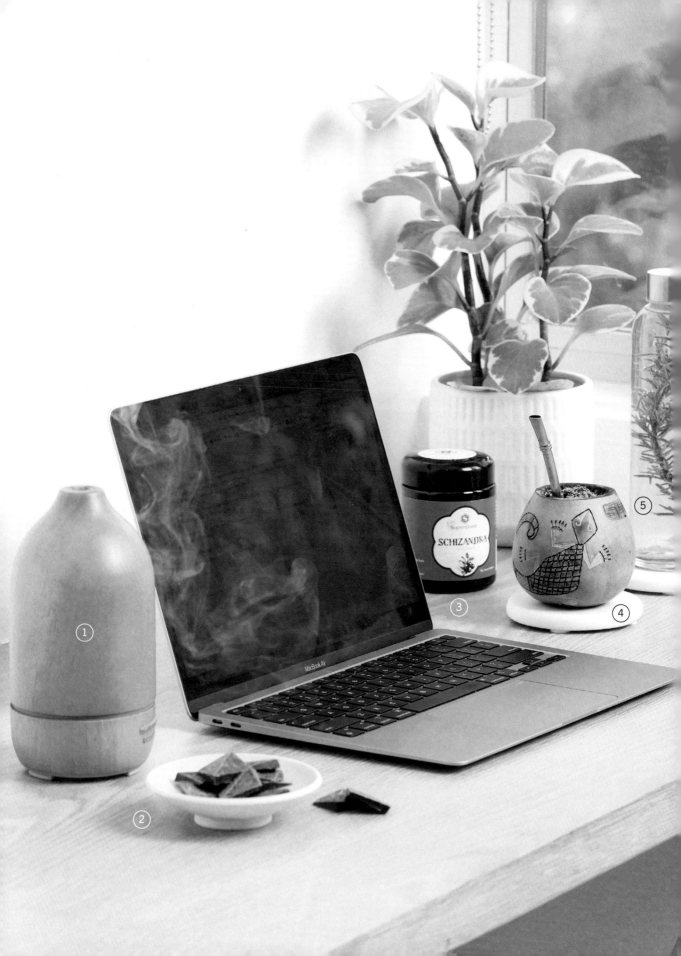

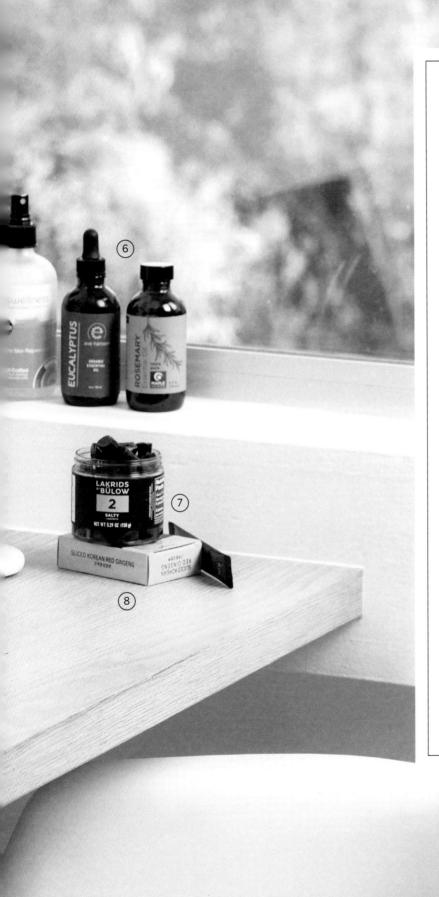

The Desk

1) Yes, another diffuser, with essential oils to support focus and clarity, such as rosemary, frankincense, and lemon balm

2) Dark, raw cacao as a sustaining snack to power through the workday

3 + 8) Adaptogenic or nutritive preparations such as concentrated ginseng paste, chyawanprash, or some favorite nutritive balls to sustain energy and focus

4) Yerba maté for maintaining energy and focus

5) A light nervine or fragrant relaxant tincture or elixir to relieve tension and access higher states of creativity

6) Essential oils and hydrosols to promote clarity and focus

7) Real black licorice to stay hydrated

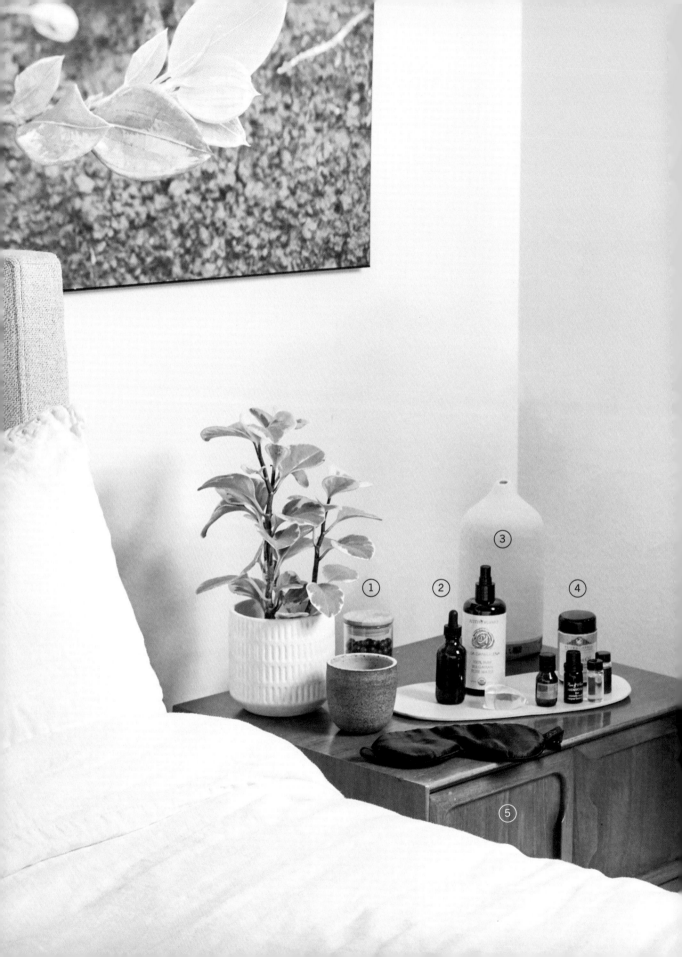

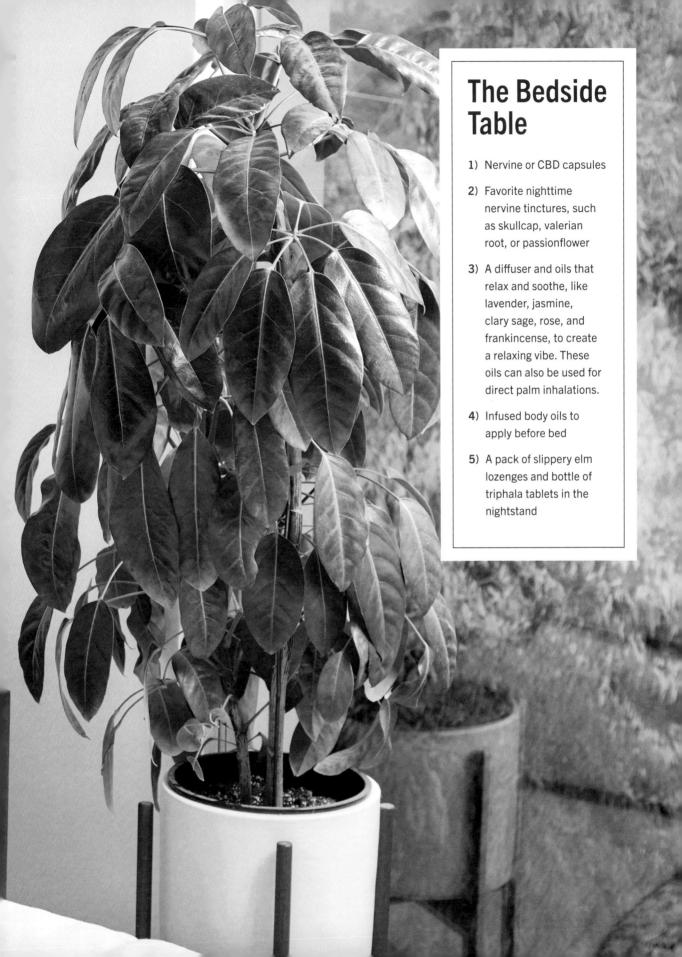

The Bedside Table

1) Nervine or CBD capsules

2) Favorite nighttime nervine tinctures, such as skullcap, valerian root, or passionflower

3) A diffuser and oils that relax and soothe, like lavender, jasmine, clary sage, rose, and frankincense, to create a relaxing vibe. These oils can also be used for direct palm inhalations.

4) Infused body oils to apply before bed

5) A pack of slippery elm lozenges and bottle of triphala tablets in the nightstand

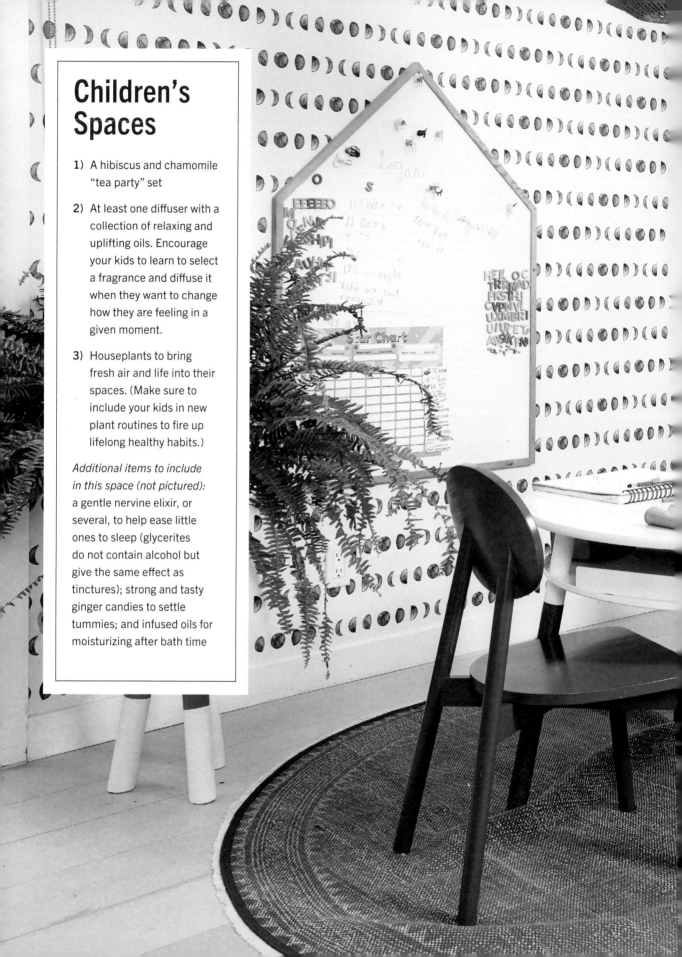

Children's Spaces

1) A hibiscus and chamomile "tea party" set

2) At least one diffuser with a collection of relaxing and uplifting oils. Encourage your kids to learn to select a fragrance and diffuse it when they want to change how they are feeling in a given moment.

3) Houseplants to bring fresh air and life into their spaces. (Make sure to include your kids in new plant routines to fire up lifelong healthy habits.)

Additional items to include in this space (not pictured): a gentle nervine elixir, or several, to help ease little ones to sleep (glycerites do not contain alcohol but give the same effect as tinctures); strong and tasty ginger candies to settle tummies; and infused oils for moisturizing after bath time

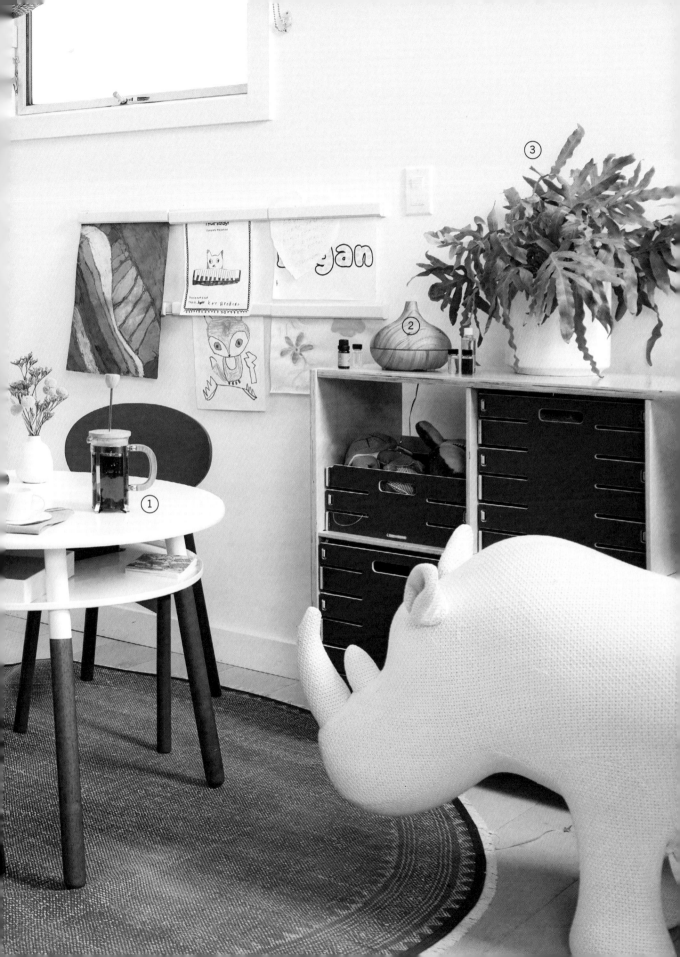

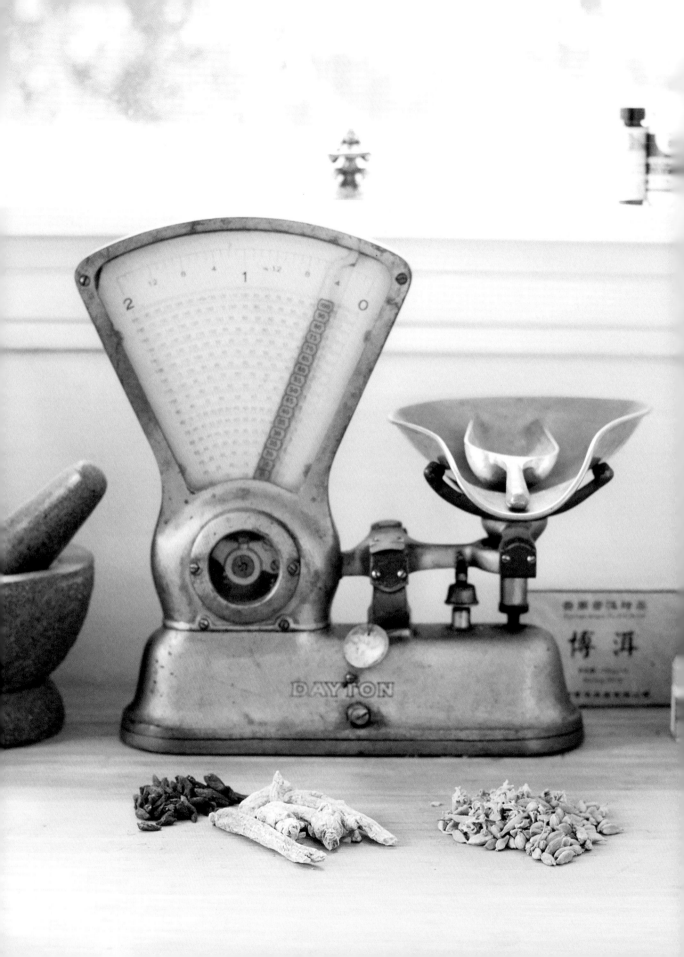

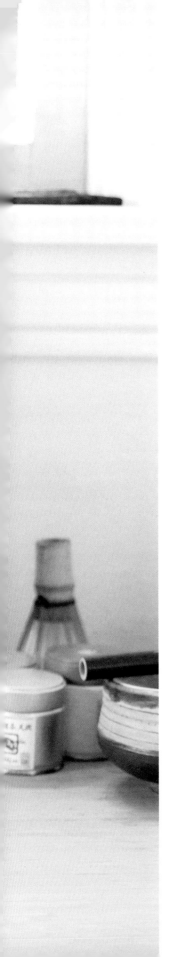

Home Apothecary

MEDICINAL PLANTS ARE THE FOUNDATION OF EVERYDAY health care for most of the world. Compared with over-the-counter pharmaceuticals, they offer a nontoxic, affordable, and environmentally sustainable option that encourages the body's natural healing mechanisms rather than merely suppress symptoms. (Failing to address the underlying issues that drive symptoms often leads to a more challenging resurgence of the problem down the road. An example of this is the chronic use of antibiotics in childhood, wreaking havoc on the gut microbiome and ultimately contributing to inflammatory conditions later in life.) This is not to say that over-the-counter medications aren't helpful in certain circumstances—simply that their excessive use by default, for conditions that are easily treated with medicinal plants, at the current, massive scale undermines both our individual and collective health. (For more on this, see the Health-Care Pyramid on page 22.)

In the following pages I'll give you an overview of common ailments and instructions for using the medicinal plants introduced throughout this book to address these issues. Often, it's simply a matter of taking the plants at higher dosages and with greater frequency to get a therapeutic effect.

Note: There are many excellent resources for furthering your understanding of how to use medicinal plants for grassroots home health care. For a list of recommended reading, see page 356.

Acid Reflux & GERD

This condition is characterized by burning sensations in the stomach, throat, and chest after eating (heartburn), regurgitating food or sour liquid, excessive belching and gas, bloating, and a lump-in-the-throat sensation. Traditional Chinese Medicine calls this upward movement a case of "rebellious qi." When these symptoms become chronic, it is classified as GERD (gastroesophageal reflux disease). The variety of factors that cause this condition are entirely rooted in diet and lifestyle. Medicinal plants can play an essential role in both reducing symptoms and correcting underlying imbalances.

Goals: Strengthen digestion, improve bile flow, soothe the lining of the GI tract, neutralize excess acid, reduce inflammation, and relax tension in the gut.

Remedies

- Add more bitter nutritive greens (like dandelion, watercress, chicory, and escarole) to your diet.

- Use bitters digestifs consistently after major meals to strengthen digestion, encourage bile flow, and cool inflammation.

- Mix individual demulcent powders or the Demulcent Powder Blend (page 189) into water and drink for immediate relief if you're experiencing acidity and heartburn. A thicker, more viscous preparation is most effective in neutralizing acid.

- Drink infusions and teas of fragrant aromatics (like chamomile, lemon balm, lavender, rose, and linden) to calm the digestive system, reduce gas and bloating, and cool inflammation.

- Eat a teaspoon of manuka honey on its own or melted into warm water two or three times a day on an empty stomach.

- Drink 2 or 3 cups (480 to 720 ml) of licorice tea and/or take DGL licorice tablets or lozenges throughout the day to reduce acidity and inflammation.

- Take turmeric capsules standardized for curcumin content and/or eat Turmeric Balls (page 123) to reduce inflammation and strengthen digestive function.

Allergies

Many of us are familiar with allergies and the uncomfortable symptoms they cause, like runny nose, itchy or watery eyes, sneezing, postnasal drip, muddled thinking, and fatigue. Whatever the trigger—pollen, cat dander, seasonal hay fever—the goal should be to reduce symptoms *and* strengthen the body's core systems to build overall resilience and lessen susceptibility to allergies.

Below are remedies that offer immediate relief. In addition, the suggestions presented in the protocol (and specifically Step 1, focused on digestion and detoxification) help reduce the body's reactive response to allergens over time. This is because allergy symptoms are an expression of the immune system's attempt to burn up a foreign substance through a histamine response. If there's an excess of preexisting inflammation in the body, reactivity to external allergens is magnified. Improving digestion and detoxification are essential ways to reduce the inflammation and toxicity that make the body more susceptible to allergies.

Goals: Eliminate mucus congestion, enhance digestion and detoxification, increase hydration, boost immune response, and neutralize opportunistic microbes.

Remedies

- Incorporate culinary spices from the hot end of the spice scale into your diet. Add minced raw garlic in olive oil to food. Grate fresh gingerroot and turmeric on your meals. Use wasabi paste, hot mustard, and sriracha as condiments.

- Make a bowl of savory, spicy miso broth using ½ teaspoon each of grated fresh gingerroot and garlic and a pinch each of dried oregano, ground black pepper, and cayenne pepper. Drink two or three bowls throughout the day.

- Add a pinch of cayenne to the Ginger Shots recipe (page 124) and take three or four shots a day when allergies kick in.

- Take trikatu tablets or powder, an Ayurvedic remedy containing three spices (black pepper, ginger, and pippali long pepper) traditionally used for allergies and mucus conditions. Take two or three tablets or ½ teaspoon powder in a small amount of water with meals.

- Increase your nutritive intake. Take freeze-dried nettles in capsule form to astringe swollen sinuses and reduce histamine reaction. Drink an overnight infusion of nettles (2 to 4 cups/480 ml to 1 L per day) as a gentle diuretic to support cleansing of inflammatory chemistry and allergens. Double or triple your daily dose of super berries or Super Berry Power Powder Blend (page 158) to get optimal amounts of immune-enhancing antioxidants and vitamin C.

- Take medicinal mushrooms (specifically reishi, maitake, turkey tail, and/or agaricus) in powdered extract form or capsules to enhance immunity and reduce histamine response. Start taking several weeks before allergy season as a preventive. During allergy season, double or triple your normal daily dose.

- Use direct palm inhalations multiple times throughout the day and/or diffuse eucalyptus, spruce, sage, pine, and/or frankincense essential oils for their antiseptic, anti-inflammatory, and decongestant effects.

Colds & Flus

Colds and flus are viral infections of the upper respiratory system. Primary symptoms include runny nose, sneezing, sinus congestion, sore throat, swollen glands, headache, chills, fever, body aches, and fatigue.

Susceptibility to colds and flu depend on a variety of factors, including—not surprisingly—the state of our innate immune system. Maintaining a high level of vitality naturally leads to a healthy immune system and is the key to defending ourselves against viruses.

Goals: Nourish core energy systems, encourage recuperative rest, boost immune response, relieve pain, and vitalize circulation.

Remedies

- Make Wei Qi Soup (page 255), a warming adaptogenic soup containing immune boosters like ginseng, warming spices, and medicinal mushrooms.

- Drink strong, hot infusions of tulsi leaf and flower tea; add slices of fresh gingerroot and a dab of manuka honey, if desired.

- Combine 1 tablespoon each loose-cut sage and cinnamon chips in a tea basket or removable infuser basket. Steep in 1 to 1½ cups (240 to 360 ml) of hot water. Add lemon juice and manuka honey to taste. Sip throughout the day to soothe a sore throat, induce sweat to cool down, and reduce symptoms generally.

- Take two or three Ginger Shots (page 124) throughout the day, adding a pinch of cayenne pepper or fresh or dried oregano for an extra immune boost.

- Drink slippery elm, marshmallow, or licorice tea, or mix the powdered form of any of those demulcents, or Demulcent Powder Blend (page 189) into room-temperature water to soothe and moisten irritated mucous membranes in the throat and promote hydration.

- Mix 5 to 10 drops of pain-relieving, circulation-enhancing peppermint essential oil with 1 tablespoon carrier oil of your choice; rub the mixture into the temples and the often tight and achy spot where your skull and neck meet at the back of your head. Keep the oil away from the eyes.

Constipation & Bloating

There are many potential causes and contributing factors that lead to constipation and bloating. For most, it is the result of one or a combination of the following: insufficient dietary fiber intake, lack of hydration, excessive tension in the gut, or lack of bile flow from the liver.

Goals: Increase plant sources of soluble fiber, hydrate and moisten the GI tract, relax tension in the gut, and increase bile flow.

Remedies

- Take a daily dose of triphala in either tablet or powder form in the morning and/or right before bed. Start with ½ teaspoon of the powder or equivalent in tablets per day and increase until you reach the desired result, usually somewhere between 3 and 6 grams.

- Eat an abundance of bitter nutritive greens for increased fiber and improved bile flow.

- Use bitters digestifs consistently after major meals to strengthen digestion and encourage bile flow.

- Consume more demulcents to hydrate the colon and as a source of prebiotic soluble fiber.

- Drink fragrant relaxant teas (like linden, chamomile, lavender, lemon balm, and peppermint) for their antispasmodic, gut-relaxing actions.

Coughs

Coughing is the body's way of clearing the lungs of congested mucus or other irritants. The goal of treating a cough with traditional plant medicine is to assist the lungs in clearing the airways by encouraging an efficient cough reflex.

Goals: Promote expectoration, soothe and hydrate the lungs and throat, reduce inflammation, and neutralize pathogens with antimicrobials.

Remedies

- Demulcents benefit all types of coughs, especially dry ones. Sip on slippery elm, marshmallow, or licorice tea; Irish moss; or slippery elm, marshmallow, or licorice powder or Demulcent Powder Blend (page 189) mixed with room-temperature water to soothe and hydrate an irritated throat, moisten the lungs, improve expectoration, and calm the cough reflex.

- For a wet cough, make a strong infusion using equal parts anise, fennel, thyme, oregano, and cardamom pods (2 or 3 tablespoons total per 1 to 1½ cups/240 to 360 ml hot water),

sweetened with 1 or 2 teaspoons manuka honey, for their antimicrobial and expectorant properties. You can also finely chop a clove of garlic and let it sit for a few minutes (to catalyze production of its potent sulfur compounds), mix with 1 teaspoon of manuka honey, and down the hatch. Repeat two or three times a day for its antimicrobial and expectorant actions.

- Add 5 to 10 drops total of eucalyptus, peppermint, lavender, spruce, pine, thyme, and/or tea tree essential oil to a pan of hot water, cover your head with a towel, and inhale deeply over the pan. This will open congested airways and promote expectoration.

- Tinctures containing nervine herbs (chamomile, California poppy, valerian root, and/or passionflower) help calm the cough reflex and ensure a restful sleep to replenish vital energy needed for healing and recovery.

Muscle Tension

Tight neck and shoulders, headaches, muscle spasms, lower-back pain, menstrual cramps, and TMJ syndrome are all potential manifestations of stress-induced tension. This type of pain usually has a dull, diffuse, achy, and throbbing quality.

Goals: Relax muscles and increase circulation, calm the nervous system, reduce inflammation.

Remedies

- Dilute 10 drops of peppermint, frankincense, helichrysum, clary sage, and/or lavender essential oil in 2 tablespoons carrier oil; massage the mixture directly onto areas of tension and pain, taking care to avoid the eyes.

- Ginger or turmeric—whether in capsules, shots, or Turmeric Balls (page 123)—invigorates circulation and reduces inflammation.

- Nervine calmatives such as California poppy, skullcap, CBD, and kava (in tincture, tablet, or capsules) help calm the nervous system, reduce pain, and decrease inflammation. Follow directions for pulse dosing on page 216.

Sore Throat

The throat is a sensitive area where pathogens often set up shop in their attempt to infiltrate the body. The soreness we experience results from the body's immune response and the associated inflammation of the mucous membranes. It's important to attend to the first signs of a sore throat to prevent the possibility of a deeper respiratory infection.

Goals: Neutralize pathogens with antimicrobials, boost local immune response, soothe inflamed mucous membranes, reduce pain and swelling.

Remedies

- Use throat sprays containing herbs with antimicrobial constituents such as sage, cinnamon, myrrh, goldenseal, or clove combined with soothing demulcents like licorice, marshmallow, or slippery elm. Do 10 to 20 sprays per day.

- Swallow a spoonful of manuka honey slowly to coat the throat a couple times a day for its soothing antimicrobial properties. Alternatively, add the honey to hot water with lemon and sip throughout the day. It's best to use honey with a UMF (Unique Manuka Factor) of 15 or above—for more on the UMF, see page 187.

- Drink slippery elm, marshmallow, or licorice tea, or Irish moss; or sip on room-temperature water mixed with the powdered form of any of the above demulcents or Demulcent Powder Blend (page 189) throughout the day to relieve soreness and irritation. Generally, the thicker, the better. By coating the throat with a layer of hydration, demulcents promote healing.

Boosting Your Immunity

Strong immunity results when all of the essential body systems are functioning optimally. In Traditional Chinese Medicine, the immune system is depicted as a force field that protects us from infiltration by outside pathogens. Each essential system we've discussed—strong digestion, proper hydration, balanced endocrine and nervous systems, and efficient detoxification of wastes and toxins—plays a vital role in generating that strong force field. In other words, the "terrain" of the body determines the vigor of our immune response. When vitality is weak and depleted due to lifestyle factors such as prolonged stress, overwork, insufficient sleep, and poor nutrition, immunity will be compromised, leaving us more vulnerable to pathogens and illness.

The immune system consists of an amazing array of cells, organs, and tissues located throughout the body. It forms physical barriers (e.g., the skin and mucous membranes) between ourselves and the outside world, keeping out pathogens (bacteria, viruses, fungi, parasites) and allergens. It maintains our body's proper pH and temperature, removes cellular wastes, governs inflammatory processes, and stimulates repair mechanisms.

All of the plants presented in this book collectively enhance immunity by supporting the key systems of the body. In addition, the novel constituents in medicinal plants strengthen the body's immune response due to the hormetic effect—the physiologic benefit of consuming small doses of compounds that mildly stimulate our biological systems to respond. It's similar to the way doing push-ups strengthens muscles by first challenging them, or the way doing mental exercises challenges the brain to keep it sharp.

Many medicinal plants are specifically beneficial to the immune system. Culinary herbs and spices contain essential oils and other compounds that are antimicrobial, neutralizing pathogens on contact, especially in the GI tract. Demulcents strengthen the barrier function of mucous membranes to prevent pathogens from infiltrating deeper into the body. Nutritives provide micronutrients that are essential for repair and regulation of the immune response. Adaptogens and medicinal mushrooms nourish the deeper aspects of the immune system, encouraging the production of important immune factors like lymphocytes, T-cells, and other antibodies. The best strategy for improving immunity is to include the widest variety of medicinal plants in your daily life, as the protocol outlines.

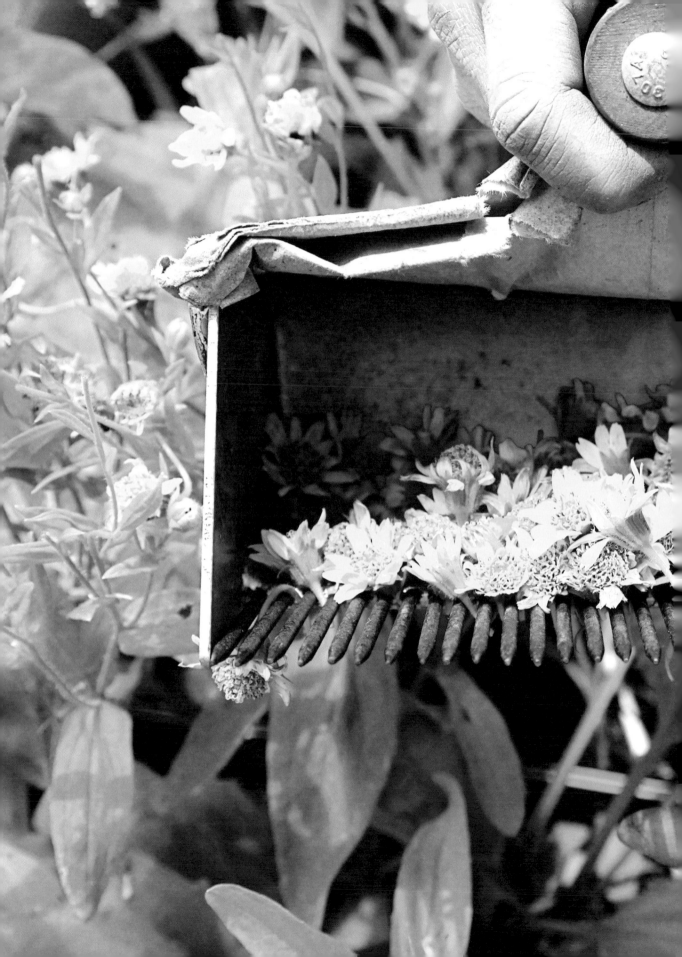

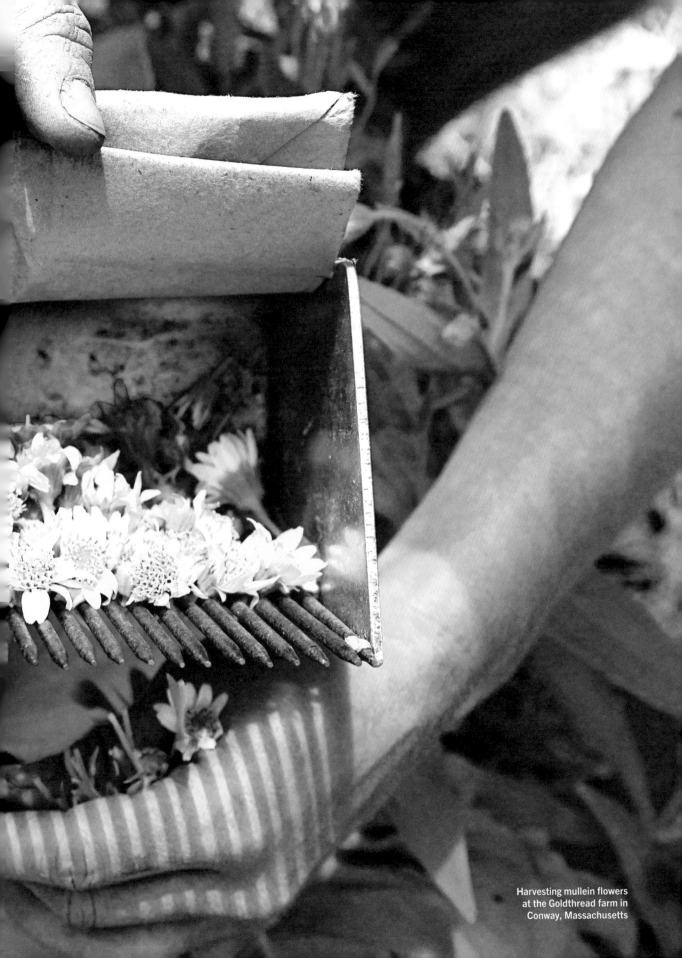

Harvesting mullein flowers
at the Goldthread farm in
Conway, Massachusetts

A Word on Kids & Medicinal Plants

In my practice, it has become increasingly common to see children with complex and entrenched health issues that previously I would have seen only in adults. This is troubling, because too many kids end up taking strong pharmaceuticals to address issues rooted in lifestyle that would resolve with dietary changes and plant-based remedies. Early on in my clinical practice, I initiated a small project with the nurse at my children's school. Like myself, our school nurse was concerned about the astronomical rise in pharmaceutical use by children and expressed a strong desire to use more natural medicine in her office.

I created a small apothecary full of loose herbs, tea blends, powders, cough syrups, elixirs, salves, and an essential oil diffuser, along with instructions on how to administer them. The goal was to exchange over-the-counter pharmaceuticals for herbal remedies, when possible, for treating common ailments like colds, flus, tummy aches, coughs, allergies, headaches, scrapes, bruises, and stings. At the outset of the project, we agreed to keep data on how often and for what conditions herbal remedies were given as well as the benefits kids were experiencing. The results we saw over the course of the year were both intriguing and inspiring.

Instead of taking aspirin and NSAIDs (nonsteroidal anti-inflammatory drugs), kids routinely drank cups of hot peppermint and chamomile tea with honey while they kicked back on the nurse's couch. They sipped on elderberry elixirs and slippery elm bark instead of over-the-counter cough suppressants. They had ginger shots and nettle infusions instead of antihistamines. Children were feeling better taking the herbal remedies, and our nurse was giving out a whole lot fewer pharmaceuticals.

In fact, she became quite popular around the school. Her office felt more like a wellness spa—kids would visit just to drink some tea

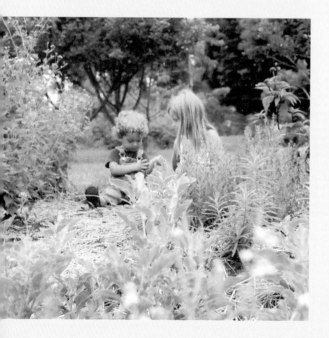

and breathe some essential oils. The ritual of taking time out to sip herbal teas and relax became an important reference point for youngsters as they began understanding the fundamentals of self-care. Taking care of themselves became associated with a pleasant experience—a great success unto itself.

The kids also started making the important connection between health and nature, which up until then was a foreign concept to many of them. We organized field trips to the farm so they could see where the herbs from the nurse's office were grown. Many started asking for teas at home, seeking them out at the grocery store, and becoming more aware of the plants growing all around them. Though this was just a small pilot project in one school, nurses offering children simple botanical remedies from school apothecaries could be transformative to our health-care system.

My own experience of raising two children, combined with twenty-plus years of clinical experience, taught me that incorporating everyday medicinal plants into kids' lifestyle at an early age creates a strong, resilient foundation of health. And it's never too early to reinforce and strengthen the key body systems. Their young bodies are full of energy and healing power, making them far more responsive to the actions of plants. The plants and remedies I've introduced in this book represent, for the most part, an expansion of our diet. Most of the herbs are appropriate for children, with some commonsense adjustments. Use the following as general guidelines when introducing kids to medicinal plants.

- Nutritives, demulcents, culinary herbs, and fragrant relaxants are all appropriate from the toddler stage and up; simply adjust the dosage based on the child's size.

- Introducing kids to bitter-flavored plants, such as bitter greens, is a good way to get them accustomed to this important taste so prevalent in medicinal plants. Stronger bitters

FURTHER READING

There are lots of great books and resources on kids and herbal nutrition and medicine, including:

Herbal Treatment of Children by Anne McIntyre

An Encyclopedia of Natural Healing for Children and Infants by Mary Bove

Kids, Herbs & Health by Linda B. White, MD, and Sunny Mavor

Naturally Healthy Babies and Children by Aviva Jill Romm

Nature's Children by Juliette de Bairacle Levy

Rosemary Gladstar's Family Herbal by Rosemary Gladstar

Rosemary Gladstar's Herbal Remedies for Children's Health by Rosemary Gladstar

for enhancing digestion can be given to kids beginning at the preteen stage, in moderation, as needed.

- Adaptogens should generally be reserved for teenagers and beyond, with some exceptions. The stimulating adaptogens, like ginseng root, rhodiola, and eleuthero, aren't appropriate for young people—they already have lots of energy! Choose milder, nourishing adaptogens, like goji berry and amla berry, or nutritive preparations like chyawanprash for children. In India and other places where adaptogens and tonics are widely used, it's common for kids to take shatavari or ashwagandha from their teenage years on.
And in Asian traditions, the entire family often consumes adaptogenic tonics in traditional dishes like Wei Qi Soup (page 255).

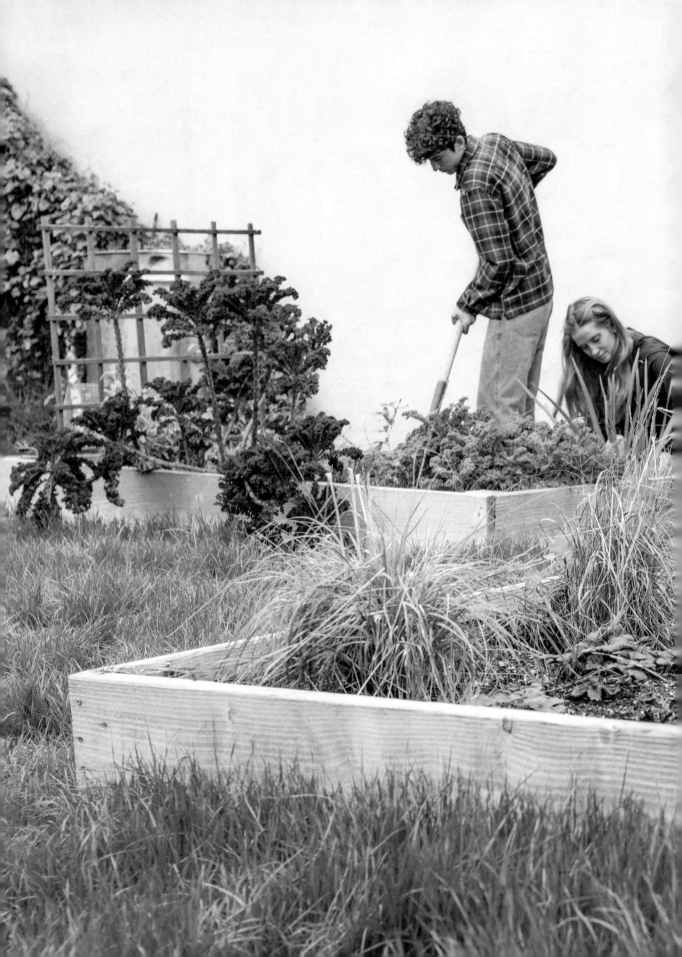

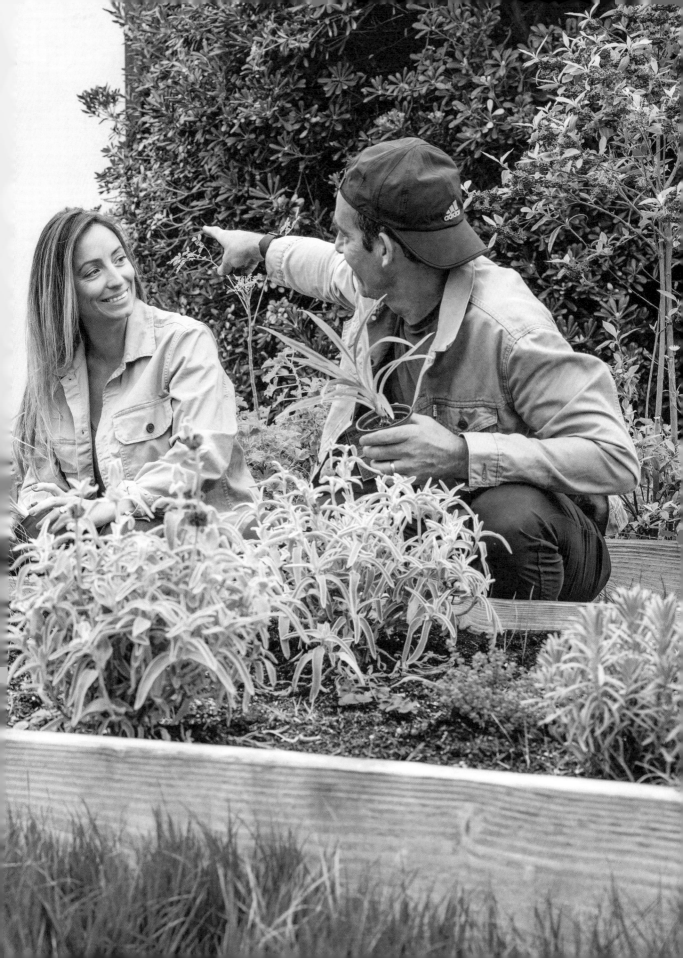

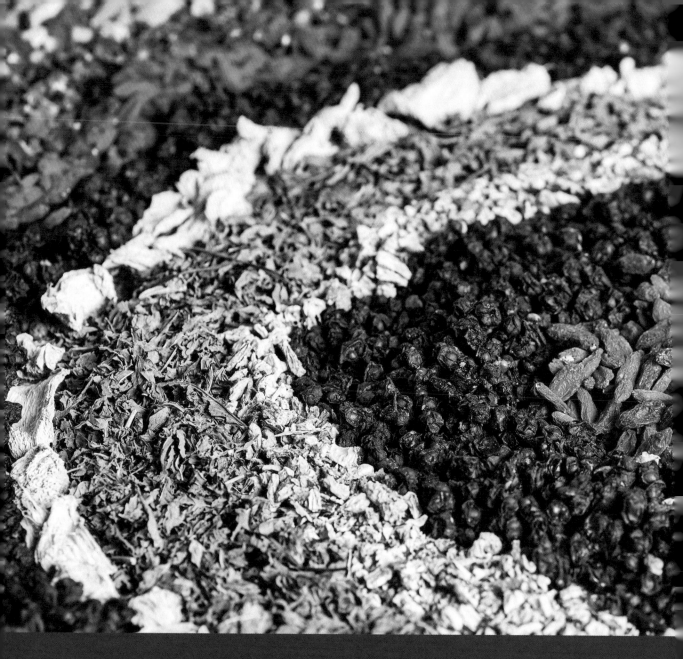

Part IV
PLANT PROFILES

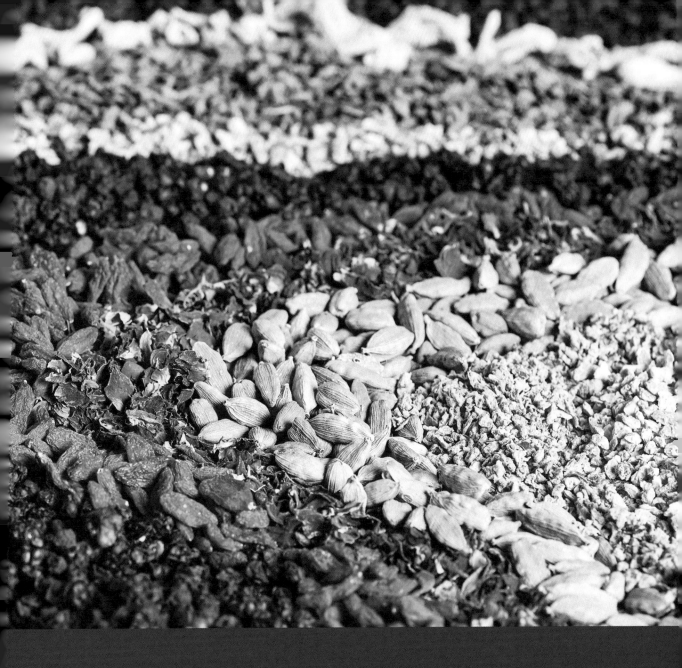

More than anything else, this book is about creating a relationship with medicinal plants. In this section, I delve a little deeper into the most essential medicinal plants from all categories—their history, traditional uses over time, and functional health benefits. At the close of each profile is a list of common ways to use the plant in your daily life.

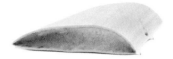

Aloe Vera
(*Aloe vera*)

DEMULCENT

This handsome North African succulent is a familiar ornamental presence in homes and gardens around the world. It thrives in hot, dry environments thanks to its ability to retain water in gel form. When consumed, this gel is deeply hydrating and nourishing to the entire system, like a spa treatment for your insides.

Aloe gel contains compounds that accelerate new cell growth and enhance the synthesis of collagen and hyaluronic acid, essentials for building healthy, moisturized skin and mucous membranes.

When applied topically, aloe vera improves the healing of wounds and scars and reduces the inflammation, itching, and swelling associated with burns, stings, bites, and virtually any other inflammatory skin issue.

Consuming aloe vera juice and/or gel on a regular basis soothes, lubricates, and revitalizes the GI tract, repairing the inevitable wear and tear, microinflammation, and occasional digestive disturbances the gut lining is subject to. Aloe is also a deeply nourishing superfood with an exceptional micronutrient profile. It's rich in iron, magnesium, potassium, zinc, and vitamins A, B_{12}, and E, along with plenty of antioxidants and healing enzymes.

How to Saturate Your Day

- The medicinal constituents in aloe vera gel are fragile and tend to degrade rapidly, so extracting fresh aloe gel directly from the leaves is by far the most potent way to get the goods—for instructions, see page 193.

- You'll find ready-to-drink aloe vera beverages in most natural food stores. Look for ones that are cold processed without preservatives, fillers, and added sugar. Preparations containing the actual gel (unprocessed) combined with extracted liquid are more potent but can be a bit thick—you can add it to water to make them drinkable.

- Concentrated liquids and gels are available as supplements.

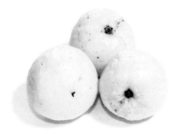

Amla Berry
(*Emblica officinalis*)

ADAPTOGEN/NUTRITIVE

Native to the Indian subcontinent, amla berries (also known as Indian gooseberries) are sour-tasting superfruits about the size of a small plum. They've been treasured in Ayurveda for millennia as a nourishing food and rejuvenating tonic—in Sanskrit they are sometimes referred to as *sarvadosha hara*, meaning "remover of all diseases," thanks to their full-spectrum, health-enhancing benefits.

Amla berries have been the subject of hundreds of studies analyzing their unique compounds and applications for enhancing health and promoting longevity. They are an extraordinarily rich source of free radical–scavenging antioxidants and essential nutrients (they contain the highest content of bioavailable vitamin C of any fruit) that boost immunity and cellular defenses. These superfruits show immense potential for improving diseases and conditions rooted in chronic inflammation, including cardiovascular issues such as elevated cholesterol and high blood pressure. In addition, they have been shown to improve vision (by preventing atrophy of the eyes due to free-radical damage), strengthen digestion, stabilize blood sugar, enhance detoxification and liver function, and reduce wrinkles and aging skin.

How to Saturate Your Day

- Dried powders and powdered extracts are readily available and the most common way to use amla berries. They have a strong sour flavor that is most palatable when blended with sweeter ingredients into antioxidant smoothies; see my Super Berry Power Powder Blend on page 158.

- Fresh amla berries are (slightly) sweeter than dried. They grow during the winter months in India, and are available online and can sometimes be found in Asian groceries in vacuum-sealed bags that preserve freshness. They are also used in juices and condiments such as chutneys and pickles. Amla berries are a primary ingredient in the Ayurvedic jam chyawanprash (page 246), a delicious and simple way to incorporate them into your daily routine.

- Amla berries are also sold in tablet and capsule forms.

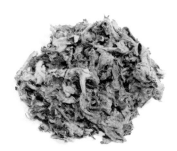

Artichoke Leaf (*Cynara scolymus*)

BITTER/DETOXIFYING

One of the world's oldest and most nutritious vegetables, artichokes are cultivated and eaten throughout the world. For medicinal purposes, the emphasis is solely on the leaves. A tea made from artichoke leaves has been used as a remedy for liver and digestive issues in Asia and the Mediterranean for centuries. Artichoke leaf is especially popular in Vietnam, where it is the main ingredient in a refreshing digestive tonic and hangover cure often consumed during hot weather known as *nước khổ qua lá dứa*, which translates to "cooling water." It's common to encounter people on the streets of Hanoi purchasing this vibrant green beverage from street vendors. The drink typically includes fresh or dried artichoke leaves, ginger or galangal, lemongrass, sugar, and pandan leaves—an aromatic tropical leaf that gives *nước khổ qua lá dứa* its tantalizing fragrance.

Like its relative milk thistle (page 331), the artichoke is a member of the thistle family and contains a host of antioxidants and other compounds that protect the liver from inflammation and oxidative stress while stimulating the regeneration of new cells. It's a rich source of vitamins A, B_6, and C as well as magnesium, iron, calcium, potassium, phosphorus, and zinc. Drinking artichoke tea is a reliable way to improve digestion, stimulate production of liver bile (thus improving the breakdown of fats and proteins), regulate cholesterol, and balance blood sugar.

How to Saturate Your Day

- Artichoke tea can be made from dried or fresh leaves. If using dry, make an infusion of loose leaves or tea bags. Fresh leaves need to be simmered or decocted (see page 94) to extract the constituents. The tea's mildly bitter, vegetal flavor is enjoyable and doesn't require sweeteners; it also blends well with other herbs and spices such as chamomile and lemongrass. For a recipe based on nước khổ qua lá dứa, see page 129.

- Artichoke leaf is also available in tincture, tablet, and capsule form. Use it for a daily detox or to treat specific issues, such as digestive disorders. When using artichoke leaf supplements, look for those standardized for cynarin and caffeoylquinic acid content.

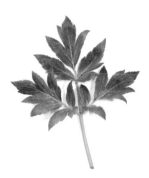

Ashitaba
(*Angelica keiskei*)

NUTRITIVE

This ancient super-nutritive plant is native to a group of volcanic islands off the coast of Japan renowned for the physical endurance and longevity of its residents. A member of the carrot family, ashitaba is considered a dietary staple on these islands and a key factor in its citizens' excellent health.

Ashitaba's name in Japanese means "tomorrow's leaf," referring to its fast-growing, energetic nature and capacity to rejuvenate those who eat it. In Japan, all parts of the plant—root, leaf, and stem—are eaten fresh, consumed as a tea (with a flavor similar to green tea), added to soba noodles and tempura, and even infused into sake.

Ashitaba contains a wide range of vitamins, minerals, and trace elements (calcium, magnesium, potassium, iron, beta-carotene, other B vitamins, vitamin C) and notable fiber content. What distinguishes it from other nutritive plants is a group of unique polyphenolic antioxidants called chalcones found in the yellow sap of ashitaba leaves and stems. Studies have found that chalcones enhance the rate at which cells remove waste and debris, a process called autophagy and one essential for cellular renewal. These findings correspond to the traditional use of ashitaba in Japanese herbal medicine as a nutrient-dense food that strengthens immunity, supports the organs of detoxification, and increases longevity.

How to Saturate Your Day

- Fresh ashitaba has a vegetal, celery-like flavor that's slightly bitter and aromatic. It can be eaten in salads, used as a garnish, or cooked into soups and stir-fries. You can often find fresh ashitaba at Japanese markets, and it's easy to grow from seed.

- Ashitaba is available dried as a cut-and-sifted herb for making infusions and for use in tea bags. You can sprinkle dried crushed leaves onto dishes as a condiment or add them to a condiment blend.

- Ashitaba as a nutritive powder can be mixed into smoothies, elixirs, or your favorite beverages (see Green Power Powder Blend, page 158).

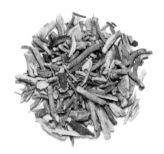

Ashwagandha Root
(*Withania somnifera*)

ADAPTOGEN

Ashwagandha is a premier adaptogen and nervous system tonic all in one. Sometimes referred to as Indian ginseng, this root is prized in Ayurvedic medicine much the same way that ginseng (page 318) is in Traditional Chinese Medicine. *Ashwagandha* means "smell of a horse" in Sanskrit, referring to both the scent of the root and its ability to give people exceptional strength and stamina. Its botanical name *somnifera* translates as "sleep enhancing," in reference to ashwagandha's calming effects. This dual action—increasing energy and endurance while providing a calming effect on the nervous system—makes ashwagandha's powerful medicinal root an ideal adaptogen when you're "wired and tired" (that is, overwhelmed by long-term stress and exhaustion coupled with anxiety and insomnia).

Taking ashwagandha root helps revitalize the system by reducing anxiety, replenishing energy reserves, balancing cortisol levels, improving cognitive function, and promoting deep, restorative sleep. In Ayurveda, ashwagandha is also used to increase muscle tone and strength; enhance libido, fertility, and reproductive hormones in both men and women; build up iron levels in the blood; and fortify immune function.

How to Saturate Your Day

- Dried ashwagandha root is easy to incorporate into your diet. It has a sweet, earthy flavor, almost like a yam or other root vegetable, and blends well with many foods.

- Whole-root powder is easy to mix into adaptogenic smoothies, foods, and beverages (see the recipes for Ashwagandha Deep Rest Replenisher on page 253 and Cacao Adaptogenic Energy Balls on page 255). The powder can be mixed into a small amount of water or a plant-based milk for a quick dose of adaptogenic nourishment.

- Ashwagandha also comes in a variety of concentrated powdered extracts, capsules, tablets, and tinctures. When using ashwagandha supplements, look for standardized content of withanolides, the main active constituents in ashwagandha. See the Resources on page 352 for recommendations.

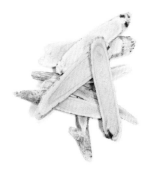

Astragalus Root (*Astragalus membranaceus*)

ADAPTOGEN

Astragalus root, an adaptogen in the same plant family as peas and beans, has been used for centuries in Asia for its powerful vitality-enhancing effects. An integral remedy in Traditional Chinese Medicine, astragalus is often combined with other tonic herbs like ginseng root (page 318), goji berry (page 319), and licorice root (page 325) into formulas for increasing energy and endurance. It is especially prized for its ability to replenish immune reserves depleted from chronic stress, overexertion, and prolonged illness.

Widely used as part of Fu Zheng therapy, a system developed in China incorporating herbs that protect the immune system and raise vitality for those undergoing intensive medical procedures, astragalus root is also commonly taken preventively in Chinese households, to improve immunity during chilly winter months and speed recovery from a lingering cold, flu, or respiratory condition. The root contains a dense concentration of immune-boosting polysaccharides, which have been shown to enhance both innate and adaptive immunity by increasing the proliferation and activity of cytokines, immunoglobulin, and a host of other immune factors.

Astragalus also acts as a healing accelerant for slow-healing wounds and injuries—the rich yellow roots get their color from an assortment of unique flavonoids that reduce inflammation and stimulate the generation of new cells.

How to Saturate Your Day

- Astragalus root, like most adaptogens, is made of tough, woody material that benefits from extended decocting to extract the active constituents (more on decoctions on page 94). In Asia, it is common to decoct whole astragalus roots to create flavorful medicinal broths to boost immune function (see Wei Qi Soup, page 255); you can also simply add astragalus root powder to the broth or soup of your choosing. Dried astragalus roots (both whole and in powder form) are available in herbal pharmacies, at Asian grocers, and online.

- Adaptogenic beverages and elixirs can be made from decoctions or infusions of the cut roots, or from astragalus powder.

- Astragalus root is available in capsules, tablets, and tinctures. When using astragalus root supplements, look for standardized content of polysaccharide.

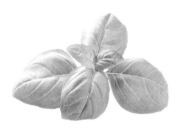

Basil Leaf
(*Ocimum basilicum*)
CULINARY

Basil is a mint-family plant native to India. The name basil comes from the Greek *basileus*, which means "king" or "royal," referring to the high esteem in which basil has long been held. Cultivation of the more than 150 different varieties of basil has spanned at least five thousand years. It is an integral ingredient in many cuisines for both its flavor and its medicinal actions, including kindling digestive fire, relaxing nerves in the gut, and enhancing the assimilation of nutrients. The polyphenols in basil are highly nourishing to the microbiome, while eugenol (a component in the essential oil) and other antimicrobial compounds help neutralize harmful bacteria without disturbing the friendly flora.

In addition to its primary role in digestive health, basil has an abundance of antioxidants that reduce inflammation throughout the body. It's beneficial for cardiovascular health, lessening oxidative stress on blood vessels, enhancing circulation, and mildly lowering blood pressure. Incorporating the flavorful trio of basil, garlic, and olive oil into your daily diet is a triple boost for optimal cardiovascular health.

The essential oils that give basil its distinctive fragrance have a long history of use for elevating mood and relaxing the nervous system, as well as stimulating blood circulation to the brain for improved clarity and mental alertness. Fresh basil is an excellent source of vitamin K, calcium, magnesium, manganese, phosphorus, and potassium.

How to Saturate Your Day

- Toss handfuls of fresh basil into dishes for a nutritional and medicinal boost, or add the dried herb, alone or in spice blends, in recipes of all kinds.

- Basil is available in both extract and capsule form for a more concentrated, medicinal dose.

- Diffuse basil essential oil to take advantage of its cognitive-enhancing effects.

Basil Seed
(*Ocimum basilicum*)
DEMULCENT

Basil seeds are a rising star in the world of medicinal foods thanks to their many health benefits (which both Ayurveda and Traditional Chinese Medicine have utilized for centuries). In India, where they are known as *sabja*, the seeds are commonly consumed in beverages with lemon and mint to rehydrate in hot weather.

Basil seeds share many of the same uses and benefits as chia seeds (page 310). Like chia, they are a rich source of dietary fiber—1 tablespoon of basil seeds provides approximately 7 to 8 g fiber. This high fiber content supports healthy digestion and elimination as well as balanced blood sugar and cholesterol levels. They're nutrient-dense, packed with iron, calcium, magnesium, potassium, and omega-3 and -6 fatty acids as well as an abundance of flavonoids, polyphenols, and other antioxidants. They are also rich in soothing mucilage, supporting gut health and providing ample prebiotic nourishment for the microbiome.

How to Saturate Your Day

• Basil seeds should be soaked before consuming. Soak 1 tablespoon basil seeds in 2 cups (480 ml) water for 5 minutes. Each seed will puff up into a demulcent gel about three times its size. If you prefer a less-viscous preparation, begin with more liquid or add more after soaking, until the desired consistency is achieved. This seedy gel makes a great base for all sorts of nutritious and refreshing beverages (see Basil Seed–Infused Water, page 182). It blends well with lemon or lime juice and

fresh mint or basil leaves. Or add it to creamy beverages and smoothies.

• Presoak the seeds in coconut or oat milk as a base for a nutrient-dense breakfast pudding; see page 194.

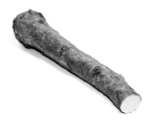

Burdock Root
(*Arctium* species)
BITTER/DETOXIFIER/NUTRITIVE

Native to Europe and northern Asia and now found growing throughout the world, burdock is a nutrient-dense, functional food that both nourishes and mildly detoxifies. It's particularly popular in Japan, where it is known as *gobo* and eaten along with other root vegetables.

Burdock is a dynamic accumulator: Its roots burrow deep into the soil, drawing up and concentrating vital minerals and trace elements. It's a nutritional supplement on your plate, rich in potassium, magnesium, selenium, riboflavin, iron, phosphorus, and vitamins C and E and high in the antioxidants luteolin and quercetin. Rich in the prebiotic fiber inulin, burdock is also soothing and beneficial to the gut, providing nourishment to the microbiome and balancing blood sugar.

In the Western herbal tradition, burdock is classified as an "alterative," a term describing a plant's ability to gradually "alter" the terrain of the body through improved detoxification. Burdock has long been used in traditional herbalism to regulate liver function and improve all manner of inflammatory skin, joint, and connective tissue conditions resulting from an accumulation of toxins.

How to Saturate Your Day

- Like a souped-up parsnip or carrot, burdock root can be prepared in similar ways: braised and cooked into stir-fries, added to miso soup, or pickled and served as an appetizer. It's the main ingredient in the famous Japanese soy-and-sake-glazed stir-fry kinpira (page 133).

- Burdock root is available as a cut, dried herb in tea bags and loose for making teas and infusions. Burdock tea has a pleasant flavor; regularly consumed, it stimulates liver and digestive functions. Dried burdock can also be added to blends with other nutritious or detoxifying herbs such as dandelion, licorice, and ginger roots and milk thistle seeds (see Spring Cleaning Tonic, page 128).

- It can also be found in tablet, capsule, and tincture form.

- Cold-pressed burdock oil is nutritious and rich in omega fatty acids, and prized for its external uses, including as a hair growth serum and in antiaging skin care. It comes in pressed oil, cream, and salve-extract formulations for these purposes.

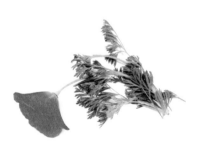

California Poppy
(*Eschscholzia californica*)

NERVINE CALMATIVE

California poppy is a beautiful orange-blossomed perennial herb native to the West Coast of the United States. The Indigenous peoples of the West used its roots, leaves, and flowers for pain relief: They chewed on the roots for toothaches and made the plant into a tea to alleviate headaches and the pain of menstruation.

A cousin of the infamous opium poppy, California poppy is far less powerful by comparison and has no morphine or other opiate alkaloids—but it is a reliable remedy for insomnia, anxiety, and pain. In fact, it first gained popularity as a nonaddictive, nonnarcotic substitute for the opium poppy. California poppy has sedative and hypnotic constituents that relax the central nervous system, and higher doses induce drowsiness and sleep. It improves sleep quality and duration without morning fatigue or dullness. Although primarily a remedy for pain and insomnia, California poppy can be used in small amounts during the day to calm anxiety and restlessness, allowing for better focus and concentration.

When it comes to treating pain, California poppy has analgesic properties that create a sort of white noise around the condition, dulling the sensation and awareness of discomfort. Antispasmodic compounds promote increased circulation and encourage relaxation and the capacity to rest.

How to Saturate Your Day

- California poppy is most commonly used in supplement form: as a tablet, capsule, or tincture. It is sold on its own or in combination with other relaxing herbs.

- The bitter taste of California poppy makes it less desirable as a beverage, but you can find it in tea bags.

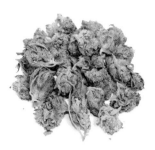

Cannabis
(*Cannabis sativa*)

NERVINE CALMATIVE

The cannabis plant originates from Central Asia, where it has a history of medicinal use among the ancient Greeks and Romans, as well as within Ayurvedic and Traditional Chinese Medicine traditions, going back some five thousand years. CBD (cannabidiol) is one of the two main cannabinoids found in the cannabis plant, with THC (tetrahydrocannabinol) being the other. CBD is a safe and reliable nonpsychoactive (i.e., it doesn't make you high) option when used on its own, and it comes in a wide variety of forms and preparations. Taken for both long- and short-term benefits, CBD exhibits no evidence for abuse or dependence according to the World Health Organization.

The human body has its own internal endocannabinoid system of neurotransmitters and receptors that play an essential role in regulating physiological functions related to mood, sleep, pain, and inflammation, among others. Our internal cannabinoids resemble the ones produced by the cannabis plant. Binding to the same receptor sites that activate our internal endocannabinoid system, CBD is highly beneficial for relaxing the nervous system, improving mood and cognitive function, relieving pain, and enhancing sleep, among many other effects.

The CBD industry has developed at breakneck speed and has a way to go when it comes to regulations and standards of efficacy. More and more foods and products are being used as delivery mechanisms for cannabidiol, and many are inadequately regulated—and concentrations vary widely, from just a small percentage all the way to 100 percent pure CBD isolates. That being said, there are reputable companies making highly efficacious products (see the Resources, page 352).

How to Saturate Your Day

- There are three primary CBD products available: Full-spectrum CBD extracts have all of the components of cannabis plants, including cannabinoids, terpenes, and a small amount of THC. Broad-spectrum CBD contains all components of cannabis except for THC. CBD isolates contain only CBD with no other components.

- CBD is available in tinctures and gummies and emulsified into carrier oil in liquid or gel caps. When taken orally, CBD preparations usually take effect in 30 to 90 minutes and tend to last for 3 to 4 hours. Dosages vary depending on the individual and the preparation, but some recent research suggests that an effective starting dose for most people is around 10 milligrams. A good guideline: Start low and work up to determine the right dosage for you.

- Smokable and vaporizable forms have a faster effect and are the quickest to be metabolized.

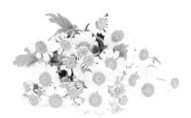

Chamomile
(*Matricaria chamomilla*)

FRAGRANT RELAXANT

Chamomile has been settling minds, easing tension, and improving digestion for over three thousand years. The plant originated in North Africa and southern Europe, but now it's possible to order up a cup of chamomile tea practically anywhere you happen to be on the globe. Of the several varieties available, German chamomile (*Matricaria chamomilla*) is best for daily use. They love it so much in Germany that they have a saying to express their appreciation—"*alles zutraut*," meaning "capable of anything."

This herb is well known for its gentle, calming effects, yet hidden within the delicate white-and-yellow flowers is a complex treasure trove of medicinal benefits. Chamomile contains hundreds of constituents all working synergistically to give it nervous-system-relaxant, antispasmodic effects that ease tension in the gut and reduce bloating, fullness, excessive gas, and painful cramping and colic. Chamomile contains, among many other beneficial compounds, the flavonoid apigenin, which has been shown to improve vagal nerve tone and activate GABA receptors—easing anxiety without creating dullness or fatigue.

A primary component of chamomile's essential oil is chamazulene, a highly anti-inflammatory and antimicrobial compound that cools overheated GI tracts, reduces nerve irritation, and neutralizes microbes. It also lessens the aches and pains from colds and flu, helps people recover more quickly from bouts of illness, and reduces hyperacidity. Chamomile's mild nature and reliable effects make it universally applicable for young and old alike.

How to Saturate Your Day

- Drinking chamomile tea throughout the day can reduce accumulated tension and enhance feelings of ease and flow. Consumed in the evening, it will encourage restful sleep. A moderately strong preparation can be made by steeping two or three tea bags or 2 to 3 teaspoons flowers in 1 to 1½ cups (240 to 360 ml) water for 10 minutes or so. Drink a cup two or three times a day.

- Chamomile is generally mild in action, but it's possible to make a more concentrated infusion for a more powerful effect. Steep 1 ounce (30 g) dried flowers in approximately 1 quart (1 L) water, covered, for 15 to 30 minutes, then strain the liquid and add honey and/or lemon juice to taste.

Remember: The darker the color of the tea, the stronger and more medicinal the effects.

- Chamomile capsules, tablets, and tinctures are all good options.

- Diffusing chamomile essential oil creates a lovely background calm.

- Mixing a few drops of chamomile essential oil into a carrier oil for topical application relaxes muscles; massage into the belly to alleviate tension and pain.

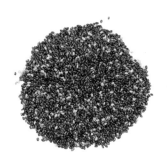

Chia Seed (*Salvia hispanica*)

DEMULCENT

Chia is the seed of a desert sage that grows from Central America and Mexico up into the American Southwest. Once a staple food of the Aztecs and Mayans, this nutrient-dense seed is an essential source of hydration for the Indigenous peoples living in these arid regions. Like other demulcent plants, chia seeds create a mucilaginous gel when combined with water. Consuming this viscous plant water facilitates deep, whole-body hydration; soothes and revitalizes the mucous membranes lining the GI tract; and provides a source of nourishment to the beneficial bacteria of the microbiome.

In his book *Born to Run*, journalist Christopher McDougall introduced readers to the Tarahumara people, indigenous to the canyons of northwestern Mexico and famous for their energy, endurance, and ultra-long-distance running. The Tarahumara make iskiate—a super-energy and hydration elixir of chia seeds, agave nectar, water, and lime juice—that powers them through their desert runs.

The chia seed is a great source of both fiber and protein—1 tablespoon provides 5 to 6 grams of mostly soluble fiber and 2 to 3 grams protein. It supports healthy digestion and elimination and helps balance blood sugar and cholesterol levels in a similar way to basil seeds (page 307). Chia seeds are a substantial source of omega-3 fatty acids and contain a trove of minerals and trace elements such as magnesium, copper, selenium, calcium, iron, and phosphorus.

How to Saturate Your Day

- Chia is a versatile food and easy to integrate into the diet. It has a nutty flavor reminiscent of sesame or poppy seeds. Sprinkle a teaspoon or two on cereals, salads, soups, stir-fries, or smoothies.

- Like basil seed (page 307), chia seed is a perfect base for any number of crowd-pleasing pudding recipes. Soak 1 tablespoon seeds in approximately 2 cups (480 ml) water for 5 minutes. Each seed will puff up into a demulcent gel about three times its size. If you prefer a less-viscous preparation, just begin with more liquid or add more after soaking, until the desired consistency is achieved.

- I have personally used and recommended a version of the Tarahumara iskiate for years (Chia-Aloe-Lime Rehydrator, page 193). Consumed first thing in the morning, this elixir is a super-rehydrating way to start the day. I add fresh aloe vera to mine for an extra boost of hydration.

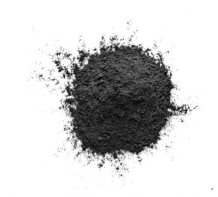

Chlorella & Spirulina (*Chlorella pyrenoidosa* & *Arthrospira platensis*)

NUTRITIVE

These microalgae are among the oldest known forms of plant life on earth and have been used as highly nutritious, rejuvenating superfoods since at least the times of the Mayan and Aztec civilizations. Both chlorella and spirulina have extraordinarily high concentrations of nutrients and antioxidants that are easy for the body to assimilate. Along with a broad spectrum of trace minerals, iron, potassium, magnesium, zinc, copper, phosphorus, folic acid, vitamins A and C, and several B vitamins, they contain plenty of fiber and omega fatty acids (particularly chlorella) as well as all nine amino acids, which makes them excellent sources of complete plant-based protein.

Chlorella and spirulina support the processes of detoxification and help the body remove toxic chemicals, including pesticide residues and heavy metals, and neutralize free radicals.

How to Saturate Your Day

- Chlorella and spirulina come in powder and extract forms that can be mixed into elixirs, smoothies, and beverages.

- They can also be found in supplement form as tablets, capsules, and gummies.

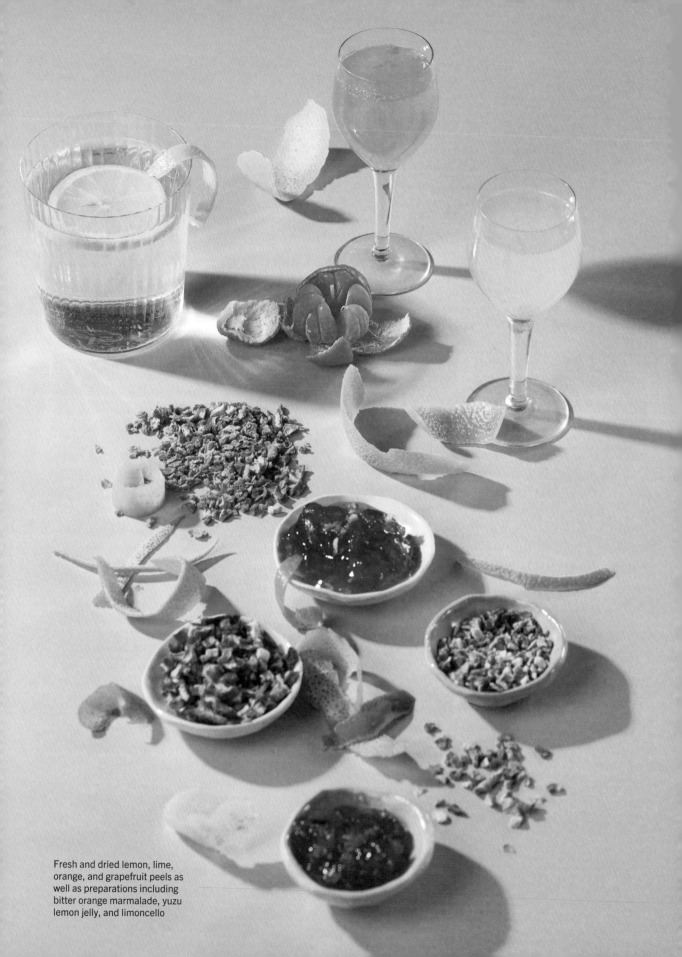

Fresh and dried lemon, lime, orange, and grapefruit peels as well as preparations including bitter orange marmalade, yuzu lemon jelly, and limoncello

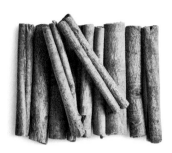

Cinnamon
(*Cinnamomum verum* & *C. cassia*)

CULINARY

Ceylon cinnamon (*Cinnamomum verum*) comes from the smooth inner bark of a medium-size evergreen native to the island of Sri Lanka; cassia cinnamon comes from the bark of the *C. cassia* tree. The bark is stripped from the branches of mature trees, cut into thin pieces, and sun-dried into "quills." Cinnamon's beautiful fragrance and medicinal benefits come from its high essential oil content.

Among the antioxidant-rich spices, cinnamon is second only to cloves when tested for ORAC value (the measure of the antioxidant capacity of plants). It is highly beneficial for cardiovascular health, reducing inflammation in blood vessels and helping to regulate cholesterol and mildly lower blood pressure.

Cinnamon also has blood-sugar-moderating effects that improve metabolic efficiency and increase energy levels, helping us maintain a healthy weight. Recent studies suggest that we can get these benefits by consuming ½ teaspoon of cinnamon powder in a small amount of water after major meals.

How to Saturate Your Day

- Cinnamon chips, sticks, and/or powder are a wonderful addition to both sweet and savory dishes.

- Drink cinnamon tea (see page 128) before, during, or after meals to kindle agni, improving the breakdown of food and assimilation of nutrients.

- Cinnamon is available as capsules and concentrated extracts.

Citrus Peels

CULINARY/DETOXIFYING

Drinking lemon water first thing in the morning is perhaps the simplest and most universal daily detox routine. The peels of lemons and all other citruses—including grapefruits, tangerines, mandarins, and oranges—contain far more vitamin C than the fruit's pulp and juice, along with synergistic flavonoids and other potent antioxidants that enhance the immune response and help fight off colds, flus, and respiratory conditions.

All citrus peels have both digestive and detoxification benefits. Citrus peels support digestion by increasing the secretion of hydrochloric acid, digestive enzymes, and bile. Peels that are sour and highly aromatic have more agni-kindling effects. The organic acids in citrus peels also help dissolve toxins in the GI tract, stimulate breakdown of cholesterol, increase fat metabolism, lower blood glucose levels, and improve liver detoxification. The more bitter the peel, like that of grapefruit and bitter orange, the stronger the detoxifying effect.

Citrus peels form the base for a wide variety of teas, elixirs, wines, jams, and marmalades. Some favorite examples include limoncello, the Italian digestif made with the zest of giant Sorrento lemons; Seville orange marmalade made in Spain from the peels of the bitter orange (*Citrus aurantium*); in Japan, lemon condiments and medicinal wines made with yuzu (*C. junos*), the unique orange-shaped lemon that contains three times more vitamin C than a typical lemon; and tangerine peel tea, a popular after-dinner beverage made from citrus grown on the tropical island of Jeju in Korea.

How to Saturate Your Day

- Use *only* organic fruits—pesticide residue tends to remain on fruit peels.

- Sprinkle grated citrus peel onto dishes.

- Add fresh zest to hot water and strain off to make a citrus peel tea.

- Add dried citrus peels to hot or cold teas and infusions.

- Gel caps of D-limonene (orange peel oil extract) offer concentrated digestive and liver function support. When using D-limonene supplements, look for products standardized to 98 percent D-limonene.

- Citrus peels in powder and powdered extract forms can be added to smoothies and other beverages.

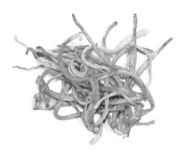

Cordyceps
(*Cordyceps sinensis* & *C. militaris*)

ADAPTOGEN

This rare and precious longevity tonic thrives above the clouds in the Himalayan mountain countries throughout Asia. Legend has it that yak herders first discovered its medicinal properties after observing increased energy and vitality in animals that grazed in meadows containing the mushrooms. In the traditional medicine of the Himalayan region, cordyceps are used to boost energy, endurance, immune function, libido, and fertility and treat a wide range of conditions, from asthma to cardiovascular disease to chronic kidney disorders.

They have long been relied upon by mountaineers for their capacity to increase oxygenation and improve acclimatization to high altitudes. In the Sikkim region around India, Nepal, and Bhutan, it is common for people to drink shots of barley wine infused with dried cordyceps to promote vigor as they advance in age.

Cordyceps's reputation as a longevity enhancer is due in part to its ability to increase the activity of superoxide dismutase, a vital enzyme responsible for breaking down free radicals and reducing inflammation, helping to protect vital organs and slow aging at a cellular level. Like other medicinal mushrooms (see page 328), cordyceps is richly concentrated in immune-enhancing polysaccharides, which increase the proliferation and activity of immune cells.

Wild Himalayan cordyceps are still harvested the traditional way, relying on people painstakingly searching through meadows by hand to find these elusive treasures—so it's not surprising that wild cordyceps are among the most expensive medicinal plants in the world today, literally worth more than their weight in gold. Cultivated cordyceps containing most of the same beneficial constituents are now widely available as a much more affordable and sustainable option.

How to Saturate Your Day

- Cordyceps' mild umami flavor makes them versatile and easy to incorporate into a variety of foods and recipes.

- They are commonly available as dried powder and powdered extract. Powders can be added to soups and broths (see Wei Qi Soup, page 255), sprinkled onto stir-fries, or blended into smoothies, coffee, cacao, and other beverages. They're also an ingredient in my Cacao Adaptogenic Energy Balls (page 255). You can purchase whole dried cordyceps online to grind into your own powder or decoct in water (more on decoctions on page 94).

- Cordyceps are available in capsules and tablets and dual-extracted tinctures (a process using a combination of hot water and alcohol, which ensures extraction of all active constituents; see page 97 for more on this method).

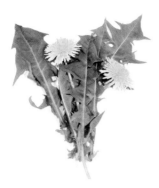

Dandelion
(*Taraxacum officinale*)

BITTER/NUTRITIVE

Although the dandelion is largely considered a lowly weed in the United States, many cultures around the world view it as an important nutrient-dense food. The Greeks make the side dish horta vrasta from dandelion greens that are briefly boiled and dressed with lemon and olive oil (see page 133). In France, dandelion greens are a complement to salads, where they are called *pissenlit*, meaning "wet the bed," owing to their mild diuretic effects.

Like burdock (page 307), dandelion has a large taproot that efficiently absorbs nutrients from deep within the soil, making it an excellent source of potassium, calcium, iron, magnesium, folate, and vitamins A, C, and E. The roots contain an abundance of inulin (40 percent by weight), a powerful prebiotic fiber that helps balance blood sugar and nourish the microbiome.

Dandelion leaves and roots contain glycosides, terpenes, tannins, and other constituents that give them their mildly bitter flavor and detoxifying actions. These compounds activate digestion and metabolism, increase bile flow in the liver, and improve elimination. Dandelion is also a gentle "potassium sparing" diuretic, meaning it enhances the kidneys' removal of nitrogenous wastes without depleting this vital electrolyte. Dandelion is one of the gentler detoxifying herbs, encouraging the organs of detox to function better without risk of irritating the body.

How to Saturate Your Day

- Wild dandelion greens are a favorite among foragers, but you can also purchase them at most grocery stores. The smaller, younger leaves are more tender and less bitter. Eat fresh spring greens raw in salads or add small amounts to supercharge a green juice blend. Dressing the greens with lemon and olive oil improves the assimilation of nutrients and helps bring out their fullest flavor. To cut down on bitterness, use half dandelion greens and half spinach.

- The tastiest way to consume dandelion roots is in a robust, nutritious dry-roasted brew that tastes coffee-ish but doesn't contain caffeine or jangle the nerves. You can find dandelion root powdered on its own or combined into coffee substitutes with other herbs (see Dandelion, Chicory, and Carob Latte, page 127). Dandelion roots can be made into a decoction (see page 94) or added to a detoxifying tea blend.

- Dandelion leaves and roots are also available as capsules, tablets, and tinctures.

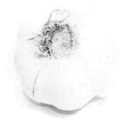

Garlic
(*Allium sativum*)

CULINARY

Garlic's health-enhancing benefits are legendary: It was given raw to Olympians in Greece to increase stamina, carried by Roman soldiers as a first-aid remedy, and used in ancient China to eradicate pathogens and purify water. It was even found in the tomb of King Tut, who apparently wanted to carry his own supply into the afterlife.

Garlic's distinctive fragrance comes from its high concentration of potent antimicrobial sulfur compounds (allicin and ajoene), which activate digestion and kill harmful bacteria, yeasts, and other microorganisms in the GI tract—all without harming the gut's friendly flora. Garlic is also a good source of glutathione; sulfur, a major constituent in glutathione, enhances detoxification functions and protects the liver from inflammation.

These sulfur compounds, along with essential nutrients like vitamins B_6 and C, magnesium, and a host of flavonoids, are also responsible for garlic's long-standing use as a tonic for the cardiovascular system, particularly in combination with olive oil. Regular consumption of garlic has been shown to reduce cholesterol, prevent formation of plaques in the vessels, enhance circulation, decrease inflammation in blood vessels, and decrease blood pressure.

How to Saturate Your Day

- Both cooked and fresh garlic have antimicrobial effects, but those actions are more concentrated when the plant is fresh. Whether eating it cooked or uncooked, crush or chop the fresh garlic and let it sit for 10 minutes before consuming. This exposure to oxygen activates the enzyme alliinase, which transforms into ajoene and allicin, the two most potent antimicrobial sulfur compounds.

- Aged garlic (aka fermented garlic), which uses proprietary processes to boost the antioxidant and anti-inflammatory activity of garlic, is recommended for cardiovascular health.

- Garlic comes in many tablet and capsule forms. When using garlic supplements, look for standardized content of sulfides and allicin, the most important active ingredients for immune benefits. Parsley or chlorophyll is sometimes added to garlic supplements to diminish the pungent odor and make the supplements gentler on digestion. You can also purchase allicin extract in capsules or tablets.

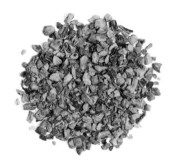

Gentian Root (*Gentiana* species)

BITTER

Gentian is among the most powerful and widely used digestive-enhancing herbs in the world, with more than three hundred species growing throughout the alpine regions of North America, Europe, and Asia. Gentian root is a primary ingredient in many bitter liquors and supplements, including the famous Angostura bitters from Argentina, a mainstay of virtually every bar in the world. It's also an important ingredient found in many Chinese and Ayurvedic medicinal formulations.

Gentian contains a host of bitter constituents that stimulate receptors on the tongue, increasing the production of saliva, hydrochloric acid, digestive enzymes, and bile from the liver and gallbladder. This results in an overall improvement in the digestive system's capacity to break down food and assimilate nutrients. Taking small amounts of gentian on a regular basis strengthens the muscle tone lining the GI tract, improving elimination. Although gentian can be used as a digestive aid on its own, it's more often found as part of a formulation designed to rejuvenate the digestive system and treat issues like poor appetite, bloating, excessive gas, hyperacidity, and constipation.

How to Saturate Your Day

- Gentian is an extremely bitter-tasting herb, mostly used as a component in bitter liquors or tinctures that are designed to be taken in small amounts before or after meals to enhance digestion.

- Gentian is also available in tablet and capsule forms. While tasting the herb amplifies its effects, bitter receptors lining the stomach stimulate the production of digestive enzymes. Chew the tablets a little before swallowing to get the most out of their constituents.

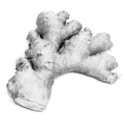

Gingerroot
(*Zingiber officinale*)

CULINARY

Native to Southeast Asia and now cultivated throughout the tropics, gingerroot (technically an underground stem, or rhizome) is widely used the world over. The earliest known record of its application as a digestive medicine was written over 2,500 years ago by Confucius, who is said to have never eaten a meal without it. In Ayurveda, ginger is called *vishwabhesaj*, or "the universal medicine"— there is virtually no health condition or constitutional type it doesn't benefit.

Ayurvedic practitioners prescribe ginger to dissolve ama, or toxins, produced as a result of poor digestion and the basis for most chronic diseases. Ginger prevents the formation of toxins by increasing metabolism and digestive power. Pungent aromatic oils and compounds found in the rhizome, called gingerols, increase circulation and warmth in the gut, invigorate the production of digestive acid and enzymes, and improve the assimilation of nutrients. Antispasmodic constituents relax the gut, helping alleviate all manner of digestive-related issues, from lack of appetite to bloating, gas, nausea, and cramping to food poisoning. And ginger's flavonoid compounds act as fertilizer to the microbiome, stimulating growth and vitality.

Modern research has identified hundreds of unique antioxidants and other compounds in ginger that offer a broad range of anti-inflammatory effects. Numerous studies have demonstrated ginger's ability to modulate COX-2 (an enzyme responsible for pain and inflammation) inflammatory pathways on par with that of NSAIDs (nonsteroidal anti-inflammatory drugs). Basically anywhere chronic inflammation is an issue, from musculoskeletal and joint issues to acute injuries and migraines all the way to core functions like cardiovascular and metabolic health, ginger can help.

How to Saturate Your Day

- Ginger (as both a fresh root and a dried powder) is a star in the kitchen and can be used in soups, stir-fries, marinades, and as a condiment or in chutneys.

- To kindle agni before a meal, take a Ginger Shot or a piece of Ginger "Pizza"; for recipes, see pages 124 and 114.

- Ginger tea prepared from fresh or dried gingerroot, honey, and lemon is an excellent combination and traditional health tonic.

- Adding ginger to any other formula—such as a tonic or elixir—improves its flavor and efficacy.

- Ginger candies and lozenges made from gingerroot help alleviate nausea and calm nervous indigestion.

- Ginger is available in capsule and tablet forms. When using ginger supplements, look for standardized content of gingerol, a good marker of efficacy.

- Tinctures and liquid ginger extracts are also available.

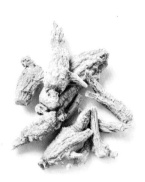

Ginseng Root
(*Panax* species)

ADAPTOGEN

Often referred to as the "king of the tonics," ginseng is perhaps the most widely known and revered of all the adaptogenic herbs. It's the remedy of choice to revitalize those dealing with long-term physical and mental exhaustion. The first recorded description of ginseng was found carved on a tortoise shell in Korea over four thousand years ago (for more on Koreans' love of ginseng, see page 243). In China, the root has been used for centuries by Taoist monks and martial artists to energize and sustain them on their path to longevity and self-mastery.

All species of ginseng are treasured for their ability to increase energy and endurance, improve cognitive function, enhance libido, and activate immunity. Modern studies have confirmed ginseng's ability to enhance mitochondrial production of ATP (the body's energy molecule) at the cellular level. Unique compounds in ginseng called ginsenosides have been shown to enhance blood circulation, increase oxygenation of working muscles, improve cardiovascular output, reduce inflammation, and accelerate repair, making it an excellent choice for enhancing athletic performance and recovery. Long-term use of ginseng also stabilizes endocrine function by reducing the output of cortisol and other stress hormones and stimulating the production of GABA, serotonin, and other mood-elevating neurochemicals.

Ginseng is a slow-growing woodland perennial that takes five to seven years to reach medicinal maturity. It has been vastly overharvested and is currently endangered in the wild. When buying ginseng, look for sustainably grown sources; see the Resources (page 352) for recommended brands.

How to Saturate Your Day

• Tough and woody, ginseng roots are often decocted and consumed in liquid form and/or added to soups and broths. Decoct whole or cut roots, using approximately ½ to 1 ounce (15 to 30 g) cut root per 1 quart (1 L) water, at a low simmer for at least 20 minutes and up to a few hours. (For more on decoction, see page 94.) Consume 1 to 2 cups (240 to 480 ml) a day.

• It's common in parts of Asia to cook ginseng with other herbs, spices, and medicinal mushrooms to make immune-boosting broths during cold and flu season (see Wei Qi Soup, page 255). Samgyetang, a powerful and delicious vitality-enhancing chicken soup using both fresh and dried ginseng roots, is a favorite in restaurants throughout Korea.

• Ginseng makes a great energizing tonic. See the recipe on page 250.

• You can find ginseng in any number of forms, including single-dose liquid pouches, liquid vials, sliced-root gummies, powder, powdered extract, capsules, and tinctures. When using ginseng supplements, look for standardized content of ginsenosides.

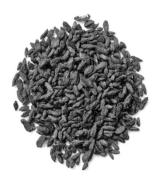

Goji Berry
(*Lycium barbarum*)

ADAPTOGEN/NUTRITIVE

Native to Mongolia and China, goji berry has been a treasured longevity tonic for over two thousand years. Legend has it that the fruit's health-promoting properties were first discovered by a traveling doctor who witnessed centenarians drinking well water surrounded by goji bushes. Upon falling into the well, the ripened berries infused the water with nutrients and vitalizing compounds, giving those who drank it extraordinary health.

In China, goji berries are a dietary staple, incorporated into a variety of dishes. They contain high levels of beta-carotene, vitamins A and C, and a host of other nutrients essential for eye health—mothers tell their children to eat their goji berries for good eyesight the same way American mothers tell their kids to finish their carrots. Antioxidants in the berries (like luteolin, zeaxanthin, and lycopene) quench free radicals, reduce inflammation, and increase circulation in the small capillaries that nourish the eyes. In Traditional Chinese Medicine, gojis are often combined in formulas with other herbs for improving night vision and blurry vision, or simply as a daily tonic for eyesight.

Goji berries increase energy and vitality by providing the body with a reliable source of essential nutrients needed to fuel physiology, including high concentrations of trace elements and minerals like zinc, magnesium, manganese, phosphorus, potassium, and iron, as well as fiber, protein, and omega fatty acids. Consuming gojis on a regular

basis has been shown to boost immune function, balance blood sugar, and improve cholesterol levels.

How to Saturate Your Day

• Gojis are sold dried in health food stores or online. They can be eaten on their own or added to trail mixes, hot or cold cereals, baked goods, soups, and stir-fries. The mild sweetness of whole dried goji berries works well in combination with a variety of medicinal plants (see Goji-Chrysanthemum-Pomegranate Eye-Brightening Elixir, page 157).

• Goji berries are also available in powder and powdered extracts, ideal for blending into elixirs and smoothies (see Peanut Butter–Maca–Goji Berry Smoothie, page 250).

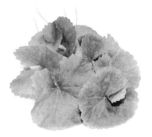

Gotu Kola
(*Centella asiatica*)

NUTRITIVE

Native to Southeast Asia, gotu kola grows in clusters of small electric-green leaves and thrives in wet jungle environments. Legend has it that observing elephants eating wild gotu kola led ancient Sri Lankan people, who revered the intelligence of the great animals, to discover its medicinal and nutritional benefits.

Gotu kola is a broad-spectrum, nutrient-dense green rich in vitamins, minerals, and antioxidants. It is a relative of parsley, celery, and carrots and has a similar flavor profile: vegetal, slightly sweet, and mildly bitter, with distinctive aromatic notes. South Asians consume the plant as a health beverage and nutritional superfood, along the lines of kale or wheatgrass.

Gotu kola is an important plant in traditional Chinese, Indonesian, and Ayurvedic medicine, revered for promoting longevity and revitalizing the nervous system. It's commonly used to sharpen memory and focus, uplift the mood, calm the mind, and enhance deep, restorative sleep. Like other nutritive tonic plants, it helps optimize the removal of metabolic wastes by supporting digestion and kidney functions.

How to Saturate Your Day

- Fresh gotu kola is a tasty, nutritious green in salads, soups, sauces, chutneys, and traditional dishes. The Sri Lankan national dish, gotu kola sambol, is a super salad with fresh gotu kola leaves, chile, lime juice, shredded coconut, shallots, and tomatoes. You can find fresh gotu kola and gotu kola beverages in many South Asian groceries. The plant is also easy to grow as an annual or as a perennial in the southern quarter of the United States—once established, it spreads like mint and you can simply snip some when you need it.

- Fresh gotu kola can be blended into green drinks and smoothies. In Vietnam, gotu kola is a key ingredient in the refreshing energy elixir nước khổ qua lá dứa (see the recipe for Gotu Kola and Lime Clarity Elixir, on page 162, for a riff on this drink). A similar Sri Lankan version, gotu kola kanda, consists of fresh gotu kola juiced or blended with coconut water, citrus, and sweetener.

- Gotu kola is also popular as a healing tea, on its own or as part of a blend.

- It's available in tablet, capsule, tincture, and powder forms as well.

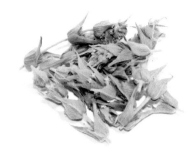

Greek Mountain Tea (*Sideritis* species)

FRAGRANT RELAXANT

The mountains of Greece provide the perfect combination of sun, soil, climate, and altitude for growing healthy medicinal plants. Of the thousands of unique species growing in this region, *tsai tou vounou*—meaning "tea of the mountain" in Greek—stands out. A highly aromatic member of the mint family, it grows in the rocky soils of wildflower meadows at high elevations (3,200 feet/975 m and above), where the air is clear and pure.

Mountain tea (aka ironwood) is easy to love for its light and aromatic flavor with notes of sage, mint, and citrus. It's said that Hippocrates, the father of modern medicine, drank copious amounts of mountain tea. It continues to be a treasured medicinal plant in daily life throughout Greece and is an essential element in the famous, health-enhancing Mediterranean diet.

Mountain tea contains hundreds of constituents with innumerable medicinal benefits. It has anti-inflammatory, immune-boosting, digestive-enhancing, and nervous-system-relaxing effects. It's an excellent source of phytonutrients and potent antioxidants, particularly flavonoids and polyphenols, which protect against free radical damage and turn on cellular defense mechanisms. The concentrations and proportions of these beneficial constituents are on par with those found in green tea (see page 136).

Mountain tea is traditionally served as a warm infusion after meals to promote digestion and calm the nervous system. The aromatic oils relax the gut, increase digestive motility, improve assimilation of nutrients, and reduce gas and bloating. When it is consumed on a regular basis, the nervine calmative actions increase cerebral blood flow, improve memory and attention, calm anxiety, and elevate mood.

How to Saturate Your Day

- Greek mountain tea is primarily used as a tea or infusion. It is most often found in whole uncut form (as stems, leaves, and flowers), which makes choosing the right amount to use subject to a little trial and error. Start off by putting a small handful of uncut Greek mountain tea (maybe four or five stems) in a pan with 1½ to 2 cups (360 to 480 ml) water. Adjust the amount of herb based on the flavor and strength you prefer—and don't worry, you can't get it wrong or overdo it. Cover the pan, place on the stove, and lightly simmer for 3 to 5 minutes. Turn off the heat and let steep for 2 to 3 minutes. Strain into a cup, then feel free to add honey and a squeeze of lemon like the Greeks do. See the Resources, page 352, for recommended sources.

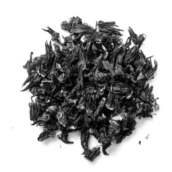

Hibiscus
(*Hibiscus sabdariffa*)

NUTRITIVE/DEMULCENT

An herbaceous shrub native to North Africa, hibiscus is now widely distributed throughout the tropics, and its common names vary regionally, including sorrel, roselle, and flor de Jamaica. Of more than three hundred species of hibiscus, only a handful, including *Hibiscus sabdariffa*, have culinary and medicinal uses.

Dried hibiscus flowers are used to make a variety of tart ruby-red nutrient- and antioxidant-rich beverages that cool and refresh. In Egypt, karkade, a popular iced hibiscus tea consumed to cool down on hot days, is said to have been a favorite drink of the pharaohs. Sorrel, a popular beverage served during holidays and celebrations in Jamaica and the West Indies, combines hibiscus with a variety of tropical spices. In Nigeria, hibiscus is the main ingredient in the favorite traditional drink zobo, which includes pineapple juice, ginger, and sliced oranges.

In addition to making a refreshing beverage and tart tea, hibiscus is a functional food with a high concentration of antioxidants and essential nutrients. It contains a wide variety of phenolic compounds, organic acids, and flavonoids: in particular, anthocyanins, the pigmented antioxidants that give hibiscus flowers their vivid magenta color. Anthocyanins quench free radicals, reduce inflammatory processes, regulate the production of cholesterol in the liver, and mildly lower blood pressure by relaxing blood vessels and increasing circulation—making hibiscus a very good cardiovascular tonic. The plant's significant vitamin C content means it has immune-enhancing benefits and helps maintain and repair the delicate inner lining of blood vessels.

Hibiscus is traditionally consumed as an infusion to help recover from colds, flus, and respiratory conditions. Similar to cranberry juice, it's also a mild diuretic and is often used to treat urinary infections—which benefit from its slight demulcent qualities (hibiscus is in the same plant family as marshmallow; see page 328).

How to Saturate Your Day

- Hibiscus is primarily enjoyed as a hot or cold infusion of dried flowers. Hibiscus combines well in tea and infusion blends containing complementary spices and fragrant relaxants such as lemon balm (page 324), peppermint (page 334), and linden (page 326).

- A significant pectin content makes hibiscus an ideal ingredient in jam or chutney.

- Powdered hibiscus works well in smoothies and berry powder blends (see Super Berry Power Powder Blend, page 158).

- If you're using hibiscus strictly as an antioxidant supplement, capsules and tablets are available.

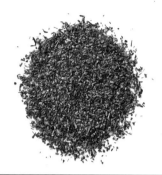

Honeybush & Rooibos (*Cyclopia intermedia* & *Aspalathus linearis*)

FRAGRANT RELAXANT

Honeybush and rooibos are two closely related medicinal plants that grow on a small slice of coastal mountains in the Cederberg region of South Africa. The indigenous Khoisan people have been gathering and using these plants since before recorded history. When the Dutch and English colonized Africa in the 1700s, they brought along their well-established tea habits and began substituting native plants, like honeybush and rooibos, for their daily brew. From there, these herbs made their way to Europe and North America.

Honeybush and rooibos have similar characteristics and health benefits: Both are delicious, noncaffeinated red teas that are low in tannins, without any bitterness regardless of how long they are steeped. Honeybush is sweeter and more floral, while rooibos has a woodier, smokier flavor.

The aromatic oils that give these herbs their sweet fragrance have antispasmodic and calmative effects that ease tension, relax the nervous system, and mildly lower blood pressure. They are frequently consumed after meals to soothe and settle digestion. Unique among the fragrant aromatics, these herbs are also nutrient-dense, packed with minerals

and trace elements including iron, magnesium, manganese, calcium, copper, and zinc. Regular consumption strengthens bones, hair, teeth, and nails. These antioxidant-rich herbs contain a vast array of flavonoids, polyphenols, xanthones, and carotenoids that act to quell inflammation, boost immunity, and turn on cellular defenses.

How to Saturate Your Day

- Both rooibos and honeybush are mainly consumed as tea, both hot and iced. The two are often combined to make a tea blend. Take 1 heaping teaspoon dried tea leaves and steep in 1 to 1½ cups (240 to 360 ml) water for 5 to 7 minutes. For iced tea, follow the same instructions, then let tea cool to room temperature and pour over ice (if you don't want to wait, double the amount of herb to create a strong brew and let the ice dilute the tea when poured in hot).

- Make a cold infusion using the same ratios as above in room-temperature or cold water and place in the fridge for 4 to 6 hours.

- Rooibos and honeybush are often integrated into special elixirs, lattes, and tonics. See Honeybush Latte, page 218.

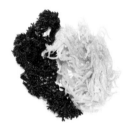

Irish Moss (*Chondrus crispus*)

DEMULCENT

Hundreds of species of sea moss can be found growing in rocky coastal areas all over the world. Among these, Irish moss is the most well known and widely used. Once considered an important food in

Ireland (where the name originated), it thrives in the cool waters on both sides of the North Atlantic, from Ireland, Europe, and the United Kingdom to the Maine coast up into Canada.

Irish moss is the most nutritious plant within the demulcent category—it provides 92 of the 102 trace minerals needed by the body, including iodine, calcium, potassium, magnesium, sulfur, zinc, phosphorus, iron, and selenium. As it is 80 percent fiber by weight, this plant also makes an excellent prebiotic for nourishing the microbiome and enhancing gastrointestinal health.

Irish moss dissolves when soaked in water, forming a thick and viscous healing gel that soothes, cools, and moistens an overheated GI tract, quelling inflammation and deeply revitalizing the entire digestive system. It's a versatile and easy demulcent preparation, with an ideal consistency that's perfect for daily use. Irish moss has a rather neutral, unremarkable flavor on its own that absorbs other flavors well, making it great for blending into smoothies and other special elixirs.

How to Saturate Your Day

- Store Irish moss gel in the fridge and scoop out a tablespoon or two for blending into smoothies, elixirs, soups, and puddings. Mix the gel with plant-based milks to accentuate its demulcent qualities. See the recipes for Irish Moss Gel and Irish Moss–Cacao Nib Elixir on page 188.

- Sea moss sourced from the warmer Caribbean waters is sometimes referred to as Irish moss, but it comes from the related *Gracilaria* species. "Moss," as it's often called there, is the main ingredient (along with milk, vanilla, cinnamon, and nutmeg) in a delicious health drink consumed throughout the Caribbean to promote libido, vitality, and energy.

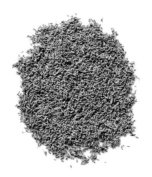

Lavender
(*Lavandula angustifolia*)

FRAGRANT RELAXANT

Lavender's uplifting fragrance and dazzling color elevate the mind and soul, washing away negativity and bad vibes. The word *lavender* derives from the Latin *lavare*, meaning to wash, and legend has it that the Egyptian queen Nefertiti loved her daily bath filled with lavender flowers.

Consuming lavender calms the agitated states of mind that come with frustration, anger, and anxiety. The herb's uniquely balancing influence on the nervous system simultaneously elevates depressive moods and calms anxious ones. It relaxes tension and increases circulation, benefiting painful conditions like tension headaches and menstrual cramps.

When taken as a tea after meals, lavender's antispasmodic constituents relax the gut, creating space for digestion and nutrient assimilation to occur. It helps reduce excess gas, bloating, and any crampy conditions related to digestive issues. Lavender is also highly anti-inflammatory and cooling to a GI tract overheated from hyperacidity or gastritis, while the herb's antiseptic constituents inhibit the growth of bacteria, yeast, and other microbes.

Using lavender during the day increases calm while still allowing for the focus and productivity necessary to get work done. In the evenings, it provides just enough sedation to usher us into a peaceful state and restful sleep.

How to Saturate Your Day

- Lavender tea is made from the herb's dried flowers. It has a strong flavor—a little goes a long way. Infuse 1 teaspoon dried flowers into 1½ cups (360 ml) water for 5 to 7 minutes.

- Lavender is used in recipes in all sorts of creative ways. Always look for organic, chemical-free varieties intended for culinary use—*Lavandula angustifolia* is the best choice. See Lavender Flower Latte, page 221.

- Lavender essential oil is primarily responsible for the herb's medicinal effects and is one of the rare essential oils that is safe for internal consumption. The oil comes in capsules made specifically for this purpose. The essential oil is also great for diffusing and direct palm inhalations. Put a couple drops on your palms, rub them together, hold your palms near your face, then take a few deep breaths: Voilà, you are at the center of a powerful, cleansing, aromatic force field.

- Lavender tincture makes for a powerful, relaxing preparation.

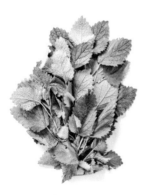

Lemon Balm
(*Melissa officinalis*)

FRAGRANT RELAXANT

This highly aromatic herb in the mint family originated in southern Europe and the Mediterranean region. Its botanical genus name, *Melissa*, comes from the Greek word for honeybee, so named because bees go crazy for it. Lemon balm is frequently planted near hives to encourage bees to feel more at home, and its potent antimicrobial and antiseptic essential oils discourage proliferation of parasitic mites and help strengthen the bees' immune systems.

To the ancients, lemon balm was considered a longevity tonic and comprehensive daily medicinal. The renowned seventeenth-century English herbalist Nicholas Culpeper said of lemon balm: "Every house should have some because it causes the heart and mind to become merry and drives away troublesome cares."

Lemon balm is first and foremost a perfect post-meal digestive. Its strong carminative and antispasmodic constituents relax nerves within the GI tract, settle digestion, improve assimilation, and relieve fullness and gas. Lemon balm provides relief for what was known in the old days as "melancholic" issues, essentially a condition characterized by poor digestion and feelings of heaviness combined with low energy and bad mood.

Lemon balm contains a whole range of unique neuroprotective antioxidants that protect the brain from inflammation and oxidative stress for long-term cognitive health. Lemon balm has the unique ability to improve alertness and concentration while simultaneously easing tension, increasing our capacity for mental work without causing dullness or fatigue. Its essential oil contains geraniol and rosmarinic acid, compounds shown to optimize the production of acetylcholine (a neurotransmitter essential for focus, memory, and alertness) and GABA (which helps calm anxiety and brightens the mood).

How to Saturate Your Day

- Drink lemon balm as a tea or infusion after meals or several times throughout the day to ease tension and promote clarity of mind. Steep 1 or 2 heaping teaspoons of loose herb (or use two or three tea bags) in 1 to 1½ cups (240 to 360 ml) water for 10 minutes. Fresh lemon balm infused into cold water also makes a refreshing beverage.

- Lemon balm extracts in capsule, tablet, or tincture form offer a convenient way to experience the benefits.

- Diffuse the essential oil in the office when working or studying to take advantage of lemon balm's cognitive-enhancing properties and mood-brightening effects.

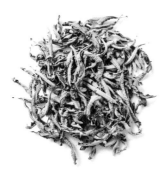

Lemon Verbena
(*Aloysia citriodora*)

FRAGRANT RELAXANT

Named for its invigorating citrusy fragrance, lemon verbena is an aromatic shrub native to South America, where it is regularly consumed as an after-meal tea for promoting digestion. I personally have been the beneficiary of its powers on many occasions. Once in the Andes, I felt groggy after overdoing it on a filling feast of heirloom corn and guinea pigs and was grateful when my hosts brought out several pots of hot tea made from lemon verbena freshly harvested from the garden. I immediately felt the fragrant essential oils relaxing the nerves in my gut, creating much-needed space for digestion to proceed.

The taste and fragrance are uniquely uplifting to the senses and promote a sense of ease, lightness, and energy flow. It's beneficial for a wide range of nervous system issues, characterized by tension, anxiety, and digestive discomfort. Lemon verbena contains hundreds of constituents working synergistically. One in particular, verbascoside, is being studied closely for its stimulation of GABA receptors in the brain, which helps to cool down anxiety and control an overexcited stress response and reduces inflammatory processes associated with neurodegenerative conditions.

How to Saturate Your Day

- A simple hot infusion of the fresh or dried leaf is the most traditional and enjoyable way to access the benefits of lemon verbena. Infuse 1 or 2 heaping teaspoons dried leaf or ¼ cup (5 g) fresh leaves in 1½ cups (360 ml) hot water for 10 to 15 minutes, then strain. Iced lemon verbena tea works well, too: Use half to two-thirds the amount of water to make the tea, chill the strained mixture, and pour over ice. Drink lemon verbena tea hot or cold after each major meal or throughout the day.

- Fresh leaves can be chopped and sprinkled onto fruit salad or added to sauces, soups, and other recipes.

- Lemon verbena is also available in tinctures, tablets, and capsules.

- Like lemon balm (opposite), lemon verbena essential oil can be diffused and shares similar relaxing and uplifting properties. It's good for improving focus and concentration as well as easing tension.

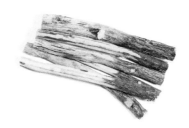

Licorice Root
(*Glycyrrhiza glabra*
& *G. uralensis*)

DEMULCENT/ADAPTOGEN

Licorice is a flowering perennial native to Asia and Southern Europe. A member of the pea family, it's used in Traditional Chinese Medicine, Ayurveda, and Western herbalism. Licorice root is fifty times sweeter than sugar, a unique property that gives this herb great versatility. In Traditional

Chinese Medicine, licorice is known as the "great harmonizer" for its ability to enhance the effects of other herbs and balance flavors. As such, it makes an excellent addition to formulas and recipes to help soften the flavor of herbs with a less-pleasant taste.

Licorice root contains a complex assortment of constituents beyond the usual moistening mucilage that characterizes most other demulcents, giving it a range of unique and complementary applications. The compounds in licorice root reduce inflammation and excess acidity in the gut and thus provide a healing balm to the entire GI tract. Licorice root is essential in any formula or preparation designed to repair the microabrasions and inflammation that occur with issues like "leaky gut." These same actions are of equal benefit for replenishing moisture within the mucous membranes of the respiratory system. Licorice soothes sore throats, moistens dry coughs, and acts as an effective expectorant. Unique among the demulcent category, licorice root also has adaptogenic actions that foster resilience in the endocrine system by lowering cortisol and other stress hormones.

Some studies show that taking large amounts of licorice over long periods of time can increase blood pressure and potentially cause water retention in those with a predisposition. It's possible to consume enough licorice to cause these issues—but that's a lot of licorice! The general guideline: Avoid taking more than 10 grams a day of licorice root for extended periods. You can also buy DGL licorice, a supplement with the glycyrrhizin removed (glycyrrhizin is the active ingredient that, in excess, can cause some of the aforementioned issues). Consuming DGL licorice still provides many beneficial actions, including moistening and rehydrating inflammation in the GI tract, albeit in a somewhat less powerful way.

How to Saturate Your Day

- Drinking licorice tea, either on its own or as part of a tea blend, is a simple and effective way to access the plant's functional benefits.

- Powdered licorice root is also beneficial, especially as a part of a demulcent powder blend recipe (like the one on page 189).

- Quality candy that uses real licorice extract is a popular treat in many Scandinavian countries (more on this on page 77).

- Licorice also comes in lozenges, capsules, and liquid extracts.

- Chewing on the whole roots is a common practice in India. If you can find them, they can be used to improve dental hygiene and as an antimicrobial restorative for the gums and mucous membranes in the mouth.

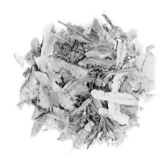

Linden
(*Tilia* species)

FRAGRANT RELAXANT/DEMULCENT

This large deciduous tree thrives in most temperate regions of the world. Highly revered in European cultures, linden trees are often found in village centers throughout the continent, where townspeople traditionally met beneath their shade to drink wine, conduct important meetings, and gather as a community.

Linden's popularity as an after-meal digestive tea in European culture is on par with that of peppermint or chamomile. Linden is unique, however, in that it combines relaxing fragrant aromatic qualities with moistening demulcent actions. (Linden is the only tree classified in the same plant family as marshmallow, known as the quintessential demulcent; see page 328.) Linden is great to use when digestive issues brought on by nervousness and anxiety combine with dryness and heat. It soothes, cools, and hydrates the GI tract, reducing irritation, hyperacidity, and inflammation.

Linden's reliable calmative effect on the nervous system makes it a valuable remedy for gently reducing anxiety and tension without sedation. Sipped in the evening, linden tea calms the nerves and promotes restful sleep.

In European traditional medicine, linden has also been used for centuries as a tonic for promoting cardiovascular health. Recent research supports this traditional use, showing that a constituent in the essential oil called farnesol can mildly lower blood pressure by increasing the flexibility of blood vessels and capacity to dilate, allowing blood to flow more freely. Linden's bright yellow color comes from its rich assortment of unique flavonoids, which protect blood vessels from inflammation and oxidative damage.

How to Saturate Your Day

- Linden tea has a deliciously sweet, floral flavor and aroma. To prepare a linden tea or infusion, steep 1 to 3 teaspoons dried leaf-and-flower mixture in 1 to 1½ cups (240 to 360 ml) water for 10 to 15 minutes. Strain and sweeten if desired.

- Linden is available in capsules and tinctures as well.

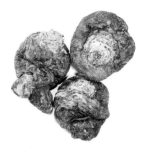

Maca Root
(*Lepidium meyenii*)

ADAPTOGEN

Maca, a small tuber in the radish family, is native to the Andes mountains of Peru. Capable of thriving in harsh conditions and altitudes up to 15,000 feet (4,500 m), this ancient superfood has been cultivated for more than two thousand years. Legend has it that Spanish conquistadors observed Incan warriors eating substantial amounts of maca root prior to battles to give them vitality and strength. Maca continues to be an important staple in the diet of highland Peruvians, and it's an increasingly essential ingredient for smoothie drinkers throughout the world.

Equal parts food and medicine, maca is an abundant source of complex carbohydrates, protein, fiber, vitamins, minerals, antioxidants, and other bioactive compounds. Consumed on a regular basis, maca helps replenish reserves of the essential nutrients we need to thrive.

In Peru, maca is revered for its aphrodisiac effects above all else. Traditional medicine systems view healthy libido and fertility as an expression of overall vitality and zest for life. Research confirms that compounds in maca root known as macamides improve hormonal and cardiovascular functions and lead to increased sexual arousal and stamina. These same compounds are also responsible for maca's ability to increase energy and endurance levels during prolonged athletic activities, aligning with its historical use as a tonic to stave off fatigue during battles and on long treks into high-altitude terrain. Like other adaptogens, maca helps restore equilibrium to the endocrine system during times of prolonged stress.

How to Saturate Your Day

- Maca root has a slightly nutty, mildly sweet flavor that blends well with a variety of foods. In Peru, it's possible to find fresh or partially dehydrated whole maca roots on the menu in some restaurants, often prepared much like a potato or yam.

- Outside of Peru, maca is most often found as powder. Look for gelatinized maca powder, made from a process that removes much of the starch content to concentrate the nutrients and active compounds, making them easier to absorb; it also gives the powder a smoother texture and sweeter flavor. Blend maca powder into hot or cold beverages, lattes, soups, and smoothies (see Peanut Butter–Maca–Goji Berry Smoothie, page 250). It's great to mix into hot cereal or energy bars, such as my Cacao Adaptogenic Energy Balls (page 255).

- Maca is also available in capsule and tablet form. When using maca supplements, look for standardized content of macamide.

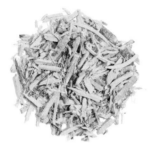

Marshmallow Root (*Althaea officinalis*)

DEMULCENT

This water-loving plant originates in Europe and western Asia, where it thrives in wetlands and other moist environments—hence the name marshmallow. The root is what is most typically used (dried, then chopped or powdered), although the leaves contain demulcent properties as well.

The ancient Egyptians combined marshmallow roots with honey to create a candy that still bears its name two thousand years later (although today's spongy white candy has no relation to the original). Marshmallow's genus name, *Althaea*, translates as "the healer," a testament to its rich mucilage content, prized for soothing all manner of respiratory and digestive issues.

Marshmallow mucilage creates a protective coating along the GI tract that cools inflammation and promotes healing and is particularly helpful for soothing heartburn, acid reflux, and other inflammatory conditions. It provides similar benefits to the respiratory, sinus, and urinary tracts. Drinking marshmallow root infusions on a regular basis strengthens the immune system by improving the integrity and barrier function of the gut lining, preventing microorganisms (and potential infections) from infiltrating.

How to Saturate Your Day

- Marshmallow water hydrates better than water alone. Simply mix 1 to 2 tablespoons marshmallow root powder in 1 quart (1 L) water. This beverage blend hydrates you in arid climates or dry seasons and during workouts and air travel. It's a reliable protective measure for respiratory passages during cold and flu season or in places where air pollution is an issue. The flavor is neutral and the texture is not too thick, but feel free to adjust the ratios to your own preferences.

- Marshmallow root is available in teas, on its own or in blends.

- You can find marshmallow as cut-and-sifted dried root for use in infusions, as well as in capsule and tincture form.

Medicinal Mushrooms

ADAPTOGEN

In nature, webs of underground mycelium and the mushrooms that sprout from them recycle decaying organic matter into nutrients that sustain plant life and vitalize the surrounding ecology. They function in a similar way in our bodies: Medicinal mushrooms activate immune functions that help the body cleanse itself of cellular wastes and debris, inflammation-causing toxins, and pathogenic microbes, liberating energy required for physiological renewal.

The medicinal mushrooms highlighted below are especially noteworthy for combining broad-spectrum immune-enhancing actions with antioxidants and essential nutrients that help reduce inflammation, balance blood sugar and cholesterol levels, enhance cognitive function, improve detoxification, and increase energy and endurance. In addition to the following, see the individual profiles on two other important medicinal mushrooms with true adaptogenic functions: reishi (page 335) and cordyceps (page 314).

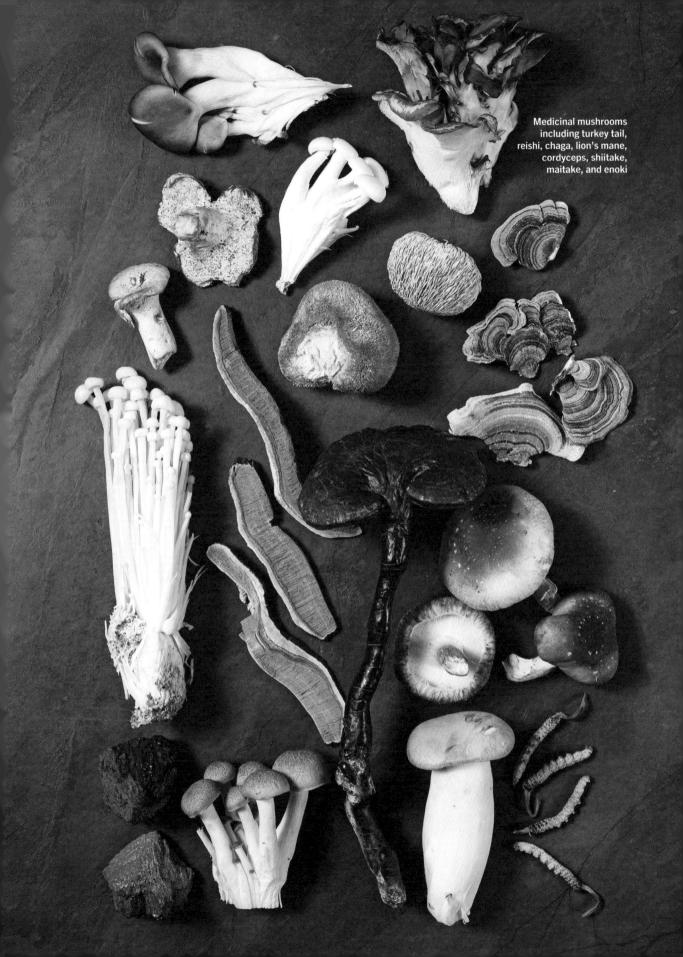

Medicinal mushrooms including turkey tail, reishi, chaga, lion's mane, cordyceps, shiitake, maitake, and enoki

Chaga (*Inonotus obliquus*): A hard, woody conk mushroom prized in Scandinavian and Russian traditional medicines, chaga looks like a chunk of burnt wood with a bright yellow core and grows almost exclusively on birch trees throughout the northern forests of North America, Scandinavia, and Asia, where it absorbs a unique constituent in the birch tree called betulinic acid. This, combined with the beta-glucans produced in the mushroom, give chaga powerful immune-enhancing and metabolic-balancing effects. The abundant antioxidants in chaga are beneficial for lowering inflammation, improving liver function, and promoting overall cellular health.

Lion's mane (*Hericium erinaceus*): These mushrooms grow on hardwood trees in forests throughout the Northern Hemisphere, where they are eaten as both food and medicine. In Japan, lion's mane is called yamabushitake and is consumed as a tea to promote calm and concentration. Traditional Chinese Medicine uses lion's mane to increase energy, ease the mind, and improve digestion. Contemporary research has revealed that certain unique compounds in lion's mane stimulate nerve growth in the brain, showing promise for improving memory and cognitive function.

Maitake (*Grifola frondosa*): Known as "hen of the woods," this mushroom grows on decaying hardwood trees throughout the Northern Hemisphere. It is prized by foragers and high-end chefs for its smoky, umami flavor. Maitake's medicinal benefits may seem like an afterthought compared with its culinary status, but this mushroom contains powerful and unique immune-enhancing compounds called D-fraction polysaccharides, which activate our host defenses and stimulate the production of macrophages, T-cells, neutrophils, and other key immune factors. In addition, the maitake's rich assortment of antioxidants improve digestive health and reduce inflammation in the gut.

Shiitake (*Lentinus edodes*): A close relative of reishi, shiitake is known as the oak mushroom in Japan, where it is a treasured medicinal food. Good for cardiovascular health, shiitakes contain a compound called eritadenine that has been found to modulate the synthesis of cholesterol in the liver. Other compounds in shiitake prevent the harmful buildup of plaque in blood vessels, encourage circulation, and moderate blood pressure. The mushroom contains lentinan (a unique immune-enhancing polysaccharide shown to increase immunoglobulin—a key immune factor) as well as a host of anti-inflammatory constituents. It's also a significant source of B vitamins.

Turkey tail (*Trametes versicolor*): Called the "mushroom of multiple colors" for its brightly colored rings, this mushroom is said to resemble the patterning on a turkey's tail feathers. With a tough, leathery exterior, this mushroom is no umami-rich shiitake. Yet what it lacks in flavor it makes up for in medicinal powers. Turkey tails are among the most potent immune enhancers of all the medicinal mushrooms, containing a highly concentrated source of protein-bound polysaccharides, shown in studies to be effective in activating a broad-spectrum immune response. These mushrooms can be found growing on decaying logs throughout the world. In folk-medicine traditions throughout Asia, the turkey tail is brewed as a strong tea for daily immune support and has been used for centuries in Traditional Chinese Medicine to strengthen digestion, respiratory health, and energy levels. The mushroom is also a good source of microbiome-nourishing prebiotic fiber.

How to Saturate Your Day

- Powdered extracts contain the full spectrum of active constituents and are the most convenient and potent way to use mushrooms for medicinal purposes. They dissolve well into liquid (no grit) and are easy to blend into smoothies and hot beverages like coffee and lattes (see Chaga Chai Latte, page 249). Tastier mushrooms like shiitake and maitake work well as a powdered condiment, sprinkled onto dishes or used as seasoning in soups and broths (a common practice in Japan).

- Fresh shiitake and maitake mushrooms are delicious in stir-fries, soups, and sauces, or grilled and served as side dishes.

- Some medicinal mushrooms, like chaga and turkey tail, can be found dried in whole form; decoct them in water (see page 94) to drink as teas and other beverages.

- Capsules, tablets, and full-spectrum tinctures are useful options. When using mushroom supplements, look for standardized content of immune-enhancing polysaccharides.

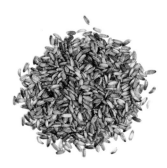

Milk Thistle
(*Silybum marianum*)

BITTER/DETOXIFYING

Milk thistle is a restorative tonic for the chronically overworked modern-day liver. Native to the Mediterranean, milk thistle has been used for centuries to alleviate "melancholic" conditions—an ancient term for physical and mental fatigue and depression, often combined with poor digestion. It's now well understood from a scientific perspective that a poorly functioning liver is often a major contributor to all manner of mood disorders.

Milk thistle gets its name from the milky white streaks running down its long spiny leaves. Historically, all parts of the milk thistle have been used as both food and medicine. The fresh, tender young leaves can be cooked and eaten as a vegetable, and the dried leaves made into bitter-tasting teas to improve digestion, lower cholesterol, and balance blood sugar. But the powerful flavonoid silymarin, responsible for milk thistle's extraordinary liver-rejuvenating effects, is found in its oily seeds.

Silymarin boosts levels of glutathione, the body's most potent antioxidant for protecting liver cells from inflammation and free-radical damage that result from its vigorous metabolic and detoxifying activities. Milk thistle seeds are especially beneficial for cooling overheated liver cells regularly exposed to alcohol, pharmaceuticals, artificial ingredients, and environmental pollutants.

How to Saturate Your Day

- Rich in nutrients and healthy fats, dried milk thistle seeds have a nutty, slightly bitter flavor, sort of a cross between hemp and sunflower seeds. Lightly toast the seeds in a skillet and add to salads or stir-fries or grind them in a coffee grinder and use as a seasoning (see Milk Thistle Detox-Enhancing Dukkah, page 135).

- Milk thistle powder or powdered extract can be blended into smoothies or other beverages.

- Milk thistle is also made into cold-pressed oil. Add the oil to smoothies and other beverages or use topically as a moisturizer to reduce dark spots and to relieve skin rashes and acne.

- Tablets, capsules, and tinctures are convenient ways to take milk thistle. When using milk thistle supplements, look for standardized content of silymarin.

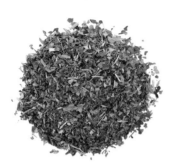

Moringa
(*Moringa oleifera*)
NUTRITIVE

This fast-growing, medium-size tree with slender branches and clusters of feathery green leaves, native to India, Nepal, and the Himalayan regions, is now widely cultivated throughout the tropics. It is drought tolerant, making it particularly valuable for regions where access to nutrition is challenging. Known as the "tree of life," moringa has been used for food and medicine for at least four thousand years. Most parts of the tree are edible, including its fruits, twigs, and seeds—but the leaf is the most commonly used part of the moringa. In Ayurvedic medicine, this highly nutritious leaf is used to boost metabolism, increase energy levels, improve digestive health, and promote detoxification.

Rich in vitamins, minerals, and trace elements (like potassium, zinc, copper, magnesium, iron, beta-carotene, B vitamins, folic acid, and vitamin C), moringa is like a green transfusion for depleted nutrient reservoirs. It has a full complement of all nine essential amino acids, making it a valuable source of plant protein. In addition, moringa contains a potent mix of antioxidants like polyphenols, flavonoids, and quercetin, which work to quench free radicals, reduce inflammation, and enhance the liver's and kidneys' ability to filter toxins. Moringa is also a significant source of both soluble and insoluble fiber, important for digestive health and balancing blood sugar.

How to Saturate Your Day

- It's possible to find fresh moringa leaves online and at international markets. They have a vegetal and slightly bitter flavor and can be minced and added to salads and stir-fries.

- Dried moringa leaves can be purchased loose or in tea bags. Infuse the leaves for iced or hot tea; add lemon and honey for an invigorating elixir. It's one of the ingredients in my Homemade Nutritive Tea Blend (page 156).

- Moringa powder can be found in natural grocers and online. Add it to smoothies and soups, or whisk it in a 50:50 ratio with matcha to make an energizing morning beverage.

- Moringa is also available in capsules and extracts.

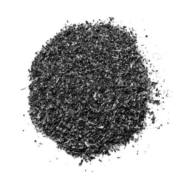

Nettles
(*Urtica dioica* & *U. urens*)
NUTRITIVE

Nettles are found growing wild in fields, streambeds, and farmlands in temperate regions around the world. They sprout in early spring, and the younger, smaller, and brighter green leaves are the best to eat—they are less fibrous and tough. These wild greens provide a highly bioavailable source of nutrients often deficient in Western diets: calcium, magnesium, manganese, and potassium, as well as vitamins A and K, beta-carotene, and folate. They contain a significant amount of plant protein and iron as well. Nettles are a dietary staple in many traditional cuisines of Europe and the Mediterranean, appearing everywhere from family kitchens to fine restaurants.

Like many nutritive plants, nettles provide dense nutrition while simultaneously enhancing detoxification pathways, helping to gently eliminate nitrogenous wastes and other metabolic toxins through the kidneys. They contain a range of antioxidants (such as flavonoids) that work to reduce inflammation and stabilize mast cells to reduce histamines in allergic and inflamed conditions.

Nettles get their name from the "needles" that blanket the leaves like tiny hairs. These hairs contain small amounts of formic acid, the same compound that gives bites from red ants their sting. When these hairs come in direct contact with skin, it causes a minor histamine response that generally goes away on its own within a few minutes. If you're harvesting your own nettles, wear heavy gardening gloves; once home, while still wearing the gloves, remove the thick stalks and wash the leaves thoroughly in a colander. Fortunately, the stinging hairs are fragile and readily dissolve when cooked or dehydrated.

How to Saturate Your Day

- Drinking 2 to 4 cups (480 ml to 1 L) of a nettles overnight infusion (see page 94) is a great way to replenish nutrient reserves and ensure a plentiful supply of needed electrolytes.

- Nettle leaves have a somewhat sweet and salty vegetal flavor, thanks to the concentration of amino acids, chlorophyll, and mineral salts. Freshly cooked nettle leaves make a tasty addition to stir-fries, simple side dishes, and soups (see Nettles Soup, page 167). Steam young, tender nettle leaves as you would spinach.

- Nettles are available as capsules, tablets, tinctures, powders, and powdered extracts.

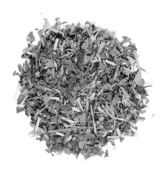

Passionflower (*Passiflora incarnata*)

NERVINE CALMATIVE

This climbing vine with cosmic purple flowers, native to the Americas, is mainly cultivated for its delicious, vitamin C–rich fruits. One unique species, *Passiflora incarnata*, has been used for centuries to reduce anxiety and promote deep and restorative sleep.

According to Traditional Chinese Medicine, excessive thinking driven by emotions heats up our brains like engines that are revving too fast. As a nervine calmative, passionflower is particularly suited to cooling and calming the worried, fretting, and anxious mind. Passionflower contains unique compounds (such as chrysin and benzoflavone) shown to increase the chemical neurotransmitter GABA and relax the central nervous system. Passionflower reliably calms emotions without dulling or sedating the mind, instead enhancing clarity and improving focus. Mild enough to be used as a subtle relaxant during the day without causing drowsiness, passionflower taken in the appropriate dose at night calms brain activity, shortening the length of time it takes to fall asleep and increasing the amount and depth of sleep one gets.

Passionflower also has antispasmodic and pain-relieving applications, especially when muscle tension causes insomnia and mental agitation.

How to Saturate Your Day

- To make passionflower tea, steep 1 to 3 heaping teaspoons cut-and-sifted herb (or two or three tea bags) in 1 to 1½ cups (240 to 360 ml) water for 10 to 15 minutes. The longer the steeping, the stronger the preparation.

- Passionflower tincture is convenient and works well to ease tension and promote sleep. It's a good preparation to keep at one's bedside.

- Passionflower is also available in tablet and capsule forms.

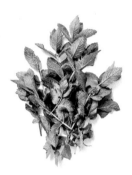

Peppermint & Spearmint (*Mentha* × *piperita* & *M. spicata*)

FRAGRANT RELAXANT

Peppermint and spearmint are the most popular varieties among the dozens of unique mint species and cultivars used in herbal traditions. Mint's characteristic cooling sensation comes from its abundance of menthol, the constituent that gives these herbs their distinctive fragrance, flavor, and beneficial effects. Peppermint and spearmint share similar medicinal actions and therapeutic benefits, so which mint to choose depends mostly on individual preferences and tastes.

Drinking mint tea after meals relaxes the nerves in the gut and creates space in the GI tract for digestive processes to efficiently transform food into energy. Mint's relaxant effects help relieve congestion, fullness, gas, cramping, nausea, bloating, and tightness throughout the entire digestive system.

Mint's expansive aromatic compounds invigorate the circulation of blood and energy throughout the body, increasing alertness, deepening breathing, and sharpening cognitive functions. Drinking mint tea and breathing mint essential oil are surprisingly

effective at waking us up and getting us going. Mint's invigorating properties bring more oxygen to the brain and nervous system to help us stay focused.

How to Saturate Your Day

- To make mint tea, steep 1 or 2 teaspoons dried loose herb in 1 to 1½ cups (240 to 360 ml) water, covered, for 10 minutes. Add fresh mint to cold water for a cold infusion (see page 94).

- Fresh mint leaves are great for cooking and can be used as garnishes.

- Mint is a common ingredient in elixirs that promote good digestion and soothe nausea and indigestion.

- Peppermint spirits and extracts are excellent, convenient options (see Peppermint Elixir, page 210). Peppermint oil capsules and tablets are also available.

- Peppermint essential oil diluted with a carrier oil of your choice applied topically to the temples and back of the head can be used to relieve tension headaches.

Psyllium Husk (*Plantago ovata*)

DEMULCENT

Psyllium husks are the fibrous coating covering the seeds of several species of plants in the *Plantago* genus. These simple green herbs with spikes of white flowers are native to the Mediterranean region and now cultivated throughout the world.

Psyllium husks contain up to 30 percent pure mucilage and are a major source of soluble fiber—a unique combination that is the perfect recipe for gut health. They increase motility in the intestines and are an excellent source of nourishment for the microbiome. They are highly water absorptive, enhancing the moisture balance in the intestines. They also help heal the gut lining, bind up toxins, and are mildly laxative—all of which improve intestinal function. When used consistently, their high fiber content is a useful strategy to help balance blood sugar and lower cholesterol.

How to Saturate Your Day

• Psyllium husk is the main ingredient in over-the-counter formulas used as bulking laxatives for GI complaints, including Metamucil (introduced by G.D. Searle and Company in 1934, back when most OTC medicines were derived from medicinal plants).

• Use psyllium husks in capsule, whole, or powder form as part of a comprehensive fiber formula for digestive health. Stir 1 tablespoon whole psyllium husks or powder into 1 cup (240 ml) apple juice or other beverage, then follow with 1 cup (240 ml) more liquid, once or twice a day on an empty stomach. See the fiber formula containing psyllium husks on page 194.

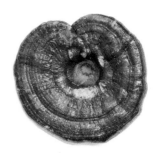

Reishi
(*Ganoderma lucidum*)
ADAPTOGEN

This elusive forest mushroom can be found growing atop decaying hardwood trees in temperate regions throughout the world. Known as the "elixir of immortality," reishi (aka lingzhi) was considered the most powerful of all tonics by Taoist monks in their quest for longevity. The classic text of Traditional Chinese Medicine, *Shen Nong Ben Cao Jing*, in descriptions dating back more than two thousand years, states that the use of reishi "increases vital energy, refreshes the mind, and enables one to live a long life."

Like all medicinal mushrooms (see page 328), reishi is a potent immune enhancer, effective for both acute conditions like colds and flus and protecting against long-term immune challenges. It has the unique capacity to regulate and balance immune activity, calming it down when hyperactive (as in autoimmune conditions) or nourishing it when depleted.

Reishi contains dozens of powerful anti-inflammatory triterpene compounds that improve acute and chronic respiratory issues such as allergies, coughs, and asthma. Reishi promotes cardiovascular health by increasing circulation, lowering blood pressure, and improving cholesterol levels. It also has well-researched beneficial effects for the liver, working to significantly reduce inflammation and oxidative damage in hepatocytes, balance enzyme levels, and boost the production of glutathione.

In traditional Chinese and Japanese medicine, reishi is said to "calm the spirit" for its ability to balance the stress response, relax the nervous system, improve sleep, and elevate mood. Reishi is an excellent daily tonic for the mind, containing potent compounds that protect brain cells from inflammation and oxidative processes and stimulate the growth of new neurons. This last effect promotes improved cognitive elasticity, longevity, and learning capacity, aligning with reishi's traditional use as an aid to concentration.

How to Saturate Your Day

- Powdered extracts are the most versatile option for using reishi because they blend well into hot or cold beverages like coffee and cacao (see Cacao-Reishi-Cordyceps Latte, page 249). Tablets and capsules made from powdered extracts are also available.

- Dried whole reishi can be decocted into a strong tea. (See page 94 for more on decoction.)

- If using tincture of reishi, be sure to look for products utilizing a dual-extraction method (a combination of hot water and alcohol, which ensures extraction of all active constituents).

- Reishi spores are the most powerful part of the mushroom, and spore oil is particularly good for the immune system. A special process used to crack the spores and extract the oil generates 500 to 700 percent more potency than regular reishi extract. You can find spore oil in liquid and capsule form.

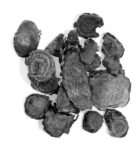

Rhodiola
(*Rhodiola rosea*)
ADAPTOGEN

Named for the characteristic rose-like aroma released from its sliced roots, rhodiola is a small succulent that grows in the Arctic and subarctic regions of Europe, Asia, and North America. It has been used for centuries to promote strength, endurance, and resilience by those living in the harsh and challenging regions where it grows. Siberian newlyweds were traditionally given a bouquet of rhodiola's yellow blooms as a gift to promote fertility. The Vikings are said to have consumed copious quantities of rhodiola ale to psyche them up before raids. The Inuit from eastern Canada relied on rhodiola for energy during long hunting expeditions. More recently, Olympic athletes and astronauts using rhodiola have shown improved performance, endurance, and recovery time, and it has been an important part of Himalayan traditional medicine systems for centuries.

Rhodiola is an excellent choice to help restore and refresh a brittle nervous system exhausted by long-term stress. Depending on the dosage, it can act as either a mild stimulant or a sedative. Small amounts increase serotonin, dopamine, and endorphin levels (our "feel-good" chemistry), which improves cognitive function, elevates the mood, and keeps energy levels up during intense mental work. In larger doses, rhodiola helps calm an overactive nervous system, reducing anxiety and promoting physiological equilibrium. Rhodiola can be used both as a short-term cognitive enhancer and to balance endocrine functions and improve resilience during long-term stress. It's useful to experiment with varying dosages and length of administration to determine what works best for you.

Rhodiola is one of the first adaptogens to consider for increasing physical energy and endurance. In several studies, it has been shown to boost muscle power and enhance oxygenation during athletic activities as well as accelerate recovery between workouts.

How to Saturate Your Day

- Rhodiola powder or powdered extracts make a nice addition to smoothies, lattes, tonics, and elixirs.

- Rhodiola capsules, tablets, and tinctures all work well. When using rhodiola supplements, look for standardized content of rosavins, one of the main active compounds used as a biomarker for potency.

- With a woody texture and an aromatically sweet, slightly bitter, and astringent flavor, dried rhodiola root can be decocted (see page 94) to drink as a medicinal tonic, with a natural sweetener of your choice added to improve the flavor.

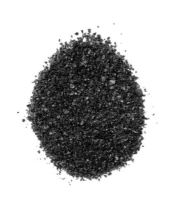

Rose Hip
(*Rosa canina* & *R. rugosa*)
NUTRITIVE

The fruits of various rose species, rose hips have a delicious, tart flavor and have been consumed in syrups, jams, wines, tonics, and elixirs for centuries—most commonly using the fruit of the wild dog rose (*Rosa canina*) and Japanese beach rose (*R. rugosa*), both of which can be found growing in temperate regions around the globe. Evidence of their use has been discovered at prehistoric sites, and they were a lifesaver for many people during World War II when vitamin C deficiency was a serious issue. Rose hips contain a host of synergistic flavonoids that support and enhance the absorption of its rich allotment of vitamin C, amplifying its effects. Flavonoids and vitamin C are essential in activating cellular immunity and increasing the body's healing and repair functions. They are also necessary for building collagen, capillaries, cartilage, and muscle.

Rose hips contain hundreds of antioxidants; vitamins A, B, and K; and beta-carotene. They are a rich source of pectin that soothes the digestive system and nourishes the microbiome. The oil obtained from the pressed seed of the rose hip is prized for its hydrating, regenerative properties and is a common ingredient in many cosmetics and skin-care products. Rose hip oil is used to promote healing in various inflammatory skin conditions such as acne, burns, and scarring.

How to Saturate Your Day

- Dried rose hips (with the seeds and hair removed) are used to make delicately flavored infusions and teas. Dried rose hips are also the base for nutritive jams; see the recipe for Rose Hips Super Berry Antioxidant Jam on page 163.

- Rose hip powder makes an excellent vitamin C–rich boost for smoothies and other beverages.

- Fresh rose hips can be gathered in season: Peel, remove the seeds, and incorporate into various elixirs and recipes. In Sweden, a delicious traditional soup made from fresh or dried rose hips, nyponsoppa (see page 165), is a source of much-needed immune-boosting vitamins and antioxidants during the long winter months.

- Rose hips are available as capsules and tablets or incorporated into vitamin C–rich supplements.

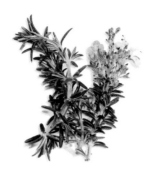

Rosemary
(*Rosmarinus officinalis*)
CULINARY/FRAGRANT RELAXANT

The town of Acciaroli, on the Mediterranean coast of Italy, is home to a unique variety of rosemary that grows wild in the surrounding hills and is ubiquitous in the local diet. Acciaroli is also home to a higher-than-average population of people in their eighties and nineties in excellent cognitive health compared to people of similar age in other Western countries. Researchers studying the town elders believe that regular consumption of this pungent local rosemary has a lot to do with their uncommon health and longevity.

Shakespeare referred to rosemary as "the herb of remembrance," alluding to its long history of use as a tonic for the brain and cognitive function. Research has identified several unique compounds in rosemary that affirm this traditional use: One of its main constituents, carnosic acid, has been shown to specifically reduce oxidative damage in brain cells and stimulate the growth of new neurons. A constituent in rosemary essential oil known as 1,8 cineole has been shown to enhance concentration and free recall (short-term memory) when inhaled by exam-taking students.

Like other culinary herbs, rosemary is excellent at promoting good digestion thanks to its pungent, agni-enhancing aromatic oils. It contains an assortment of antimicrobial, immune-boosting compounds, including rosmarinic acid, which also supports digestive function and acts as a circulatory enhancer—making this herb beneficial for cardiovascular function, stimulating hair growth, warming up cold hands and feet, relieving headaches, and easing muscle tension.

How to Saturate Your Day

- Rosemary infused as tea or in tonics, elixirs, and other beverages works to improve appetite and metabolism. In Acciaroli, some of the town elders I spent time with drank several glasses of rosemary-infused water every day. To make your own: Chop 1 tablespoon fresh rosemary and add to 2 cups (480 ml) water (regular or sparkling); stir in 1 teaspoon lemon juice. Let soak for about 30 minutes, stir, strain, and drink. Or try a refreshing Sparkling Rosemary Limeade (page 126).

- Fresh or dried, rosemary is a standout culinary herb and an ingredient in the famed French blend herbes de Provence.

- Rosemary tablets and capsules can be taken for a more targeted approach to improving cognitive health or for their anti-inflammatory and antioxidant compounds. When using rosemary supplements, look for standardized content of carnosic and rosmarinic acids and 1,8 cineole.

- Diffusing rosemary essential oil or doing direct palm inhalations helps improve alertness, clarity, and concentration.

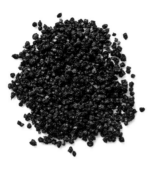

Schisandra Berry (*Schisandra chinensis*)

ADAPTOGEN

Schisandra berries are the bright red fruits of a climbing vine related to magnolia that originates in the temperate forests of northern Asia. Schisandra was classified as a "superior herb" in the ancient Chinese medicinal text *Shen Nong Ben Cao Jing*—a designation reserved for a rare group of herbs with extraordinary effects on the entire body. Its name in Traditional Chinese Medicine is *wu we zi*, meaning "five-flavored berry": The skin is sour, the pulp is sweet, the seeds are bitter and pungent, and the entire berry has hints of saltiness. According to TCM, hidden within these five primary flavors is a complex and diverse array of unique compounds and constituents.

Like many adaptogens, schisandra has paradoxical effects, simultaneously increasing energy levels and endurance while also grounding and relaxing the nervous system. Research has confirmed its capacity to increase resilience during stress, normalize cortisol levels, and boost serotonin. During the day, it improves cognitive performance, reduces anxiety, and elevates the mood. At night, it encourages healthy, restorative sleep.

Schisandra berries are rich in potent antioxidant compounds called lignins, which protect the liver from free radical damage, reduce inflammation, stimulate regeneration of damaged cells, and enhance the production of detoxification enzymes.

The ancient Chinese texts claimed that the unique sour astringency of the schisandra berry worked to "consolidate the qi." In Asia, the berry is often consumed during hot weather or after strong physical exertion to tighten pores, prevent excessive fluid loss through sweat, and provide a source of essential electrolytes.

How to Saturate Your Day

• Schisandra berries' taste is similar to a sour cranberry: delicious and enlivening. Dried berries work well for making refreshing teas, elixirs, and tonics (see Schisandra Berry–Rose Energizing Lemonade, page 253). Schisandra berries are popular in Korea, where they are called *omija* and often made into lightly sweetened beverages to start off the day and as an energy boost before a workout or replenisher afterward.

• Schisandra works well as a tincture, powdered extract, capsule, or tablet.

Sea Vegetables

NUTRITIVE

Sea vegetables draw their nourishing power from the ocean, the planet's great repository of essential minerals and trace elements like iron, potassium, copper, magnesium, chromium, zinc, manganese, selenium, calcium, and sulfur. They are a highly bioavailable source of vitamins A, B, C, D, E, and K as well as essential fatty acids (DHA and EPA), and they provide a natural source of iodine, which is essential for the functioning of the endocrine system, especially the thyroid. In addition, sea vegetables support healthy digestion and detoxification with their abundant fiber and presence of phycocolloids, compounds that help remove heavy metals, radioactive isotopes, and other chemical pollutants from the GI tract.

It's no surprise, then, that many cultures include sea vegetables as part of their diets and nutritional strategy. And eating these vegetables is an ever more relevant way to support the environment and practice sustainability: They are easy to farm, don't require pesticides, and improve the health of the oceans.

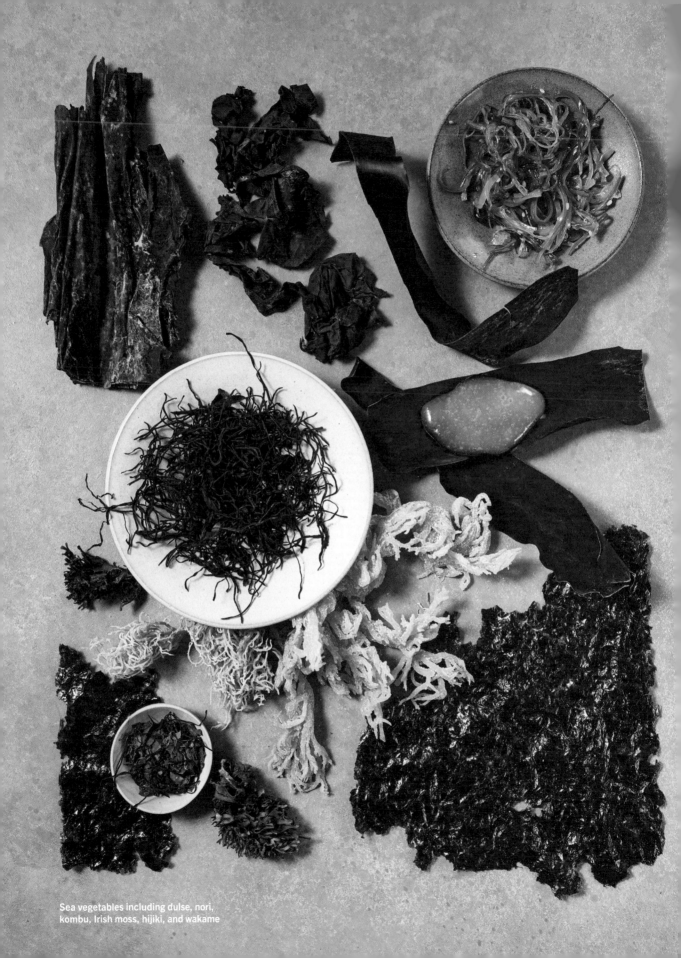

Sea vegetables including dulse, nori, kombu, Irish moss, hijiki, and wakame

There's a wide variety of sea vegetables to choose from, each with its own unique nutrient profile, flavor, and texture. All the sea vegetables below contain essential minerals, trace elements, and vitamins, so you can mix and match knowing you're getting everything you need—try to consume 3 to 5 grams of seaweed per day (20 to 30 g per week). In addition to the sea vegetables described below, see Irish moss (page 322).

Dulse (*Palmaria palmata*): This red sea vegetable is found in the North Pacific and Atlantic. Some of the best dulse comes from the craggy shores of coastal Maine, Ireland, and the Pacific Northwest, where it's harvested by hand from rocks at low tide. Dulse's genus name, *Palmaria*, refers to the fanlike shape of its fronds. Evidence of its use as a food source dates back several thousand years but likely far exceeds that. In Ireland and Scotland, dulse was sometimes chewed like tobacco and then swallowed, and it was once used as a cure for scurvy in the British Isles, thanks to its high vitamin C content. You can still find dried flakes served with a salty snack like peanuts in some remote Irish and British pubs. High levels of vitamin A make dulse extremely beneficial for maintaining eye health. Dulse is also rich in B_{12}, an essential vitamin that's often difficult to get enough of, especially for those following vegetarian or vegan diets. Dulse is very high in fiber (35 percent by weight), making it good for digestive health. Like other sea vegetables, dulse contains unique fibrous polysaccharides such as alginic acid that bind to heavy metals and radioactive isotopes to help remove them from the body.

Kombu (*Laminaria* species): Kombu, aka kelp, is a brown seaweed in a large family of thirty or more varieties of sea vegetables, including wakame. It is the origin of the famed umami flavor, and in Japan most people eat kombu every day in one form or another. Remains of kombu have been found in Japanese ruins dating back at least fourteen thousand years. Kombu is an essential food in the famed Okinawa diet, the traditional cuisine in Japan's Ryukyu Islands, where the Indigenous population is known for their amazing health and

longevity. The seaweed contains calcium and has the highest concentration of iodine of all the sea vegetables. High levels of iron make it beneficial for treating anemia. Because kombu contains enzymes that help break down raffinose sugar in beans, adding a small strip of kombu to bean dishes during the cooking process makes it easier to digest them and reduces gas.

Nori (*Pyropia yezoensis* and *P. tenera*): Chances are, your first seaweed encounter was with nori. This gateway sea vegetable is a central ingredient in sushi rolls. It's also become a popular snack food, roasted and coated with olive oil, sesame seeds, or wasabi. Nori is a type of red algae that grows in intertidal zones in temperate regions throughout the world. It's a daily essential in Japan, Korea, and China and has been harvested in Japan since prehistoric times. Battling samurai used moistened nori sheets as bandages. Nori was consumed as a thick paste until the 1700s, when a method was developed to make nori into sheets by shredding and drying it on racks (similar to the way paper is made). Nori contains up to 50 percent protein by dried weight, with all nine amino acids, including glutamate, which is responsible for nori's umami flavor.

How to Saturate Your Day

- Dulse has a chewy texture and is often added in flake form to salads. You can lightly toast it in a pan and mix into mashed potatoes or a bowl of oatmeal for a savory boost. Dulse is delicious panfried and added to various dishes.

- Kombu is a key ingredient in dashi broth. It flavors soup stock and is added as seasoning strips to salads and pastas. Kelp noodles and jerky are other popular options. Powdered kelp in small amounts is a great nutritional boost in smoothies. In Japan, dried kombu is infused into a hot seaweed tea called kombucha (*cha* means "tea")—different from the kombucha we Westerners may be familiar with. It is sold fresh in Asian grocery stores, and you can also find it in dried form at many health food stores.

- Nori sheets are used for sushi rolls and can be enjoyed on their own as a snack food. Ground-up nori flakes are combined with toasted sesame seeds, red pepper flakes, shiitake mushroom powder, poppy seeds, and miso powder to make the popular condiment furikake.

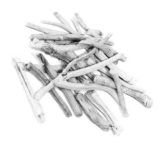

Shatavari Root
(*Asparagus racemosus*)

ADAPTOGEN/DEMULCENT

This wild species of asparagus is one of Ayurveda's premier rejuvenating tonics for women. A native of India's tropical grasslands, this nourishing adaptogen has been used for centuries to enhance all phases of female reproductive health. Shatavari root's unique compounds increase production of essential hormones that boost fertility, increase libido, balance menstruation, and alleviate discomforts related to menopause. Shatavari's reputation for improving women's reproductive health is so legendary that its name translates as "woman with a hundred husbands."

In Ayurveda, shatavari is classified as a *rasayanana*, a Sanskrit term referring to herbs or substances that replenish the vital sap responsible for our vitality and longevity. This aligns with the Western classification of adaptogens' ability to increase resilience to stress while boosting energy and endurance. Shatavari is also said to increase *ojas*, an Ayurvedic word for the subtle nutritive essence responsible for maintaining and promoting youthfulness, immunity, and emotional balance.

Shatavari contains substantial amounts of vitamins, minerals, fiber, and protein. Unique in the category of adaptogens, it's also a mucilage-rich, deeply hydrating demulcent, the perfect remedy for when stress is literally heating us up and drying us out. Shatavari helps moisten and cool the delicate mucous membranes lining the digestive, respiratory, urinary, and reproductive systems; nourish the skin and hair; provide the microbiome with a source of prebiotic-rich soluble fiber; and calm aggravated nerves. Although traditionally prized by women, shatavari's many benefits extend to men as well.

How to Saturate Your Day

- Shatavari root powder has a mild flavor and a fine texture, making it perfect for blending into smoothies and creamy drinks (see Strawberry Shatavari Smoothie, page 251), mixing into beverages containing ingredients that accentuate its cooling and/or nourishing properties (adding 1 heaping teaspoon shatavari powder to 1½ to 2 cups (360 to 480 ml) coconut water or plant-based milk, for example), or combining with other herbs (see Cacao Adaptogenic Energy Balls, page 255, and Demulcent Powder Blend, page 189).

- Shatavari is available as capsules, tablets, and powdered extracts.

- It's often a primary ingredient in various Ayurvedic replenishing formulations such as chyawanprash, the nutrient-rich Ayurvedic jam (see page 246).

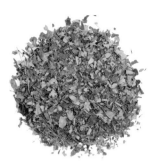

Skullcap
(*Scutellaria lateriflora*)

NERVINE CALMATIVE

This water-loving member of the mint family is most frequently found growing in moist meadows and forests and along riverbanks. The herb's tiny purple flowers resemble miniature helmets—hence its name. A native of North America, skullcap has been used for centuries by Indigenous peoples to treat a wide range of conditions. They shared many of these uses with early Anglo-American doctors known as physiomedicalists, who took a special interest in skullcap's beneficial actions on the nervous system.

Skullcap acts as both relaxant and restorative. For acute nervous system imbalances, taking skullcap is a reliable way to calm anxiety and bring about sleep during periods of intermittent insomnia. Unlike many sedatives, skullcap promotes deep, restful sleep without leaving you feeling groggy or fatigued the next morning.

Taking skullcap for extended periods can help restore and rejuvenate a nervous system that's been under chronic, unproductive stress—that classic "wired and tired" scenario, characterized by a hypervigilant nervous system and compensatory tension that short-circuits the body's ability to properly rest and restore itself. Skullcap's antispasmodic compounds ease muscle tension that gets locked into places like the neck, shoulders, jaw, and back, allowing the nervous system to gradually disarm and relax. Creating a consistent sense of ease and relaxation slowly retrains the nervous system to reclaim the energy lost to tension.

Additional uses for skullcap include easing the pain and discomfort of menstrual cramps, headaches, and nerve pain.

How to Saturate Your Day

- Skullcap works well in tincture or capsule form.

- You can take skullcap as a tea or infusion. The taste isn't spectacular, but the effects are worth it. To make a tea, steep 2 or 3 teaspoons finely cut dry herb in 1 to 1½ cups (240 to 360 ml) water for 10 to 15 minutes.

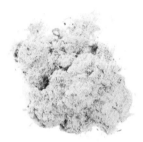

Slippery Elm
(*Ulmus rubra*)

DEMULCENT

Growing up to 60 feet (18 m) tall and living as long as two hundred years, this North American tree gets its name from the mucilage-rich inner bark found in its branches and stems. Indigenous peoples prized the bark of the slippery elm for medicine, to alleviate thirst, and as a nutritious food source, usages they taught to the Europeans. Legend has it that during the siege of Valley Forge in the winter of 1777, George Washington and his starving troops had to survive on slippery elm bark porridge for twelve days. If true, you could say that without slippery elm there would be no United States.

Slippery elm powder is a hardworking demulcent, thanks to its high mucilage content. When blended with water, it swells to many times its volume, creating a thick, viscous solution that has a flavor similar to oatmeal. Drinking slippery elm deeply hydrates and soothes the mucous membranes lining the digestive and respiratory systems. It alleviates inflammatory GI issues and serves as a soothing antacid for gastritis and GERD. It provides a valuable source of prebiotic fiber to nourish the microbiome, absorbs toxins in the GI tract, and is a bulking laxative. Slippery elm is also used to soothe and moisten sore throats and dry coughs.

Slippery elm is a threatened species in the wild from the decimation of native trees in America and Europe by Dutch elm disease, a fungal parasite. The good news is that there are plenty of sustainably grown and harvested slippery elm sources available for purchase; see the Resources, page 352.

How to Saturate Your Day

- For a simple hydrating beverage, mix 1 to 2 teaspoons slippery elm powder in 1 quart (1 L) water.

- Slippery elm is a key ingredient in a variety of demulcent preparations. See Demulcent Hydration Balls (page 189) and Prebiotic Fiber Blend (page 194).

- The shredded bark of the slippery elm can be used to make hot or cold tea.

- Slippery elm also comes in powder, capsule, and lozenge form.

Super Berries

NUTRITIVE

The term *super berry* has been coined to describe berries that are extraordinarily high in vitamins, antioxidants, and other health-enhancing constituents, and to distinguish them from the berries we ordinarily eat as part of a healthy diet. The higher concentration of vitamins and antioxidants in super berries—like polyphenols, anthocyanins, flavonoids, and vitamin C—gives them stronger flavors and makes them more medicinal in their applications and effects.

These powerful superfoods are an integral part of both diet and medicine in traditional cultures. Super berries enhance immunity, improve circulatory and

cardiovascular as well as eye health, help maintain stable blood sugar, increase energy, and reduce inflammation. Their delicious flavors make them an enjoyable way to get much-needed nutrients and antioxidants.

The super berries group includes nutritious fruits like acai berry, elderberry, camu camu, lingonberry, aronia, maqui berry, amla berry (see page 302), and goji berry (see page 319). Here's a spotlight on four important super berries.

Acai berry (*Euterpe oleracea*): Native to the rain forests of South America, this dark purple berry is the grape-size fruit of the acai palm tree. It's used extensively as both food and medicine among many Indigenous peoples, frequently added to meals and even eaten as a pulpy porridge. Because acai is delicate and only lasts a short time post-harvest before its constituents begin to degrade, it's often sold as dried powders or extracts, and can sometimes be found frozen.

Elderberry (*Sambucus canadensis* and *S. nigra*): Elderberries grow on virtually every continent and have a long history of use in traditional European and North American herbal medicine, where they are a treasured ingredient in elixirs, syrups, jams, and medicinal wines. Hippocrates referred to elderberries as "nature's medicine chest" due to the extensive list of health conditions they benefit. The delicious, juicy berries contain a host of unique antioxidants that enhance immunity and respiratory health. Traditionally they have been used to speed recovery from allergies, colds, flu, and minor coughs, and they are currently the focus of many scientific trials confirming these applications.

Lingonberry (*Vaccinium vitis-idaea*): This small, cold-loving, ruby-red berry grows wild in forests throughout the Northern Hemisphere. Lingonberry is still primarily wild harvested rather than cultivated. It's especially popular in Sweden, where it's the Scandinavian equivalent of cranberries and an integral part of the diet, eaten as an accompaniment in many meals as condiments, jams, and syrups. Lingonberry has a primarily sour

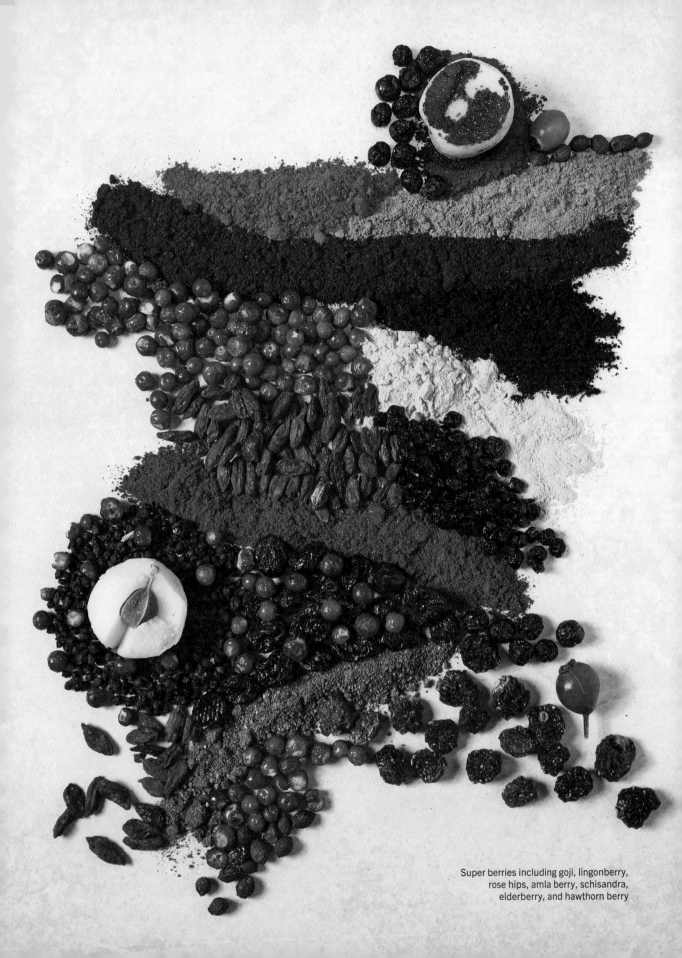

Super berries including goji, lingonberry, rose hips, amla berry, schisandra, elderberry, and hawthorn berry

taste with a hint of sweetness and is rarely eaten raw. It's also available in freeze-dried powders and juices.

Maqui berry (*Aristotelia chilensis*): Maqui is the dark purple berry of a large bush native to central and southern Chile. The leaves, stems, and berries are used extensively as both food and medicine by the indigenous Mapuche people to promote vigor and health. The antioxidant concentration of the maqui berry has been shown to be several times higher than the same quantity of blackberries, raspberries, or blueberries. Look for it in freeze-dried powders and juices.

How to Saturate Your Day

- Whole super berries are available both fresh and frozen and used in condiments, chutneys, relishes, and sauces (see Rose Hips Super Berry Antioxidant Jam, page 163).

- Super berries come in liquid concentrates, extracts, and herbal tea blends.

- Powdered formulations are great for adding to smoothies (see Super Berry Power Powder Blend, page 158).

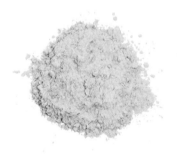

Triphala

BITTER/DETOXIFYING

Triphala is a famous Ayurvedic formula consisting of three medicinal fruits native to India and Southeast Asia: amla berry (*Emblica officinalis*), bibhitaki (*Terminalia bellirica*), and haritaki (*Terminalia chebula*). It is ubiquitous in Indian households as a daily detoxification remedy and a vitality-enhancing

tonic that removes and prevents the accumulation of ama (the Ayurvedic term for toxins) in the GI tract.

Triphala has a gentle, non–habit forming laxative effect that supports healthy elimination, kindles agni, and increases digestive power. Its unique astringency tones the villi in the small intestine, increasing their capacity to absorb nutrients. Triphala also helps balance the microbiome by neutralizing pathogenic yeasts and bacteria in the gut and supporting the growth of healthy microflora. Taken at night, triphala assists the body in its nighttime cleansing functions and encourages morning elimination. In the morning, the benefits are focused on increasing digestive fire, improving assimilation, and boosting metabolism.

Triphala supports the immune system thanks to its high vitamin C and flavonoid content. It enhances liver detoxification, reduces inflammation and other signs of excess toxins in the system, and even improves vision and dental health. This formulation is so highly respected and appreciated for its health-enhancing actions that in Ayurveda it's said, "Triphala is second only to a good mother."

How to Saturate Your Day

- Triphala is available as a powder or tablet. Mix ½ teaspoon powder in 1 to 1½ cups (240 to 360 ml) warm water and drink 2 hours after eating dinner or an hour or so before breakfast (it's best on an empty stomach). To take triphala in both the morning and evening, simply split the overall daily dosage in two. Follow the same timing using tablets or capsules in the equivalent amount. Its flavors are underwhelming, so drink it down quickly!

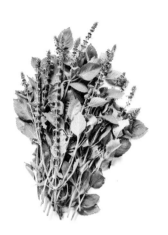

Tulsi
(*Ocimum sanctum*)

ADAPTOGEN/NERVINE

Tulsi translates as "the incomparable one" in Sanskrit and is among the most sacred herbs in all of Ayurvedic medicine. A member of the mint family, tulsi, aka holy basil, holds an important place in Hindu rituals and celebrations throughout the year. It is commonly grown in and around homes and holy places for its atmosphere-purifying effects.

Tulsi has a long and impressive list of beneficial actions that enhance functioning in virtually all essential body systems. As an adaptogen, tulsi enhances resilience to stress, increases energy, improves immunity, reduces inflammation, and promotes longevity. Its aromatic compounds vitalize nerve flow, easing tension, improving cognitive functioning, and promoting a calm, elevated state of mind.

Tulsi's warming and stimulating nature activates the respiratory system, improving breathing and increasing oxygenation. It clears congestion in the sinuses, reduces coughing, and boosts immunity during colds and flus. Like other basils, tulsi is an excellent digestive remedy for conditions characterized by low digestive fire, gas, bloating, damp stagnation, and general sluggishness. Tulsi also benefits cardiovascular health by helping to maintain balanced blood sugar and lipid levels, increasing circulation, mildly lowering blood pressure, and reducing inflammation.

How to Saturate Your Day

- Tulsi is frequently consumed as an infusion, elixir, or tea (see Tulsi Rose Chai, page 127).

- Use fresh leaves and flowers to make aromatic water (see page 210).

- Add tulsi powder or powdered extract to smoothies or powder blends.

- Tulsi also comes in tablet, capsule, and tincture forms.

- Diffuse tulsi essential oil for its calming nervine qualities.

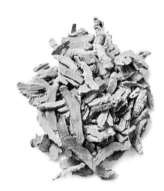

Turmeric
(*Curcuma longa*)

CULINARY

Native to southwest India, turmeric is a close relative of ginger and shares many of the same uses and benefits. It improves metabolism, enhances digestion, reduces gas and bloating, neutralizes harmful microbes, and nourishes healthy gut flora. This combined with its delicious flavor and electric orange color make turmeric one of the most beloved and widely used spices in curries throughout Asia. In India, it's called the "queen of all herbs" and imbued with great spiritual significance.

Though turmeric has been used for over five thousand years, there has been a recent resurgence of interest in its health-enhancing potential. The timing couldn't be better, as our society is contending with a massive increase in chronic disease driven by inflammation run amok. In the hunt for safe and effective natural medicines, many roads lead back to "the golden spice."

Turmeric's underground stem (rhizome) is packed with hundreds of powerful anti-inflammatory, antioxidant constituents—most notably a group of flavonoids called curcuminoids, which are responsible for its bright orange color. One of them, curcumin, has been shown to significantly increase the activity of cellular antioxidants that work to clean up free radicals and address the cause of inflammation. Turmeric is therefore invaluable for a whole host of conditions with inflammation at the root: arthritis, inflammatory gut problems, cardiovascular issues, acne, rashes, allergies, and more. It's equally beneficial to consume turmeric on a regular basis for prevention and optimization. Consistent use will create an overall improvement in essential metabolic and cellular functions while keeping inflammatory processes functional and contained.

How to Saturate Your Day

- Curcumin is poorly absorbed in the gut on its own. Combining turmeric with a small amount of black pepper has been shown to boost curcumin absorption rates up to 2,000 percent.

- Adding turmeric (either fresh or dried) to your diet a few times a week delivers antioxidants and anti-inflammatory compounds in a slow-drip fashion that will accumulate benefits over time.

- Fresh or dried turmeric can also be used to make tonics, elixirs, and lattes (see Turmeric Golden Milk Latte, page 127).

- Shots of fresh turmeric juice taken prior to meals help kindle agni (see page 40).

- Turmeric Balls (page 123) maximize absorption of the spice's active constituents.

- Turmeric can be purchased as gummies, capsules, and standardized extract tablets for convenience and potency. Curcumin is also available as an isolated compound in tablet or capsule form.

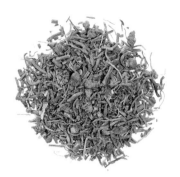

Valerian Root
(*Valeriana officinalis*)
NERVINE CALMATIVE

Valerian's name derives from the Latin *valere*, which means "to be in good health." Originally from Europe and Asia, valerian is now found growing throughout the world. Of the hundreds of valerian species, only a few are used as medicine. The species most often used in the United States and Europe, *Valeriana officinalis*, is a tried-and-true remedy for treating insomnia and anxiety.

Valerian root is rich in essential-oil constituents called valepotriates that help increase drowsiness and deepen sleep. Among them, valerenic acid and valerenol have been shown to increase the levels of GABA in the brain and prolong GABA's presence by diminishing the enzymes responsible for destroying it. This reduces anxiety and promotes worry-free sleep. Valerian is not purely sedative in action, however; taken over a period of time, it helps revitalize a weakened and depleted nervous system.

Although the flowers also contain medicinal qualities, it is the roots of valerian that are of primary use. The essential oils in valerian roots have antispasmodic effects on smooth muscles, valuable in relaxing menstrual cramps and tension-related digestive disorders such as IBS.

How to Saturate Your Day

- Drying accentuates the warming qualities of valerian root, and for some people drinking valerian tea made with the dried root can have a paradoxical energizing effect on the nervous system. Valerian tincture is mostly made from the fresh roots, which tend not to have this same effect.

• Valerian is most often used in tincture, tablet, or capsule form.

• To make a valerian tea, place ½ to 1 teaspoon cut-and-sifted dried root (or one to three tea bags) in 1 to 1½ cups (240 to 360 ml) hot water and let sit, covered, for 10 to 15 minutes.

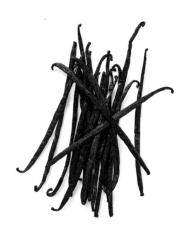

Vanilla
(*Vanilla planifolia*)
CULINARY/FRAGRANT RELAXANT

Vanilla comes from the seedpod of a jungle orchid native to Central America and southern Mexico. It was first cultivated by the Totonac people, who lived on Mexico's gulf coast. Aztecs called the plant "black flower" and included it as a key ingredient in their ancient cacao drink xocoatl (more on this on page 168).

Today, vanilla is widely cultivated in tropical countries throughout the world, including Madagascar, Indonesia, Papua New Guinea, and Tahiti. It's second only to saffron as the most expensive spice in the world. Most vanilla is turned into extract by soaking the beans in a mixture of alcohol and water to release the active constituents. The extract is available in various concentrations, denoted by the number of folds—the more folds, the higher the concentration.

Vanilla has a complex chemistry, containing more than two hundred compounds responsible for its singular aroma and flavor. Vanillin, the most well-researched constituent in vanilla, is a phenolic compound with powerful antioxidant and anti-inflammatory properties. And anyone who has ever smelled vanilla's sweet, euphoric fragrance can attest to its calming effect on the nervous system. The bean has a long history of use as a mood elevator, aphrodisiac, and fertility enhancer. Vanilla's calming effects also extend to the digestive system, where it relaxes tension in the gut, relieves excess gas and bloating, improves assimilation of nutrients, and increases appetite.

How to Saturate Your Day

• Vanilla can be consumed as a hot beverage for medicinal effects: Cut 1 vanilla bean in half per cup. Slice open the bean so the seeds and paste inside are exposed. Infuse directly into 1½ cups (360 ml) hot water for 10 minutes. Remove the bean. (You can also substitute 1 teaspoon pure vanilla extract for the vanilla bean and drink immediately.) Vanilla tastes slightly bitter—feel free to add honey or a natural sweetener of your choice to taste.

• Vanilla can be found in tea blends with other herbs.

• Diffusing vanilla essential oil calms the nervous system and elevates the mood.

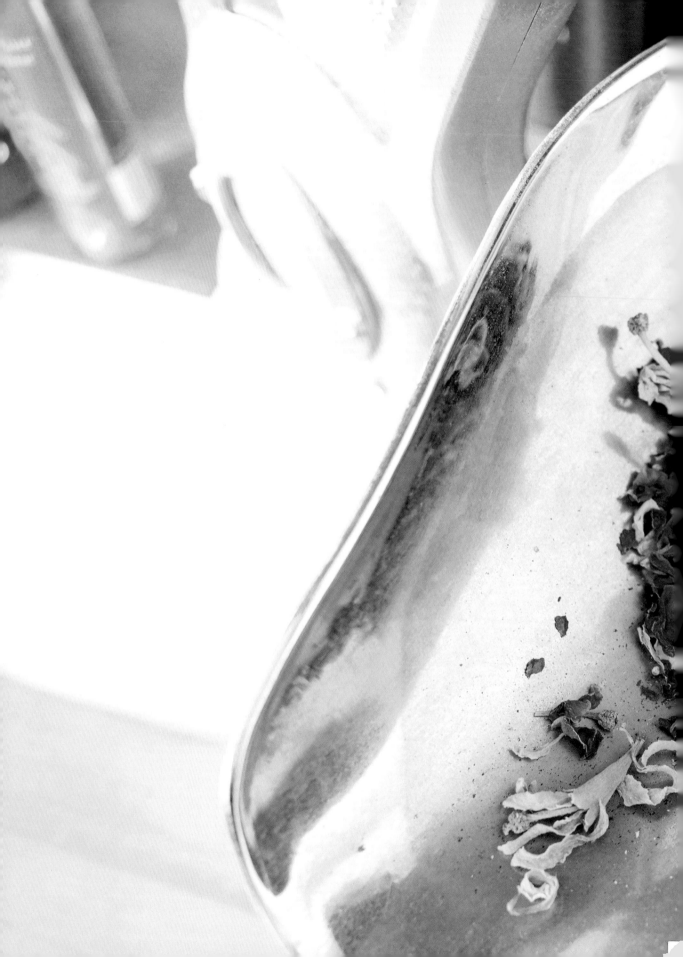

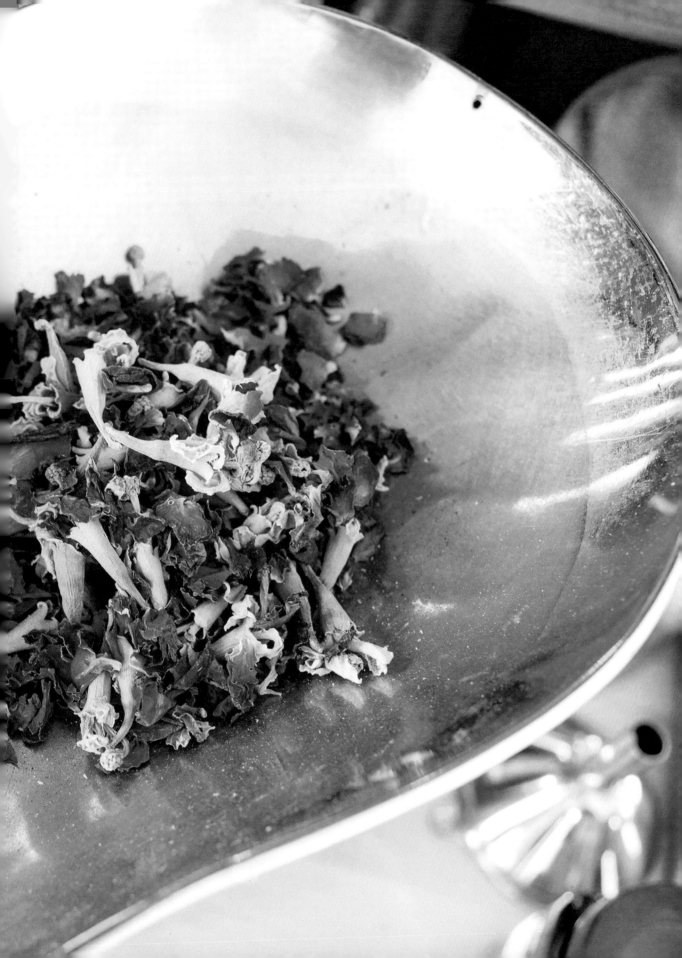

Resources

ADAPTOGENS

Four Sigmatic
us.foursigmatic.com
*Medicinal mushroom powdered extracts
and capsules*

Fungi Perfecti
fungi.com
*Medicinal mushroom powdered extracts
and capsules*

Korea Ginseng Corp
kgcus.com
Ginseng liquid packets and pastes and capsules

Kotuku Elixirs
kotukuelixirs.com
*Medicinal mushroom powdered extracts
and capsules*

Mushroom Science
mushroomscience.com
*Medicinal mushroom powdered extracts
and capsules*

Natura
naturahealthproducts.com
Adaptogenic formulas

The Tibetan Goji Berry Company
gojiberry.com
Goji berries

AYURVEDIC FORMULAS

Ayurvedic Institute
store.ayurveda.com
Drakshas

Banyan Botanicals
banyanbotanicals.com
*Chyawanprash and other Ayurvedic herbs
and supplements*

Hanah Life
hanahlife.com
Portable chyawanprash packs

Maharishi Ayurveda
mapi.com
Ayurvedic herbs and products

Mapi
mapi.com
Amrit chyawanprash

Organic India
organicindiausa.com
Teas and Ayurvedic formulations

BITTERS

Dandy Blend
dandyblend.com
Coffee alternative

Healthy Hildegard
healthyhildegard.com
Original digestive bitters tablets

Nature's Way
naturesway.com
Swedish bitters

Planetary Herbals
planetaryherbals.com
Digestive grape bitters

Urban Moonshine
urbanmoonshine.com
Digestive bitters

CACAO

Dandelion Chocolate
dandelionchocolate.com
*Large 100% cacao chunks
and nibs*

Taza Chocolate
tazachocolate.com
*Traditional stone-ground chocolate discs for cacao
beverages, including xocoatl (see page 168)*

DEMULCENTS

Lakrids by Bülow
lakridsbybulow.com
Licorice candy

New Zealand Honey Co.
newzealandhoneyco.com
Manuka honey

Planetary Herbals
planetaryherbals.com
Tri-cleanse fiber formula

Pure Encapsulations
pureencapsulationspro.com
DGL licorice

Thorne
thorne.com
FiberMend demulcent formula

ESSENTIAL OILS, RESINS & AROMATIC WOODS

Böswellness
boswellness.com
Frankincense essential oils, resins, and hydrosols

Floracopeia Botanical Treasures
floracopeia.com
*Essential oils plus ceramic bowls, charcoal, and
other equipment for diffusing and burning resins*

GREEN TEA & MATCHA

Hibiki-An
hibiki-an.com
Japanese green tea

Matcha Kari
matcha.com
Matcha

NERVINES

Bula Kava House
bulakavahouse.com
*Powdered kava, micronized kava powder,
and kava drinking supplies*

Gaia Herbs
gaiaherbs.com
Nervine tablets and capsules

Integrative Therapeutics
integrativepro.com
*D-limonene and lavender
oil capsules*

Kalm with Kava
kalmwithkava.com
Powdered kava and liquid concentrates

Klio
kliotea.com
*Greek mountain tea
and more*

New Chapter
newchapter.com
Lemon balm capsules

Papa & Barkley
papaandbarkley.com
CBD

Root of Happiness
rootofhappinesskava.com
Kava

Watkins
watkins1868.com
Peppermint extract

NUTRITIVES

Ace Ashitaba
aceashitaba.com
*Ashitaba liquid, powder, tea, and capsules,
organically grown in volcanic soil of the Izu
Islands of Japan*

Ironbound Island Seaweed
ironboundisland.com
*Sustainable wild seaweed from Maine's
Schoodic Peninsula*

Maine Coast Sea Vegetables
seaveg.com
*Sustainably harvested sea vegetables
from the coast of Maine*

Nutrex Research
nutrex.com
Hawaiian spirulina powder and tablets

Sunfood SuperFoods
sunfood.com
*Organic chlorella, moringa, and other nutritive
powders, capsules, and extracts*

PLANT-BASED TONICS

Goldthread Tonics
drinkgoldthread.com
*Plant-based tonics formulated to support the
essential systems of the body with 14 grams of
medicinal plants in each bottle*

Mastiqua
greekflavours.com
Sparkling water infused with Greek mastic

TINCTURES & SUPPLEMENTS

Gaia Herbs
gaiaherbs.com
*Adaptogenic capsules, digestive capsules, and
capsules to aid in sleep, plus individual herb
tinctures and capsules*

Herb Pharm
herb-pharm.com
*Adaptogenic capsules, digestive capsules, and
capsules to aid in sleep, plus individual herb
tinctures and capsules*

Herbalist and Alchemist
herbalist-alchemist.com
*Adaptogenic capsules, digestive capsules, and
capsules to aid in sleep, plus individual herb
tinctures and capsules*

Integrative Therapeutics
integrativepro.com
D-limonene orange peel extract capsules, curcumin capsules, lavender essential oil capsules, and peppermint essential oil capsules

New Chapter
newchapter.com
Cinnamon, elderberry, ginger, holy basil, lemon balm, rhodiola, and turmeric capsules, plus elderberry gummies

Planetary Herbals
planetaryherbals.com
Digestive grape bitters, amla and triphala capsules, as well as various other capsule formulations and liquid herbal extracts

Thorne
thorne.com
Turmeric and concentrated curcumin capsules

TRADITIONAL CHINESE FORMULAS

Kan Herb Company
kanherb.com
Traditional Chinese Medicine formulas in capsule and liquid extract form, for both adults and children

Mayway
mayway.com
Bulk loose herbs such as astragalus, reishi, he shou wu, and others, as well as a range of supplements and patent formulations

WHOLE HERBS, POWDERS & POWDERED EXTRACTS

From Great Origins
fromgreatorigins.com
Tea bags

Frontier Herbs
frontiercoop.com
Bulk whole loose herbs, powders, and tea bags

Microingredients
microingredients.com
Super-berry and green powdered extracts and tablets, adaptogens, and medicinal mushroom extract powders

Mountain Rose Herbs
mountainroseherbs.com
Bulk whole loose herbs, powders, and tea bags

Pacific Botanicals
pacificbotanicals.com
Bulk whole loose herbs, powders, and tea bags

Starwest Botanicals
starwest-botanicals.com
Bulk whole loose herbs, powders, and tea bags

Traditional Medicinals
traditionalmedicinals.com
Tea bags

Zack Woods Herb Farm
zackwoodsherbs.com
Bulk whole loose herbs and powders

Further Reading

Adaptogens: Herbs for Strength, Stamina, and Stress Relief by David Winston and Steven Maimes

Ayurveda, Nature's Medicine by Dr. David Frawley and Dr. Subhash Ranade

Ayurveda: The Science of Self-Healing by Dr. Vasant Lad

Christopher Hobbs's Medicinal Mushrooms: The Essential Guide by Christopher Hobbs, LAc

Foundations of Health: Healing with Herbs by Christopher Hobbs, LAc

The Healing Power of Minerals, Special Nutrients, and Trace Elements by Paul Bergner

Healing Spices: How to Use 50 Everyday and Exotic Spices to Boost Health and Beat Disease by Dr. Bharat B. Aggarwal with Debora Yost

The Herbal Handbook: A User's Guide to Medical Herbalism by David Hoffmann

Herbal Recipes for Vibrant Health: 175 Teas, Tonics, Oils, Salves, Tinctures, and Other Natural Remedies for the Entire Family by Rosemary Gladstar

Herbs for Common Ailments: How to Make and Use Herbal Remedies for Home Health Care by Rosemary Gladstar

In Search of the Medicine Buddha: A Himalayan Journey by David Crow

Newcomb's Wildflower Guide by Lawrence Newcomb

Planetary Herbology: An Integration of Western Herbs into the Traditional Chinese and Ayurvedic Systems by Michael Tierra, LAc, OMD

The Way of Herbs by Michael Tierra, LAc, OMD

The Web That Has No Weaver: Understanding Chinese Medicine by Ted J. Kaptchuk, OMD

Acknowledgments

My name may be on the front cover, yet the truth is that the information contained in this book—about the many benefits readers will surely get from including medicinal plants in their lives—is the end result of many, many people's support, wisdom, generosity, patience, and hard work. I am immensely grateful to all of them for inspiring me and teaching me what I needed to know to write this book. The first mention has to go to my friends and family for cheering me on every day and understanding my periodic disappearing acts. You know who you are!

Hazel and Caleb, thank you for your spirit of adventure, curiosity, and belief in me, and for always being up for chewing on some spilanthes buds.

I have to thank everyone who has been a student of mine over the years. You challenged me to develop, refine, organize, and express this subject with ever-greater clarity and usefulness.

Thank you to my Ayurvedic sensei, my co-conspirator in the grassroots herbal health-care revolution, and the man I'll always be willing to go on a spruce chase with, David Crow. Many of the ideas in this book were inspired by his brilliance and commitment and our long days working together on the farm.

To the dedicated and talented Goldthread team, you guys rock! There is no crew I'd rather be on the front lines with. You all have made our vision of medicinal plants being widely accessible and mainstream a reality with your tireless hard work, determination, and passion.

I would like to thank Edith and Dennis Mehiel for their immense support and mentorship, without which I would never have had the opportunity to get this book from my mind onto the page.

Thanks to Mark Plotkin, my longtime hero and friend from down in the Bayou. You never stop working tirelessly and with good humor to protect the places where plants and people intersect. Having you recognize me as a fellow ethnobotanist is a high honor indeed.

Many, many thanks to my community of fellow plant people around the world (some pictured on page 358). It's a privilege to spend time with and learn from those who love medicinal plants as much as I do! I have been fortunate enough to see firsthand so many of the inspiring projects and so much of the work you are doing to cultivate and gather the plants we rely on to keep us healthy, and to pass on the knowledge about how to use them best.

Thank you to my book whisperer and agent, Stephanie Tade, the first person to jump on board with me when I was just a wildly enthusiastic guy who knew how to help people get healthy with medicinal plants. Thanks for picking me up off the mat when I needed it and always being the steadying force that helped me stay the course.

Thank you to Danielle Claro for giving the book its liftoff and compass heading. You created a simple, elegant, and cogent outline that got this whole thing started.

I always knew that bringing this subject to life visually was a vital part of communicating the subject matter of this book, but I had no idea that a photo shoot could be a mind-blowing, life-altering experience! Thank you so much Kelsey Fugere, Monika Bukowska, Baxley Andresen, and Jeffrey Fountain for giving medicinal plants the supermodel treatment and capturing their beauty and magic so masterfully. Getting a front-row seat to true artists at work for those two weeks was electric, inspiring, hilarious, and utterly exhausting in the best way!

Special thanks to Alexis Lipsitz for her incredible skill as a writer/editor/coach all in one. The work we did together was the most productive and intense time of the whole

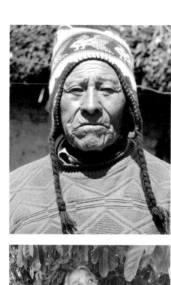
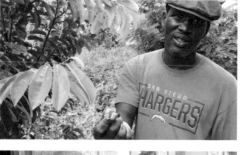
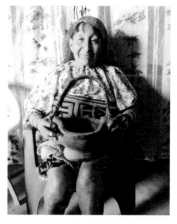
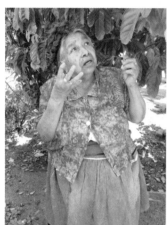
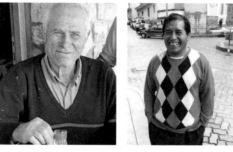
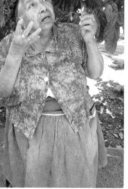
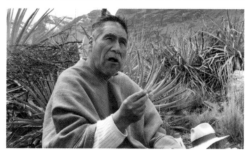
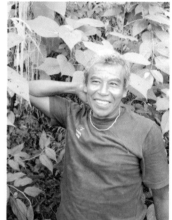
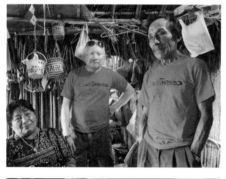
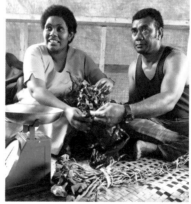
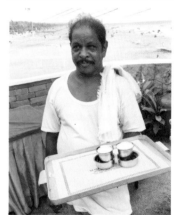
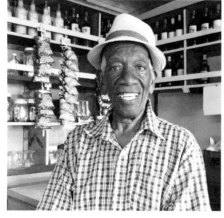
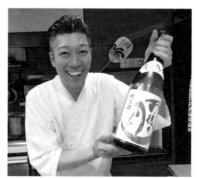
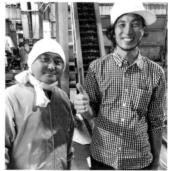

project, and I will always be grateful to you for literally dragging me to the finish line of this manuscript. Your positivity from our first phone call to the last page made all the difference. Thank you for being so patient as we turned an amorphous blob of inspiration into clear, useful information.

They say it takes a village, and the whole Artisan team was mine. Lia Ronnen, visionary and literary genius, your belief in me and the Plant Medicine Protocol gave me the confidence to shoot for the stars. You gave me the space and support to do whatever it took to make the best book possible. Thank you for taking a chance on this project and so generously sharing your invaluable insight and wisdom.

It is difficult to convey how amazing and essential my tireless and talented editor, Bridget Monroe Itkin, has been to this project. You were the expert Sherpa guiding me up the mountain of this enormous endeavor. Your eye for detail, organization, and precision were indispensable, keeping me on track and literally crossing my t's and dotting my i's. I'll be forever grateful for all the work you put into making this book become a reality.

The Artisan design team—Suet Chong, Nina Simoneaux, and Erica Heitman-Ford—absolutely crushed it, managing endless feedback, revisions, and tight deadlines. Thanks for working so diligently and rising to the challenge of designing a book with so many complex elements and themes that people can actually use. You brought everything to life so thoughtfully, beautifully, and with great style.

And thanks to the rest of my publishing team: Laura Cherkas, Sibylle Kazeroid, Sara Vigneri, Diana Valcárcel, Annie O'Donnell, Maggie Byrd, Nancy Murray, Donna Brown, Erica Huang, Zach Greenwald, Rebecca Carlisle, Moira Kerrigan, and Cindy Lee.

There is literally no way in hell that I would have completed this book without Edith, my beautiful, talented, genius wife and partner. Throughout every adventure, every photo, every word on every page, she has been right there with me, working with superhuman dedication, perseverance, and good humor on what were often thankless, frustrating, and time-consuming tasks. Her commitment to the mission of getting plants to people and willingness to do the hard work without any expectation of recognition or accolades is truly amazing to me. I say without a trace of hyperbole that I can only aspire to be as loving, generous, and supportive as she is to me on a daily basis. I am a truly lucky man to travel the rough road of life with a woman like her by my side.

I'll conclude with a salute to my green friends. Because of the plants, I've seen the world, met amazing people, and had priceless experiences. I always feel the healthiest and happiest when I am full of phytochemicals, and if I can do even half as good a job on their behalf as they have done for me, I will consider it a success.

Notes

Preface

8 most well-researched compounds, piperine: Haq, Iahtisham-UI, et al. "Piperine: a review of its biological effects." *Phytotherapy research* 35, 2 (2021): 680–700. doi:10.1002/ptr.6855.

Introduction

17 clear factors in their longevity: Johnson, Adiv A., et al. "Human age reversal: fact or fiction?" *Aging cell* 21, 8 (2022): e13664. doi:10.1111/acel.13664.

PART I:
NATURAL MEDICINE FUNDAMENTALS

27 According to the World Health Organization: WHO. "Traditional, Complementary and Integrative Medicine." Accessed October 25, 2022. https://www.who.int/health-topics/traditional-complementary-and-integrative-medicine.

40 The lymph glands lining our GI tract: West, Christina E., et al. "The gut microbiota and inflammatory noncommunicable diseases: associations and potentials for gut microbiota therapies." *Journal of allergy and clinical immunology* 135, 1 (2015): 3–13; quiz 14. doi:10.1016/j.jaci.2014.11.012.

48 people who have a high HRV: Manresa-Rocamora, Agustín, et al. "Heart rate variability-guided training for enhancing cardiac-vagal modulation, aerobic fitness, and endurance performance: a methodological systematic review with meta-analysis." *International journal of environmental research and public health* 18, 19 (29 Sep. 2021): 10299. doi:10.3390/ijerph181910299.

da Estrela, Chelsea, et al. "Heart rate variability, sleep quality, and depression in the context of chronic stress." *Annals of behavioral medicine* 55, 2 (2021): 155–64. doi:10.1093/abm/kaaa039.

Schiweck, Carmen, et al. "Heart rate and high frequency heart rate variability during stress as biomarker for clinical depression: a systematic review." *Psychological medicine* 49, 2 (2019): 200–211. doi:10.1017/S0033291718001988.

52 a 1 to 2 percent decrease in the body's water: Szinnai, G., et al. "Effect of dehydration and rehydration on cognitive performance and mood among male college students." *Journal of cognitive neuroscience*: 17, 2 (2005): 143–52.

58 Science has discovered more than twenty-five thousand: Minich, D. M. "A review of the science of colorful, plant-based food and practical strategies for 'eating the rainbow.'" *Journal of nutrition and metabolism* 2019 (2 Jun. 2019): 2125070. doi:10.1155/2019/2125070.

61 immune-boosting mushrooms: Ahmad, Rizwan, et al. "*Ganoderma lucidum* (reishi) an edible mushroom; a comprehensive and critical review of its nutritional, cosmeceutical, mycochemical, pharmacological, clinical, and toxicological properties." *Phytotherapy research* 35, 11 (2021): 6030–62. doi:10.1002/ptr.7215.

Motta, Francesca, et al. "Mushrooms and immunity." *Journal of autoimmunity* 117 (2021): 102576. doi:10.1016/j.jaut.2020.102576.

61 echinacea and andrographis, are used primarily: Ogal, Mercedes, et al. "Echinacea reduces antibiotic usage in children through respiratory tract infection prevention: a randomized, blinded, controlled clinical trial." *European journal of medical research* 26, 1 (8 Apr. 2021): 33. doi:10.1186/s40001-021-00499-6.

Hu, Xiao-Yang, et al. "*Andrographis paniculata* (chuān xīn lián) for symptomatic relief of acute respiratory tract infections in adults and children: a systematic review and meta-analysis." *PLOS one* 12, 8 (4 Aug. 2017): e0181780. doi:10.1371/journal.pone.0181780.

63 Having daily doses of spices: Serafini, Mauro, et al. "Functional foods for health: the interrelated antioxidant and anti-inflammatory role of fruits, vegetables, herbs, spices and cocoa in humans." *Current pharmaceutical design* 22, 44 (2016): 6701–15. doi:10.2174/1381612823666161123094235.

El-Saber Batiha, Gaber, et al. "Chemical constituents and pharmacological activities of garlic (*Allium sativum* L.): a review." *Nutrients* 12, 3 (24 Mar. 2020): 872. doi:10.3390/nu12030872.

Ranasinghe, Priyanga, et al. "Medicinal properties of 'true' cinnamon (*Cinnamomum zeylanicum*): a systematic review." *BMC complementary and alternative medicine* 13, 275 (22 Oct. 2013). doi:10.1186/1472-6882-13-275.

78 Herbs like chamomile: El Mihyaoui, Amina, et al. "Chamomile (*Matricaria chamomilla* L.): a review of ethnomedicinal use, phytochemistry and pharmacological uses." *Life* (Basel, Switzerland) 12, 4 (25 Mar. 2022): 479. doi:10.3390/life12040479.

Zam, Wissam, et al. "An updated review on the properties of *Melissa officinalis* L.: not exclusively anti-anxiety." *Frontiers in bioscience* (scholar edition) 14, 2 (2022): 16. doi:10.31083/j.fbs1402016.

82 **Adaptogens help regulate the stress response:** Panossian, Alexander, et al. "Effects of adaptogens on the central nervous system and the molecular mechanisms associated with their stress-protective activity." *Pharmaceuticals* (Basel, Switzerland) 3, 1 (19 Jan. 2010) 188–224. doi:10.3390/ph3010188.

82 **fortify the immune system by simmering:** Zhang, Jianqin, et al. "Astragaloside IV derived from *Astragalus membranaceus*: a research review on the pharmacological effects." *Advances in pharmacology* (San Diego, Calif.) 87 (2020): 89–112. doi:10.1016/bs.apha.2019.08.002.

82 **If the goal is enhanced athletic performance:** Sellami, Maha, et al. "Herbal medicine for sports: a review." *Journal of the international society of sports nutrition* 15, 14 (15 Mar. 2018). doi:10.1186/s12970-018-0218-y.

PART II:
THE PLANT PROTOCOL

Step One: Culinary Herbs, Spices, and Bitters

115 **confirm it has a positive effect:** Allen, Robert W., et al. "Cinnamon use in type 2 diabetes: an updated systematic review and meta-analysis." *Annals of family medicine* 11, 5 (2013): 452–59. doi:10.1370/afm.1517.

117 **support the functioning of our liver:** Tsai, Yu-Ling, et al. "Probiotics, prebiotics and amelioration of diseases." *Journal of biomedical science* 26, 1 (4 Jan. 2019) 3. doi:10.1186/s12929-018-0493-6.

136 **Green tea has proven medicinal benefits:** Khan, Naghma, et al. "Tea polyphenols in promotion of human health." *Nutrients* 11, 1 (2018 Dec. 25): 39. doi:10.3390/nu11010039.

139 **increasing the amino acid L-theanine:** Owen, Gail N., et al. "The combined effects of L-theanine and caffeine on cognitive performance and mood." *Nutritional neuroscience* 11, 4 (2008): 193–98. doi:10.1179/147683008X301513.

Step Two: Nutritives

153 **to improve vision and ease eye:** Kan, Juntao, et al. "A novel botanical formula improves eye fatigue and dry eye: a randomized, double-blind, placebo-controlled study." *American journal of clinical nutrition* 112, 2 (2020): 334–42. doi:10.1093/ajcn/nqaa139.

168 **wide range of polyphenolic flavonoids:** Ellam, Samantha, et al. "Cocoa and human health." *Annual review of nutrition* 33 (2013): 105–28. doi:10.1146/annurev-nutr-071811-150642.

168 **Compounds such as theobromine, caffeine:** Nehlig, Astrid. "The neuroprotective effects of cocoa flavanol and its influence on cognitive performance." *British journal of clinical pharmacology* 75, 3 (2013): 716–27. doi:10.1111/j.1365-2125.2012.04378.x.

170 **Harvard researchers that concluded:** Bayard, V., et al. "Does flavanol intake influence mortality from nitric oxide-dependent processes? Ischemic heart disease, stroke, diabetes mellitus, and cancer in Panama." *International journal of medical sciences* 4, 1 (20071): 53–58. doi:10.7150/ijms.4.53.

Step Three: Demulcents

176 **are high in mucilage content and therefore:** Szentmihályi, Klára, et al. "[Mineral content of some herbs and plant extracts with anti-inflammatory effect used in gastrointestinal diseases]." *Orvosi hetilap* 154, 14 (2013): 538–43. doi:10.1556/OH.2013.29578.

183 **plantain leaf, which has a unique:** Adom, Muhammad Bahrain, et al. "Chemical constituents and medical benefits of *Plantago major*." *Biomedicine & pharmacotherapy* 96 (2017): 348–60. doi:10.1016/j.biopha.2017.09.152.

186 **olive oil has demulcent properties:** Millman, Jasmine F., et al. "Extra-virgin olive oil and the gut-brain axis: influence on gut microbiota, mucosal immunity, and cardiometabolic and cognitive health." *Nutrition reviews* 79, 12 (2021): 1362–74. doi:10.1093/nutrit/nuaa148.

186 **manuka stands out among them for:** Johnston, Matthew, et al. "Antibacterial activity of manuka honey and its components: an overview." *AIMS microbiology* 4, 4 (27 Nov. 2018): 655–64. doi:10.3934/microbiol.2018.4.655.

Step Four: Nervines

200 **with cooling, anti-inflammatory actions:** Pandur, Edina, et al. "Anti-inflammatory effect of lavender (*Lavandula angustifolia* Mill.) essential oil prepared during different plant phenophases on THP-1 macrophages." *BMC complementary medicine and therapies* 21, 1 (24 Nov. 2021): 287. doi:10.1186/s12906-021-03461-5.

200 **improve sleep quality:** Yıldırım, Dilek, et al. "The effect of lavender oil on sleep quality and vital signs in palliative care: a randomized clinical trial."

Complementary medicine research 27, 5 (2020): 328–35. doi:10.1159/000507319.

200 **lavender oil is beneficial when applied topically:** Ben Djemaa, Ferdaous Ghrab, et al. "Antioxidant and wound healing activity of *Lavandula aspic* L. ointment." *Journal of tissue viability* 25, 4 (2016): 193–200. doi:10.1016/j.jtv.2016.10.002.

200 **anti-inflammatory, blood-vitalizing, and antimicrobial actions:** Antunes Viegas, Daniel, et al. "*Helichrysum italicum*: from traditional use to scientific data." *Journal of ethnopharmacology* 151, 1 (2014): 54–65. doi:10.1016/j.jep.2013.11.005.

200 **jatamansi has relaxing and hypnotic qualities:** Panara, Kalpesh, et al. "Central nervous system depressant activity of jatamansi (*Nardostachys jatamansi* DC.) rhizome." *Ayu* 41, 4 (2020): 250–54. doi:10.4103/ayu.AYU_251_20.

201 **when applied topically, frankincense has significant:** Li, Xiao-Jun, et al. "α-Pinene, linalool, and 1-octanol contribute to the topical anti-inflammatory and analgesic activities of frankincense by inhibiting COX-2." *Journal of ethnopharmacology* 179 (2016): 22–26. doi:10.1016/j.jep.2015.12.039.

208 **Mountain tea relaxes tension:** Brankovic, Suzana, et al. "Spasmolytic activity of the ethanol extract of *Sideritis raeseri* spp. *raeseri* Boiss. & Heldr. on the isolated rat ileum contractions." *Journal of medicinal food* 14, 5 (2011): 495–98. doi:10.1089/jmf.2010.0036.

211 **Drinking this frothy green beverage:** Baba, Yoshitake, et al. "Matcha consumption maintains attentional function following a mild acute psychological stress without affecting a feeling of fatigue: a randomized placebo-controlled study in young adults." *Nutrition research* (New York, NY) 88 (2021): 44–52. doi:10.1016/j.nutres.2020.12.024.

211 **Packed with antioxidants:** Jakubczyk, Karolina, et al. "Antioxidant properties and nutritional composition of matcha green tea." *Foods* (Basel, Switzerland) 9, 4 (12 Apr. 2020): 483. doi:10.3390/foods9040483.

211 **magnesium, a vital mineral for improving:** Mah, Jasmine, et al. "Oral magnesium supplementation for insomnia in older adults: a systematic review & meta-analysis." *BMC complementary medicine and therapies* 21, 1 (17 Apr. 2021): 125. doi:10.1186/s12906-021-03297-z.

215 *abhyanga*, **delivers the calming:** Basler, Annetrin Jytte. "Pilot study investigating the effects of Ayurvedic abhyanga massage on subjective stress experience." *Journal of alternative and complementary medicine* (New York, NY) 17, 5 (2011): 435–40. doi:10.1089/acm.2010.0281.

226 **kavalactones, are responsible for its relaxing:** Wang, Yingli, et al. "Biological activity, hepatotoxicity, and structure-activity relationship of kavalactones and flavokavins, the two main bioactive components in kava (*Piper methysticum*)." *Evidence-based complementary and alternative medicine* 2021 (20 Aug. 2021): 6851798. doi:10.1155/2021/6851798.

PART IV: PLANT PROFILES

302 **ALOE VERA (*Aloe vera*):** Gao, Yan, et al. "Biomedical applications of *Aloe vera*." *Critical reviews in food science and nutrition* 59, sup1 (2019): S244–56. doi:10.1080/10408398.2018.1496320.

Hekmatpou, Davood, et al. "The effect of *Aloe vera* clinical trials on prevention and healing of skin wound: a systematic review." *Iranian journal of medical sciences* 44, 1 (2019): 1–9.

Sánchez, Marta, et al. "Pharmacological update properties of *Aloe vera* and its major active constituents." *Molecules* (Basel, Switzerland) 25, 6 (13 Mar. 2020): 1324. doi:10.3390/molecules25061324.

302 **AMLA BERRY (*Emblica officinalis*):** Akhtar, Muhammad Shoaib, et al. "Effect of amla fruit (*Emblica officinalis* Gaertn.) on blood glucose and lipid profile of normal subjects and type 2 diabetic patients." *International journal of food sciences and nutrition* 62, 6 (2011): 609–16. doi:10.3109/09637486.2011.560565.

Ghaffari, Samad, et al. "A randomized, triple-blind, placebo-controlled, add-on clinical trial to evaluate the efficacy of *Emblica officinalis* in uncontrolled hypertension." *Evidence-based complementary and alternative medicine* (7 Oct. 2020): 8592869. doi:10.1155/2020/8592869.

Krishnaveni, Mani, et al. "Therapeutic potential of *Phyllanthus emblica* (amla): the Ayurvedic wonder." *Journal of basic and clinical physiology and pharmacology* 21, 1 (2010): 93–105. doi:10.1515/jbcpp.2010.21.1.93.

Yadav, Suraj Singh, et al. "Traditional knowledge to clinical trials: a review on therapeutic actions of *Emblica officinalis*." *Biomedicine & pharmacotherapy* 93 (2017): 1292–1302. doi:10.1016/j.biopha.2017.07.065.

302 **Amla berries have been the subject:** Variya, Bhavesh C., et al. "*Emblica officinalis* (amla): a review for its phytochemistry, ethnomedicinal uses and medicinal potentials with respect to molecular mechanisms." *Pharmacological research* 111 (2016): 180–200. doi:10.1016/j.phrs.2016.06.013.

303 **ARTICHOKE LEAF (*Cynara scolymus*):** Ben Salem, Maryem, et al. "Pharmacological studies of artichoke leaf extract and their health benefits." *Plant foods for human nutrition* (Dordrecht, Netherlands) 70, 4 (2015): 441–53. doi:10.1007/s11130-015-0503-8.

Moradi, Sajjad, et al. "The effects of *Cynara scolymus* L. supplementation on liver enzymes: a systematic review and meta-analysis." *International journal of clinical practice* 75, 11 (2021): e14726. doi:10.1111 /ijcp.14726.

304 **ASHITABA (*Angelica keiskei*):** Kil, Yun-Seo, et al. "*Angelica keiskei*, an emerging medicinal herb with various bioactive constituents and biological activities." *Archives of pharmacal research* 40, 6 (2017): 655–75. doi:10.1007/s12272-017-0892-3.

304 **chalcones enhance the rate at which cells:** Chang, Chia-Ting, et al. "Chalcone flavokawain B induces autophagic-cell death via reactive oxygen species-mediated signaling pathways in human gastric carcinoma and suppresses tumor growth in nude mice." *Archives of toxicology* 91, 10 (2017): 3341–64.

304 **ASHWAGANDHA ROOT (*Withania somnifera*):** Mandlik Ingawale, et al. "Pharmacological evaluation of ashwagandha highlighting its healthcare claims, safety, and toxicity aspects." *Journal of dietary supplements* 18, 2 (2021): 183–226. doi:10.1080 /19390211.2020.1741484.

Mishra, L. C., et al. "Scientific basis for the therapeutic use of *Withania somnifera* (ashwagandha): a review." *Alternative medicine review* 5, 4 (2000): 334–46.

Paul, Subhabrata, et al. "*Withania somnifera* (L.) dunal (ashwagandha): a comprehensive review on ethnopharmacology, pharmacotherapeutics, biomedicinal and toxicological aspects." *Biomedicine & pharmacotherapy* 143 (2021): 112175. doi:10.1016/j.biopha.2021.112175.

Speers, Alex B., et al. "Effects of *Withania somnifera* (ashwagandha) on stress and the stress-related neuropsychiatric disorders anxiety, depression, and insomnia." *Current neuropharmacology* 19, 9 (2021): 1468–95. doi:10.2174/157015 9X19666210712151556.

Wankhede, Sachin, et al. "Examining the effect of *Withania somnifera* supplementation on muscle strength and recovery: a randomized controlled trial." *Journal of the international society of sports nutrition* 12 (25 Nov. 2015): 43. doi:10.1186/ s12970-015-0104-9.

305 **ASTRAGALUS ROOT (*Astragalus membranaceus*):** Fu, Juan, et al. "Review of the botanical characteristics, phytochemistry, and pharmacology of *Astragalus membranaceus* (huangqi)." *Phytotherapy research* 28, 9 (2014): 1275–83. doi:10.1002/ptr.5188.

Li, Chun-Xiao, et al. "Astragalus polysaccharide: a review of its immunomodulatory effect." *Archives of pharmacal research* 45, 6 (2022): 367–89. doi:10.1007/s12272-022-01393-3.

Qi, Yan, et al. "Anti-inflammatory and immunostimulatory activities of astragalosides." *American journal of Chinese medicine* 45, 6 (2017): 1157–67. doi:10.1142/S0192415X1750063X.

Zheng, Yijun, et al. "A review of the pharmacological action of astragalus polysaccharide." *Frontiers in pharmacology* 11 (24 Mar. 2020): 349. doi:10.3389 /fphar.2020.00349.

306 **BASIL LEAF (*Ocimum basilicum*):** Sestili, Piero, et al. "The potential effects of *Ocimum basilicum* on health: a review of pharmacological and toxicological studies." *Expert opinion on drug metabolism & toxicology* 14, 7 (2018): 679–92. doi:10.1080/1742 5255.2018.1484450.

Teofilovic, Branislava, et al. "Pharmacological effects of novel microvesicles of basil, on blood glucose and the lipid profile: a preclinical study." *Scientific reports* 11, 1 (11 Nov. 2021): 22123. doi:10.1038/s41598 -021-01713-5.

307 **BASIL SEED (*Ocimum basilicum*):** Calderón Bravo, Héctor, et al. "Basil seeds as a novel food, source of nutrients and functional ingredients with beneficial properties: a review." *Foods* (Basel, Switzerland) 10, 7 (24 Jun. 2021): 1467. doi:10.3390/ foods10071467.

Martínez, Rosario, et al. "Bioavailability and biotransformation of linolenic acid from basil seed oil as a novel source of omega-3 fatty acids tested on a rat experimental model." *Food & function* 13, 14 (18 Jul. 2022): 7614–28. doi:10.1039/d2fo00672c.

307 **BURDOCK ROOT (*Arctium* species):** Chan, Yuk-Shing, et al. "A review of the pharmacological effects of *Arctium lappa* (burdock)." *Inflammopharmacology* 19, 5 (2011): 245–54. doi:10.1007/s10787-010-0062-4.

de Souza, Ariádine Reder Custodio, et al. "Phytochemicals and biological activities of burdock (*Arctium lappa* L.) extracts: a review." *Chemistry & biodiversity* (5 Oct. 2022): e202200615. doi:10.1002/cbdv.202200615.

Li, Dandan, et al. "Prebiotic effectiveness of inulin extracted from edible burdock." *Anaerobe* 14, 1 (2008): 29–34. doi:10.1016/j. anaerobe.2007.10.002.

308 **CALIFORNIA POPPY (*Eschscholzia californica*):** Rolland, A., et al. "Behavioural effects of the American traditional plant *Eschscholzia californica*: sedative and anxiolytic properties." *Planta medica* 57, 3 (1991): 212–16. doi:10.1055/s-2006-960076.

309 **CANNABIS (*Cannabis sativa*):** Aviram, J., et al. "Efficacy of cannabis-based medicines for pain management: a systematic review and meta-analysis of randomized controlled trials." *Pain physician* 20, 6 (2017): E755–96.

Bonini, Sara Anna, et al. "*Cannabis sativa*: a comprehensive ethnopharmacological review of a medicinal plant with a long history." *Journal of ethnopharmacology* 227 (2018): 300–315. doi:10.1016/j.jep.2018.09.004.

Farinon, Barbara, et al. "The seed of industrial hemp (*Cannabis sativa* L.): nutritional quality and potential functionality for human health and nutrition." *Nutrients* 12, 7 (29 Jun. 2020): 1935. doi:10.3390/nu12071935.

Sarris, Jerome, et al. "Medicinal cannabis for psychiatric disorders: a clinically-focused systematic review." *BMC psychiatry* 20, 1 (16 Jan. 2020): 24. doi:10.1186/s12888-019-2409-8.

309 **CHAMOMILE (*Matricaria chamomilla*):** Amsterdam, Jay D., et al. "Putative antidepressant effect of chamomile (*Matricaria chamomilla* L.) oral extract in subjects with comorbid generalized anxiety disorder and depression." *Journal of alternative and complementary medicine* (New York, NY) 26, 9 (2020): 813–19. doi:10.1089/acm.2019.0252.

McKay, Diane L., et al. "A review of the bioactivity and potential health benefits of chamomile tea (*Matricaria recutita* L.)." *Phytotherapy research* 20, 7 (2006): 519–30. doi:10.1002/ptr.1900.

310 **CHIA SEED (*Salvia hispanica*):** Parker, John, et al. "Therapeutic perspectives on chia seed and its oil: a review." *Planta medica* 84, 9–10 (2018): 606–12. doi:10.1055/a-0586-4711.

Valdivia-López, Ma Ángeles, et al. "Chia (*Salvia hispanica*): a review of native Mexican seed and its nutritional and functional properties." *Advances in food and nutrition research* 75 (2015): 53–75. doi:10.1016/bs.afnr.2015.06.002.

Vega Joubert, Michelle Berenice, et al. "*Salvia hispanica* L. (chia) seed improves liver inflammation and endothelial dysfunction in an experimental model of metabolic syndrome." *Food & function* 13, 21 (31 Oct. 2022): 11249–61. doi:10.1039/d2fo02216h.

311 **CHLORELLA & SPIRULINA:** Bito, Tomohiro, et al. "Potential of *Chlorella* as a dietary supplement to promote human health." *Nutrients* 12, 9 (20 Aug. 2020): 2524. doi:10.3390/nu12092524.

Ko, Seok-Chun, et al. "Protective effect of a novel antioxidative peptide purified from a marine *Chlorella ellipsoidea* protein against free radical-induced oxidative stress." *Food and chemical toxicology* 50, 7 (2012): 2294–302. doi:10.1016/j.fct.2012.04.022.

Panahi, Yunes, et al. "*Chlorella vulgaris*: a multifunctional dietary supplement with diverse medicinal properties." *Current pharmaceutical design* 22, 2 (2016): 164–73. doi:10.2174/1381612822666151112145226.

Wu, Qinghua, et al. "The antioxidant, immunomodulatory, and anti-inflammatory activities of spirulina: an overview." *Archives of toxicology* 90, 8 (2016): 1817–0. doi:10.1007/s00204-016-1744-5.

313 **CINNAMON (*Cinnamomum verum*):** Ghavami, Abed, et al. "What is the impact of cinnamon supplementation on blood pressure? A systematic review and meta-analysis." *Endocrine, metabolic & immune disorders drug targets* 21, 5 (2021): 956–65. doi:10.2174/1871530320666200729143614.

Mollazadeh, Hamid, et al. "Cinnamon effects on metabolic syndrome: a review based on its mechanisms." *Iranian journal of basic medical sciences* 19, 12 (2016): 1258–70. doi:10.22038/ijbms.2016.7906.

Singh, Neetu, et al. "Phytochemical and pharmacological review of *Cinnamomum verum* J. Presl—a versatile spice used in food and nutrition." *Food chemistry* 338 (2021): 127773. doi:10.1016/j.foodchem.2020.127773.

313 **Cinnamon also has blood-sugar moderating effects:** Gruenwald, Joerg, et al. "Cinnamon and health." *Critical reviews in food science and nutrition* 50, 9 (2010): 822–34. doi:10.1080/10408390902773052.

313 **by consuming ½ teaspoon of cinnamon:** Allen, Robert W., et al. "Cinnamon use in type 2 diabetes: an updated systematic review and meta-analysis." *Annals of family medicine* 11, 5 (2013): 452–59. doi:10.1370/afm.1517.

313 **CITRUS PEELS:** Liu, Na, et al. "A review of chemical constituents and health-promoting effects of citrus peels." *Food chemistry* 365 (2021): 130585. doi:10.1016/j.foodchem.2021.130585.

Parmar, Hamendra Singh, et al. "Medicinal values of fruit peels from *Citrus sinensis*, *Punica granatum*, and *Musa paradisiaca* with respect to alterations in tissue lipid peroxidation and serum concentration of glucose, insulin, and thyroid hormones." *Journal of medicinal food* 11, 2 (2008): 376–81. doi:10.1089/jmf.2006.010.

Singh, Balwinder, et al. "Phenolic composition, antioxidant potential and health benefits of citrus peel." *Food research international* (Ottawa, Ont.) 132 (2020): 109114. doi:10.1016/j.foodres.2020.109114.

Terpstra, A. H. M., et al. "The hypocholesterolemic effect of lemon peels, lemon pectin, and the waste stream material of lemon peels in hybrid F1B hamsters." *European journal of nutrition* 41, 1 (2002): 19–26. doi:10.1007/s003940200002

314 **CORDYCEPS** (*Cordyceps sinensis* & *C. militaris*): Das, Gitishree, et al. "*Cordyceps* spp.: a review on its immune-stimulatory and other biological potentials." *Frontiers in pharmacology* 11 (8 Feb. 2021): 602364. doi:10.3389/fphar.2020.602364.

Ji, Deng-Bo, et al. "Antiaging effect of *Cordyceps sinensis* extract." *Phytotherapy research* 23, 1 (2009): 116–22. doi:10.1002/ptr.2576.

Olatunji, Opeyemi Joshua, et al. "The genus *Cordyceps*: an extensive review of its traditional uses, phytochemistry and pharmacology." *Fitoterapia* 129 (2018): 293–316. doi:10.1016/j.fitote.2018.05.010.

Zhang, Hong Wei, et al. "*Cordyceps sinensis* (a traditional Chinese medicine) for treating chronic kidney disease." *Cochrane database of systematic reviews* 12 (18 Dec. 2014): CD008353. doi:10.1002/14651858.CD008353.pub2.

315 **DANDELION** (*Taraxacum officinale*): González-Castejón, Marta, et al. "Diverse biological activities of dandelion." *Nutrition reviews* 70, 9 (2012): 534–47. doi:10.1111/j.1753-4887.2012.00509.x.

Li, Yanni, et al. "The potential of dandelion in the fight against gastrointestinal diseases: a review." *Journal of ethnopharmacology* 293 (2022): 115272. doi:10.1016/j.jep.2022.115272.

Schütz, Katrin, et al. "*Taraxacum*—a review on its phytochemical and pharmacological profile." *Journal of ethnopharmacology* 107, 3 (2006): 313–23. doi:10.1016/j.jep.2006.07.021.

315 **GARLIC** (*Allium sativum*): Dorrigiv, Mahyar, et al. "Garlic (*Allium sativum*) as an antidote or a protective agent against natural or chemical toxicities: a comprehensive update review." *Phytotherapy research* 34, 8 (2020): 1770–97. doi:10.1002/ptr.6645.

Shang, Ao, et al. "Bioactive compounds and biological functions of garlic (*Allium sativum* L.)." *Foods* (Basel, Switzerland) 8, 7 (5 Jul. 2019): 246. doi:10.3390/foods8070246.

316 **GENTIAN ROOT** (*Gentiana* species): Li, Jie, et al. "Phytochemistry and pharmacological activities of the genus *Swertia* (Gentianaceae): a review." *American journal of Chinese medicine* 45, 4 (2017): 667–736. doi:10.1142/S0192415X17500380.

317 **GINGERROOT** (*Zingiber officinale*): Akinyemi, Ayodele Jacob, et al. "Inhibition of angiotensin-1-converting enzyme activity by two varieties of ginger (*Zingiber officinale*) in rats fed a high cholesterol diet." *Journal of medicinal food* 17, 3 (2014): 317–23. doi:10.1089/jmf.2012.0264.

Ali, Badreldin H., et al. "Some phytochemical, pharmacological and toxicological properties of ginger (*Zingiber officinale* Roscoe): a review of recent research." *Food and chemical toxicology* 46, 2 (2008): 409–20. doi:10.1016/j.fct.2007.09.085.

Haniadka, Raghavendra, et al. "A review of the gastroprotective effects of ginger (*Zingiber officinale* Roscoe)." *Food & function* 4, 6 (2013): 845–55. doi:10.1039/c3fo30337c.

Mao, Qian-Qian, et al. "Bioactive compounds and bioactivities of ginger (*Zingiber officinale* Roscoe)." *Foods* (Basel, Switzerland) 8, 6 (30 May 2019): 185. doi:10.3390/foods8060185.

317 **ginger's ability to modulate COX-2:** Grzanna, Reinhard, et al. "Ginger—an herbal medicinal product with broad anti-inflammatory actions." *Journal of medicinal food* 8, 2 (2005): 125–32. doi:10.1089/jmf.2005.8.125.

318 **GINSENG ROOT** (*Panax* species): de Oliveira Zanuso, Bárbara, et al. "*Panax ginseng* and aging related disorders: a systematic review." *Experimental gerontology* 161 (2022): 111731. doi:10.1016/j.exger.2022.111731.

Flanagan, Shawn D., et al. "The effects of a Korean ginseng, GINST15, on hypo-pituitary-adrenal and oxidative activity induced by intense work stress." *Journal of medicinal food* 21, 1 (2018): 104–12. doi:10.1089/jmf.2017.0071.

Jung, Dong-Hyuk, et al. "Effects of ginseng on peripheral blood mitochondrial DNA copy number and hormones in men with metabolic syndrome: a randomized clinical and pilot study." *Complementary therapies in medicine* 24 (2016): 40–46. doi:10.1016/j.ctim.2015.12.001.

Kiefer, David, et al. "*Panax ginseng.*" *American family physician* 68, 8 (2003): 1539–42.

Shergis, Johannah L., et al. "*Panax ginseng* in randomised controlled trials: a systematic review." *Phytotherapy research* 27, 7 (2013): 949–65. doi:10.1002/ptr.4832.

318 **ginseng's ability to enhance mitochondrial:** Luo, John Zeqi, et al. "American ginseng stimulates insulin production and prevents apoptosis through regulation of uncoupling protein-2 in cultured beta cells." *Evidence-based complementary and alternative medicine* 3, 3 (2006): 365–72. doi:10.1093/ecam/nel026.

319 **GOJI BERRY (*Lycium barbarum*):** Gao, Yanjie, et al. "*Lycium barbarum*: a traditional Chinese herb and a promising anti-aging agent." *Aging and disease* 8, 6 (Dec. 2017): 778–91. doi:10.14336/AD.2017.0725.

Kan, Juntao, et al. "A novel botanical formula improves eye fatigue and dry eye: a randomized, double-blind, placebo-controlled study." *American journal of clinical nutrition* 112, 2 (2020): 334–42. doi:10.1093/ajcn/nqaa139.

Tian, Xiaojing, et al. "Extraction, structural characterization, and biological functions of *Lycium barbarum* polysaccharides: a review." *Biomolecules* 9, 9 (21 Aug. 2019): 389. doi:10.3390/biom9090389.

Yang, Chunhong, et al. "Effects of *Lycium barbarum* L. polysaccharides on vascular retinopathy: an insight review." *Molecules* (Basel, Switzerland) 27, 17 (31 Aug. 2022): 5628. doi:10.3390/molecules27175628.

319 **GOTU KOLA (*Centella asiatica*):** Chandrika, Udumalagala Gamage, et al. "Gotu kola (*Centella asiatica*): nutritional properties and plausible health benefits." *Advances in food and nutrition research* 76 (2015): 125–57. doi:10.1016/bs.afnr.2015.08.001.

Puttarak, Panupong, et al. "Effects of *Centella asiatica* (L.) Urb. on cognitive function and mood related outcomes: a systematic review and meta-analysis." *Scientific reports* 7, 1 (6 Sep. 2017): 10646. doi:10.1038/s41598-017-09823-9.

Sun, Boju, et al. "Therapeutic potential of *Centella asiatica* and its triterpenes: a review." *Frontiers in pharmacology* 11 (4 Sep. 2020): 568032. doi:10.3389/fphar.2020.568032.

Torbati, Farshad Abedi, et al. "Ethnobotany, phytochemistry and pharmacological features of *Centella asiatica*: a comprehensive review." *Advances in experimental medicine and biology* 1308 (2021): 451–99. doi:10.1007/978-3-030-64872-5_25.ß

320 **commonly used to sharpen memory and focus:** Wong, Jia Hui, et al. "Mitoprotective effects of *Centella asiatica* (L.) urb.: anti-inflammatory and neuroprotective opportunities in neurodegenerative disease." *Frontiers in pharmacology* 12 (29 Jun. 2021): 687935. doi:10.3389/fphar.2021.687935.

320 **GREEK MOUNTAIN TEA (*Sideritis* species):** Tadić, Vanja M., et al. "Anti-inflammatory, gastroprotective, and cytotoxic effects of *Sideritis scardica* extracts." *Planta medica* 78, 5 (2012): 415–27. doi:10.1055/s-0031-1298172.

Todorova, Milka, et al. "*Sideritis scardica* Griseb., an endemic species of Balkan peninsula: traditional uses, cultivation, chemical composition, biological activity." *Journal of ethnopharmacology* 152, 2 (2014): 256–65. doi:10.1016/j.jep.2014.01.022.

Wightman, Emma L., et al. "The acute and chronic cognitive and cerebral blood flow effects of a *Sideritis scardica* (Greek mountain tea) extract: a double blind, randomized, placebo controlled, parallel groups study in healthy humans." *Nutrients* 10, 8 (24 Jul. 2018): 955.

321 **HIBISCUS (*Hibiscus sabdariffa*):** Abdelmonem, Mohamed, et al. "Efficacy of *Hibiscus sabdariffa* on reducing blood pressure in patients with mild-to-moderate hypertension: a systematic review and meta-analysis of published randomized controlled trials." *Journal of cardiovascular pharmacology* 79, 1 (2022): e64–74. doi:10.1097/FJC.0000000000001161.

Ali, Badreldin H., et al. "Phytochemical, pharmacological and toxicological aspects of *Hibiscus sabdariffa* L.: a review." *Phytotherapy research* 19, 5 (2005): 369–75. doi:10.1002/ptr.1628.

Da-Costa-Rocha, Inês, et al. "*Hibiscus sabdariffa* L.—a phytochemical and pharmacological review." *Food chemistry* 165 (2014): 424–43. doi:10.1016/j.foodchem.2014.05.002.

Guardiola, Soledad, et al. ["Therapeutic potential of *Hibiscus sabdariffa*: a review of the scientific evidence."] *Endocrinologia y nutricion* 61, 5 (2014): 274–95. doi:10.1016/j.endonu.2013.10.012.

Riaz, Ghazala, et al. "A review on phytochemistry and therapeutic uses of *Hibiscus sabdariffa* L." *Biomedicine & pharmacotherapy* 102 (2018): 575–86. doi:10.1016/j.biopha.2018.03.023.

321 **lower blood pressure by relaxing blood vessels:** Serban, Corina, et al. "Effect of sour tea (*Hibiscus sabdariffa* L.) on arterial hypertension: a systematic review and meta-analysis of randomized controlled trials." *Journal of hypertension* 33, 6 (2015): 1119–27. doi:10.1097/HJH.0000000000000585.

322 **HONEYBUSH & ROOIBOS:** Marnewick, Jeanine L., et al. "Effects of rooibos (*Aspalathus linearis*) on oxidative stress and biochemical parameters in adults at risk for cardiovascular disease." *Journal of ethnopharmacology* 133, 1 (2011): 46–52. doi:10.1016/j.jep.2010.08.061.

Choi, Sun Young, et al. "Protective effects of fermented honeybush (*Cyclopia intermedia*) extract (HU-018) against skin aging: a randomized, double-blinded, placebo-controlled study." *Journal of cosmetic and laser therapy* 20, 5 (2018): 313–18. doi:10.1080/14764172.2017.1418512.

McKay, Diane L., et al. "A review of the bioactivity of South African herbal teas: rooibos (*Aspalathus linearis*) and honeybush (*Cyclopia intermedia*)." *Phytotherapy research* 21, 1 (2007): 1–16. doi:10.1002/ptr.1992.

323 **IRISH MOSS (*Chondrus crispus*):** Liu, Jinghua, et al. "Prebiotic effects of diet supplemented with the cultivated red seaweed *Chondrus crispus* or with fructo-oligo-saccharide on host immunity, colonic microbiota and gut microbial metabolites." *BMC complementary and alternative medicine* 15 (14 Aug. 2015): 279. doi:10.1186/s12906-015-0802-5.

Robertson, Ruairi C., et al. "The anti-inflammatory effect of algae-derived lipid extracts on lipopolysaccharide (LPS)-stimulated human THP-1 macrophages." *Marine drugs* 13, 8 (20 Aug. 2015): 5402-24. doi:10.3390/md13085402.

323 **LAVENDER (*Lavendula angustifolia*):** Cavanagh, H. M. A., et al. "Biological activities of lavender essential oil." *Phytotherapy research* 16, 4 (2002): 301–8. doi:10.1002/ptr.1103.

Firoozeei, Toktam Sadat, et al. "The antidepressant effects of lavender (*Lavandula angustifolia* Mill.): a systematic review and meta-analysis of randomized controlled clinical trials." *Complementary therapies in medicine* 59 (2021): 102679. doi:10.1016/j.ctim.2021.102679.

Karan, Nazife Begüm. "Influence of lavender oil inhalation on vital signs and anxiety: a randomized clinical trial." *Physiology & behavior* 211 (2019): 112676. doi:10.1016/j.physbeh.2019.112676.

323 **lavender calms the agitated states:** Donelli, Davide, et al. "Effects of lavender on anxiety: a systematic review and meta-analysis." *Phytomedicine* 65 (2019): 153099. doi:10.1016/j.phymed.2019.153099.

324 **LEMON BALM (*Melissa officinalis*):** Ghazizadeh, Javid, et al. "The effects of lemon balm (*Melissa officinalis* L.) on depression and anxiety in clinical trials: a systematic review and meta-analysis." *Phytotherapy research* 35, 12 (2021): 6690–705. doi:10.1002/ptr.7252.

Miraj, Sepide, et al. "*Melissa officinalis* L.: a review study with an antioxidant prospective." *Journal of evidence-based complementary & alternative medicine* 22, 3 (2017): 385–94. doi:10.1177/2156587216663433.

Sadraei, H., et al. "Relaxant effect of essential oil of *Melissa officinalis* and citral on rat ileum contractions." *Fitoterapia* 74, 5 (2003): 445–52. doi:10.1016/s0367-326x(03)00109-6.

Shakeri, Abolfazl, et al. "*Melissa officinalis* L.—a review of its traditional uses, phytochemistry and pharmacology." *Journal of ethnopharmacology* 188 (2016): 204–28. doi:10.1016/j.jep.2016.05.010.

Shekarriz, Zahra, et al. "Effect of *Melissa officinalis* on systolic and diastolic blood pressures in essential hypertension: a double-blind crossover clinical trial." *Phytotherapy research* 35, 12 (2021): 6883–92. doi:10.1002/ptr.7251.

324 **Its essential oil contains geraniol:** Petrisor, Gabriela, et al. "*Melissa officinalis*: composition, pharmacological effects and derived release systems—a review." *International journal of molecular sciences* 23, 7 (25 Mar. 2022): 3591. doi:10.3390/ijms23073591.

325 **LEMON VERBENA (*Aloysia citriodora*):** Bahramsoltani, Roodabeh, et al. "*Aloysia citriodora* Paláu (lemon verbena): a review of phytochemistry and pharmacology." *Journal of ethnopharmacology* 222 (2018): 34–51. doi:10.1016/j.jep.2018.04.021.

325 **verbascoside, is being studied closely:** Daels-Rakotoarison, D. A., et al. "Neurosedative and antioxidant activities of phenylpropanoids from *Ballota nigra*." *Arzneimittel-Forschung* 50, 1 (2000): 16–23. doi:10.1055/s-0031-1300158.

325 **LICORICE ROOT (*Glychrizzia glabra*):** Murugan, Sasi Kumar, et al. "A flavonoid rich standardized extract of *Glycyrrhiza glabra* protects intestinal epithelial barrier function and regulates the tight-junction proteins expression." *BMC complementary medicine and therapies* 22,1 (7 Feb. 2022): 38. doi:10.1186/s12906-021-03500-1.

Pastorino, Giulia, et al. "Liquorice (*Glycyrrhiza glabra*): a phytochemical and pharmacological review." *Phytotherapy research* 32, 12 (2018): 2323–39. doi:10.1002/ptr.6178.

Wahab, Shadma, et al. "*Glycyrrhiza glabra* (licorice): a comprehensive review on its phytochemistry, biological activities, clinical evidence and toxicology." *Plants* (Basel, Switzerland) 10, 12 (14 Dec. 2021): 2751. doi:10.3390/plants10122751.

326 **licorice over long periods of time:** Penninkilampi, R., et al. "The association between consistent licorice ingestion, hypertension and hypokalaemia: a systematic review and meta-analysis." *Journal of human hypertension* 31, 11 (2017): 699–707. doi:10.1038/jhh.2017.45.

326 **potentially cause water retention:** Celik, M. M., et al. "Licorice induced hypokalemia, edema, and thrombocytopenia." *Human & experimental toxicology* 31, 12 (2012): 1295–98. doi:10.1177/0960327112446843.

326 **LINDEN (*Tilia* species.):** Angeles-López, Guadalupe E., et al. "Neuroprotective evaluation of *Tilia americana* and *Annona diversifolia* in the neuronal damage induced by intestinal ischemia." *Neurochemical research* 38, 8 (2013): 1632–40. doi:10.1007/s11064-013-1065-5.

327 **farnesol can mildly lower blood pressure:** Silva, E. A. P., et al. "Cardiovascular effects of farnesol and its β-cyclodextrin complex in normotensive and hypertensive rats." *European journal of pharmacology* 901 (2021): 174060. doi:10.1016/j.ejphar.2021.174060.

327 **protect blood vessels from inflammation:** Calderón-Montaño, J. M., et al. "A review on the dietary flavonoid kaempferol." *Mini reviews in medicinal chemistry* 11, 4 (2011): 298–344. doi:10.2174/138955711795305335.

327 **MACA ROOT (*Lepidium meyenii*):** Colareda, Germán A., et al. "*Lepidium meyenii* (maca) and soy isoflavones reduce cardiac stunning of ischemia-reperfusion in rats by mitochondrial mechanisms." *Journal of traditional and complementary medicine* 11, 6 (2 Apr. 2021): 471–80. doi:10.1016/j.jtcme.2021.03.004.

da Silva Leitão Peres, Natália, et al. "Medicinal effects of Peruvian maca (*Lepidium meyenii*): a review." *Food & function* 11, 1 (2020): 83–92. doi:10.1039/c9fo02732g.

Wang, Sunan, et al. "Chemical composition and health effects of maca (*Lepidium meyenii*)." *Food chemistry* 288 (2019): 422–43. doi:10.1016/j.foodchem.2019.02.071.

Zhu, Hongkang, et al. "Anti-fatigue effect of *Lepidium meyenii* Walp. (maca) on preventing mitochondria-mediated muscle damage and oxidative stress in vivo and vitro." *Food & function* 12, 7 (2021): 3132–41. doi:10.1039/d1fo00383f.

327 **compounds in maca root:** Shin, Byung-Cheul, et al. "Maca (*L. meyenii*) for improving sexual function: a systematic review." *BMC complementary and alternative medicine* 10 (2010): 44. doi:10.1186/1472-6882-10-44.

328 **MARSHMALLOW ROOT (*Althaea officinalis*):** Bonaterra, Gabriel A., et al. "Anti-inflammatory and anti-oxidative effects of Phytohustil and root extract of *Althaea officinalis* L. on macrophages in vitro." *Frontiers in pharmacology* 11 (17 Mar. 2020): 290. doi:10.3389/fphar.2020.00290.

Xue, Tao-Tao, et al. "Evaluation of antioxidant, enzyme inhibition, nitric oxide production inhibitory activities and chemical profiles of the active extracts from the medicinal and edible plant *Althaea officinalis*." *Food research international* (Ottawa, Ont.) 156 (2022): 111166. doi:10.1016/j.foodres.2022.111166.

330 **Chaga (*Inonotus obliquus*):** Szychowski, Konrad A., et al. "*Inonotus obliquus*—from folk medicine to clinical use." *Journal of traditional and complementary medicine* 11, 4 (22 Aug. 2020): 293–302. doi:10.1016/j.jtcme.2020.08.003.

Zhao, Yanxia, et al. "Deciphering the antitumoral potential of the bioactive metabolites from medicinal mushroom *Inonotus obliquus*." *Journal of ethnopharmacology* 265 (2021): 113321. doi:10.1016/j.jep.2020.113321.

330 **Lion's mane (*Hericium erinaceous*):** He, Xirui, et al. "Structures, biological activities, and industrial applications of the polysaccharides from *Hericium erinaceus* (lion's mane) mushroom: a review." *International journal of biological macromolecules* 97 (2017): 228–37. doi:10.1016/j.ijbiomac.2017.01.040.

Khan, Md Asaduzzaman, et al. "*Hericium erinaceus*: an edible mushroom with medicinal values." *Journal of complementary & integrative medicine* 10, 1 (24 May 2013). doi:10.1515/jcim-2013-0001.

Mori, Koichiro, et al. "Improving effects of the mushroom yamabushitake (*Hericium erinaceus*) on mild cognitive impairment: a double-blind placebo-controlled clinical trial." *Phytotherapy research* 23, 3 (2009): 367–72. doi:10.1002/ptr.2634.

Saitsu, Yuusuke, et al. "Improvement of cognitive functions by oral intake of *Hericium erinaceus*." *Biomedical research* (Tokyo, Japan) 40, 4 (2019): 125–31. doi:10.2220/biomedres.40.125.

330 **unique compounds in lion's mane:** Gregory, et al. "Neuroprotective herbs for the management of Alzheimer's disease." *Biomolecules* 11, 4 (8 Apr. 2021): 543. doi:10.3390/biom11040543.

330 **Maitake (*Grifola frondosa*):** Li, Qian, et al. "Purification, characterization and immunomodulatory activity of a novel polysaccharide from *Grifola frondosa*." *International journal of biological macromolecules* 111 (2018): 1293–303. doi:10.1016/j.ijbiomac.2018.01.090.

Ulbricht, Catherine, et al. "Maitake mushroom (*Grifola frondosa*): systematic review by the natural standard research collaboration." *Journal of the society for integrative oncology* 7, 2 (2009): 66–72.

Wu, Jian-Yong, et al. "Bioactive ingredients and medicinal values of *Grifola frondosa* (maitake)." *Foods* (Basel, Switzerland) 10, 1 (5 Jan. 2021): 95. doi:10.3390/foods10010095.

330 **Shiitake (*Lentinus edodes*):** Assemie, Anmut, et al. "The effect of edible mushroom on health and their biochemistry." *International journal of microbiology* 2022 (23 Mar. 2022): 8744788. doi:10.1155/2022/8744788.

Bisen, P. S., et al. "*Lentinus edodes*: a macrofungus with pharmacological activities." *Current medicinal chemistry* 17, 22 (2010): 2419–30. doi:10.2174/092986710791698495.

Kabir, Y., et al. "Effect of shiitake (*Lentinus edodes*) and maitake (*Grifola frondosa*) mushrooms on blood pressure and plasma lipids of spontaneously hypertensive rats." *Journal of nutritional science and vitaminology* 33, 5 (1987): 341–46. doi:10.3177/jnsv.33.341.

330 **Turkey tail (*Trametes versicolor*):** Benson, Kathleen F., et al. "The mycelium of the *Trametes versicolor* (turkey tail) mushroom and its fermented substrate each show potent and complementary immune activating properties in vitro." *BMC complementary and alternative medicine* 19, 1 (2 Dec. 2019): 342.

Chu, Kevin K. W., et al. "*Coriolus versicolor*: a medicinal mushroom with promising immunotherapeutic values." *Journal of clinical pharmacology* 42, 9 (2002): 976–84.

330 **effective in activating a broad-spectrum immune:** Ren, Lu, et al. "Antitumor activity of mushroom polysaccharides: a review." *Food & function* 3, 11 (2012): 1118–30. doi:10.1039/c2fo10279j.

331 **MILK THISTLE (*Silybum marianum*):** Shaker, E., et al. "Silymarin, the antioxidant component and *Silybum marianum* extracts prevent liver damage." *Food and chemical toxicology* 48, 3 (2010): 803–6. doi:10.1016/j.fct.2009.12.011.

Skottová, N., et al. "Silymarin as a potential hypocholesterolaemic drug." *Physiological research* 47, 1 (1998): 1–7.

Soleimani, Vahid, et al. "Safety and toxicity of silymarin, the major constituent of milk thistle extract: an updated review." *Phytotherapy research* 33, 6 (2019): 1627–38. doi:10.1002/ptr.6361.

Wang, Xin, et al. "Health benefits of *Silybum marianum*: phytochemistry, pharmacology, and applications." *Journal of agricultural and food chemistry* 68, 42 (2020): 11644. doi:10.1021/acs.jafc.0c04791.

332 **MORINGA (*Moringa oleifera*):** Abdull Razis, Ahmad Faizal, et al. "Health benefits of *Moringa oleifera*." *Asian Pacific journal of cancer prevention* 15, 20 (2014): 8571–76. doi:10.7314/apjcp.2014.15.20.8571.

Anwar, Farooq, et al. "*Moringa oleifera*: a food plant with multiple medicinal uses." *Phytotherapy research* 21, 1 (2007): 17–25. doi:10.1002/ptr.2023.

Kou, Xianjuan, et al. "Nutraceutical or pharmacological potential of *Moringa oleifera* Lam." *Nutrients* 10, 3 (12 Mar. 2018): 343. doi:10.3390/nu10030343.

Watanabe, Shihori, et al. "*Moringa oleifera* Lam. in diabetes mellitus: a systematic review and meta-analysis." *Molecules* (Basel, Switzerland) 26, 12 (9 Jun. 2021): 3513. doi:10.3390/molecules26123513.

332 **kidneys' ability to filter toxins:** Akter, Tanzina, et al. "Prospects for protective potential of *Moringa oleifera* against kidney diseases." *Plants* (Basel, Switzerland) 10, 12 (20 Dec. 2021): 2818. doi:10.3390/plants10122818.

332 **Moringa is also a significant source:** Ahmad, Jamil, et al. "*Moringa oleifera* and glycemic control: a review of current evidence and possible mechanisms." *Phytotherapy research* 33, 11 (2019): 2841–48. doi:10.1002/ptr.6473.

332 **NETTLES (*Urtica dioica* and *U. urens*):** Dhouibi, Raouia, et al. "Screening of pharmacological uses of *Urtica dioica* and other benefits." *Progress in biophysics and molecular biology* 150 (2020): 67–77. doi:10.1016/j.pbiomolbio.2019.05.008.

Hajihashemi, Saeed, et al. "Ameliorative effect of cotreatment with the methanolic leaf extract of *Urtica dioica* on acute kidney injury induced by gentamicin in rats." *Avicenna journal of phytomedicine* 10, 3 (2020): 273–86.

Kregiel, Dorota, et al. "*Urtica* spp.: ordinary plants with extraordinary properties." *Molecules* (Basel, Switzerland) 23, 7 (9 Jul. 2018): 1664. doi:10.3390/molecules23071664.

333 **PASSIONFLOWER (*Passiflora incarnata*):** Appel, Kurt, et al. "Modulation of the γ-aminobutyric acid (GABA) system by *Passiflora incarnata* L." *Phytotherapy research* 25, 6 (2011): 838–43. doi:10.1002/ptr.3352.

Miroddi, M., et al. "*Passiflora incarnata* L.: ethnopharmacology, clinical application, safety and evaluation of clinical trials." *Journal of ethnopharmacology* 150, 3 (2013): 791–804. doi:10.1016/j.jep.2013.09.047.

333 ***Passiflora incarnata*, has been used for centuries:** Miyasaka, L. S., et al. "Passiflora for anxiety disorder." *Cochrane database of systematic reviews* 1 (24 Jan. 2007): CD004518. doi:10.1002/14651858.CD004518.pub2.

334 **PEPPERMINT & SPEARMINT:** Chumpitazi, B. P., et al. "Review article: the physiological effects and safety of peppermint oil and its efficacy in irritable bowel syndrome and other functional disorders." *Alimentary pharmacology & therapeutics* 47, 6 (2018): 738–52. doi:10.1111/apt.14519.

Kennedy, David, et al. "Volatile terpenes and brain function: investigation of the cognitive and mood effects of *Mentha × piperita* L. essential oil with in vitro properties relevant to central nervous system function." *Nutrients* 10, 8 (7 Aug. 2018): 1029. doi:10.3390/nu10081029.

Mahboubi, Mohaddese. "*Mentha spicata* L. essential oil, phytochemistry and its effectiveness in flatulence." *Journal of traditional and complementary medicine* 11, 2 (28 Sep. 2018): 75–81. doi:10.1016/j. jtcme.2017.08.011.

Mahendran, Ganesan, et al. "The traditional uses, phytochemistry and pharmacology of spearmint (*Mentha spicata* L.): a review." *Journal of ethnopharmacology* 278 (2021): 114266. doi:10.1016/j.jep.2021.114266.

McKay, Diane L., et al. "A review of the bioactivity and potential health benefits of peppermint tea (*Mentha piperita* L.)." *Phytotherapy research* 20, 8 (2006): 619–33. doi:10.1002/ptr.1936.

Zhang, Lu-Lu, et al. "Bioactive properties of the aromatic molecules of spearmint (*Mentha spicata* L.) essential oil: a review." *Food & function* 13, 6 (21 Mar. 2022): 3110–2. doi:10.1039/d1fo04080d.

334 **PSYLLIUM HUSK (*Plantago ovata*):** Fierascu, Radu Claudiu, et al. "*Plantago media* L.—explored and potential applications of an underutilized plant." *Plants* (Basel, Switzerland) 10, 2 (30 Jan. 2021): 265. doi:10.3390/plants10020265.

Jovanovski, Elena, et al. "Effect of psyllium (*Plantago ovata*) fiber on LDL cholesterol and alternative lipid targets, non-HDL cholesterol and apolipoprotein B: a systematic review and meta-analysis of randomized controlled trials." *American journal of clinical nutrition* 108, 5 (2018): 922–32. doi:10.1093/ajcn/nqy115.

Sarfraz, Rai Muhammad, et al. "*Plantago ovata*: a comprehensive review on cultivation, biochemical, pharmaceutical and pharmacological aspects." *Acta poloniae pharmaceutica* 74, 3 (2017): 739–46.

335 **REISHI (*Ganoderma lucidum*):** Ahmad, Md Faruque, et al. "*Ganoderma lucidum*: a potential source to surmount viral infections through β-glucans immunomodulatory and triterpenoids antiviral properties." *International journal of biological macromolecules* 187 (2021): 769–79. doi:10.1016 /j.ijbiomac.2021.06.122.

Chan, Sze Wa, et al. "The beneficial effects of *Ganoderma lucidum* on cardiovascular and metabolic disease risk." *Pharmaceutical biology* 59, 1 (2021): 1161–71. doi:10.1080/13880209.2021. 1969413.

Meng, Jia, et al. "Protective effect of *Ganoderma* (lingzhi) on cardiovascular system." *Advances in experimental medicine and biology* 1182 (2019): 181–99. doi:10.1007/978-981-32-9421-9_7.

Sanodiya, Bhagwan S., et al. "*Ganoderma lucidum*: a potent pharmacological macrofungus." *Current pharmaceutical biotechnology* 10, 8 (2009): 717–42. doi:10.2174/138920109789978757.

335 **also has well-researched beneficial:** Seweryn, Ewa, et al. "Health-promoting of polysaccharides extracted from *Ganoderma lucidum*." *Nutrients* 13, 8 (7 Aug. 2021): 2725. doi:10.3390/nu13082725.

336 **RHODIOLA (*Rhodiola rosea*):** Kelly, G. S. "*Rhodiola rosea*: a possible plant adaptogen." *Alternative medicine review* 6, 3 (2001): 293–302.

Cropley, Mark, et al. "The effects of *Rhodiola rosea* L. extract on anxiety, stress, cognition and other mood symptoms." *Phytotherapy research* 9, 12 (2015): 1934–39. doi:10.1002/ptr.5486.

Ma, Gou-Ping, et al. "*Rhodiola rosea* L. improves learning and memory function: preclinical evidence and possible mechanisms." *Frontiers in pharmacology* 9 (4 Dec. 2018): 1415. doi:10.3389/ fphar.2018.01415.

Panossian, A., et al. "Rosenroot (*Rhodiola rosea*): traditional use, chemical composition, pharmacology and clinical efficacy." *Phytomedicine* 17, 7 (2010): 481–93. doi:10.1016/j.phymed.2010.02.002.

337 **consider for increasing physical energy and endurance:** Olsson, Erik M., et al. "A randomised, double-blind, placebo-controlled, parallel-group study of the standardised extract shr-5 of the roots of *Rhodiola rosea* in the treatment of subjects with stress-related fatigue." *Planta medica* 75, 2 (2009): 105–12. doi:10.1055/s-0028-1088346.

337 **accelerate recovery between workouts:** Lu, Yao, et al. "Effects of *Rhodiola rosea* supplementation on exercise and sport: a systematic review." *Frontiers in nutrition* 9 (7 Apr. 2022): 856287. doi:10.3389 /fnut.2022.856287.

337 **ROSE HIP (*Rosa canina* & *R. rugosa*):** Ayati, Zahra, et al. "Phytochemistry, traditional uses and pharmacological profile of rose hip: a review." *Current pharmaceutical design* 24, 35 (2018): 4101–24. doi:10.2174/1381612824666181010151849.

Chrubasik, Cosima, et al. "A systematic review on the *Rosa canina* effect and efficacy profiles."

Phytotherapy research 22, 6 (2008): 725–33. doi:10.1002/ptr.2400.

Lei, Zhiyong, et al. "Rosehip oil promotes excisional wound healing by accelerating the phenotypic transition of macrophages." *Planta medica* 85, 7 (2019): 563–69. doi:10.1055/a-0725-8456.

Pekacar, Sultan, et al. "Anti-inflammatory and analgesic effects of rosehip in inflammatory musculoskeletal disorders and its active molecules." *Current molecular pharmacology* 14, 5 (2021): 731–45. doi:10.2174/1874467214666210804154604.

338 **ROSEMARY (*Rosmarinus officinalis*):** de Oliveira, Jonatas Rafael, et al. "*Rosmarinus officinalis* L. (rosemary) as therapeutic and prophylactic agent." *Journal of biomedical science* 26, 1 (9 Jan. 2019): 5. doi:10.1186/s12929-019-0499-8.

Murata, Kazuya, et al. "Promotion of hair growth by *Rosmarinus officinalis* leaf extract." *Phytotherapy research* 27, 2 (2013): 212–17. doi:10.1002/ptr.4712.

Zappalà, Agata, et al. "Neuroprotective effects of *Rosmarinus officinalis* L. extract in oxygen glucose deprivation (OGD)-injured human neural-like cells." *Natural product research* 35, 4 (2021): 669–75. doi: 10.1080/14786419.2019.1587428.

338 **regular consumption of this pungent local rosemary:** Brubaker, Michelle. "Remote Italian village could harbor secrets of healthy aging." Newsroom, San Diego Heath (29 Mar. 2016). https://health.ucsd.edu/news/releases/Pages/2016-03-29-remote-italian-village-may-hold-key-to-longevity.aspx.

338 **Research has identified several unique compounds:** Andrade, Joana M., et al. "*Rosmarinus officinalis* L.: an update review of its phytochemistry and biological activity." *Future science OA* 4, 4 (1 Feb. 2018): FSO283. doi:10.4155/fsoa-2017-0124.

339 **1,8 cineole has been shown to enhance:** Moss, Mark, et al. "Plasma 1,8-cineole correlates with cognitive performance following exposure to rosemary essential oil aroma." *Therapeutic advances in psychopharmacology* 2, 3 (2012): 103–13. doi:10.1177/2045125312436573.

339 **SCHISANDRA BERRY (*Schisandra chinensis*):** Che, Jinying, et al. "*Schisandra chinensis* acidic polysaccharide partially reverses acetaminophen-induced liver injury in mice." *Journal of pharmacological sciences* 140, 3 (2019): 248–54. doi:10.1016/j.jphs.2019.07.008.

Chen, Wai-Wei, et al. "Pharmacological studies on the anxiolytic effect of standardized *Schisandra lignans* extract on restraint-stressed mice." *Phytomedicine* 18, 13 (2011): 1144–47. doi:10.1016/j.phymed.2011.06.004.

Nowak, Adriana, et al. "Potential of *Schisandra chinensis* (Turcz.) Baill. in human health and nutrition: a review of current knowledge and therapeutic perspectives." *Nutrients* 11, 2 (4 Feb. 2019): 333. doi:10.3390/nu11020333.

Szopa, Agnieszka, et al. "Current knowledge of *Schisandra chinensis* (Turcz.) Baill. (Chinese magnolia vine) as a medicinal plant species: a review on the bioactive components, pharmacological properties, analytical and biotechnological studies." *Phytochemistry reviews* 16, 2 (2017): 195–218. doi:10.1007/s11101-016-9470-4.

339 **its capacity to increase resilience:** Sergeeva, Irina, et al. "Experimental studies of the effect of *Schisandra chinensis* extract on the state of adaptive capabilities of rats under chronic and general exposure to cold." *International journal of environmental research and public health* 18, 22 (10 Nov. 2021): 11780. doi:10.3390/ijerph182211780.

339 **At night it encourages healthy, restorative sleep:** Zhang, Chenning, et al. "Pharmacological evaluation of sedative and hypnotic effects of schizandrin through the modification of pentobarbital-induced sleep behaviors in mice." *European journal of pharmacology* 744 (2014): 157–63. doi:10.1016/j.ejphar.2014.09.012.

341 **Dulse (*Palmaria palmata*):** Prasher, S. O., et al. "Biosorption of heavy metals by red algae (*Palmaria palmata*)." *Environmental technology* 25, 10 (2004): 1097–106. doi:10.1080/09593332508618378.

341 **Kombu (*Laminaria* species):** Luan, Fei, et al. "Polysaccharides from *Laminaria japonica*: an insight into the current research on structural features and biological properties." *Food & function* 12, 10 (2021): 4254–83. doi:10.1039/d1fo00311a.

341 **Nori (*Pyropia yezoensis* and *P. tenera*):** Cao, Jin, et al. "*Porphyra* species: a mini-review of its pharmacological and nutritional properties." *Journal of medicinal food* 19, 2 (2016): 111–19. doi:10.1089/jmf.2015.3426.

342 **SHATAVARI ROOT (*Asparagus racemosus*):** Goyal, R. K., et al. "*Asparagus racemosus*—an update." *Indian journal of medical sciences* 57, 9 (2003): 408–14.

Majumdar, Shreyasi, et al. "Neuro-nutraceutical potential of *Asparagus racemosus*: a review." *Neurochemistry international* 145 (2021): 105013. doi:10.1016/j.neuint.2021.105013.

Pandey, Ajai K., et al. "Impact of stress on female reproductive health disorders: possible beneficial effects of shatavari (*Asparagus racemosus*)." *Biomedicine & pharmacotherapy* 103 (2018): 46–49. doi:10.1016/j.biopha.2018.04.003.

343 **SKULLCAP (*Scutellaria lateriflora*):** Awad, R., et al. "Phytochemical and biological analysis of skullcap (*Scutellaria lateriflora* L.): a medicinal plant with anxiolytic properties." *Phytomedicine* 10, 8 (2003): 640–49. doi:10.1078/0944-7113-00374.

Brock, Christine, et al. "American skullcap (*Scutellaria lateriflora*): a randomised, double-blind placebo-controlled crossover study of its effects on mood in healthy volunteers." *Phytotherapy research* 28, 5 (2014): 692–98. doi:10.1002/ptr.5044.

Lohani, Madhukar, et al. "Anti-oxidative and DNA protecting effects of flavonoids-rich *Scutellaria lateriflora*." *Natural product communications* 8, 10 (2013): 1415–18.

343 **SLIPPERY ELM (*Ulmus rubra*):** Ried, Karin, et al. "Herbal formula improves upper and lower gastrointestinal symptoms and gut health in Australian adults with digestive disorders." *Nutrition research* (New York, NY) 76 (2020): 37–51. doi:10.1016/j.nutres.2020.02.008.

344 **SUPER BERRIES:** Chang, Sui Kiat, et al. "Superfruits: phytochemicals, antioxidant efficacies, and health effects—a comprehensive review." *Critical reviews in food science and nutrition* 59, 10 (2019): 1580–604. doi:10.1080/10408398.2017.1422111.

344 **Acai berry (*Euterpe oleracea*):** Baptista, Sheyla de L., et al. "Biological activities of açaí (*Euterpe oleracea* Mart.) and juçara (*Euterpe edulis* Mart.) intake in humans: an integrative review of clinical trials." *Nutrition reviews* 79, 12 (2021): 1375–91. doi:10.1093/nutrit/nuab002.

Ulbricht, Catherine, et al. "An evidence-based systematic review of acai (*Euterpe oleracea*) by the Natural Standard Research Collaboration." *Journal of dietary supplements* 9, 2 (2012): 128–47. doi:10.3109/19390211.2012.686347.

344 **Elderberry (*Sambucus canadensis* and *S. nigra*):** Liu, Dan, et al. "Elderberry (*Sambucus nigra* L.): bioactive compounds, health functions, and applications." *Journal of agricultural and food chemistry* 70, 14 (2022): 4202–20. doi:10.1021/acs.jafc.2c00010.

Tiralongo, Evelin, et al. "Elderberry supplementation reduces cold duration and symptoms in air-travellers: a randomized, double-blind placebo-controlled clinical trial." *Nutrients* 8, 4 (24 Mar. 2016): 182. doi:10.3390/nu8040182.

Ulbricht, Catherine, et al. "An evidence-based systematic review of elderberry and elderflower (*Sambucus nigra*) by the Natural Standard Research Collaboration." *Journal of dietary supplements* 11, 1 (2014): 80–120. doi:10.3109/19390211.2013.859852.

Wieland, L Susan, et al. "Elderberry for prevention and treatment of viral respiratory illnesses: a systematic review." *BMC complementary medicine and therapies* 21, 1 (7 Apr. 2021): 112. doi:10.1186/s12906-021-03283-5.

344 **Lingonberry (*Vaccinium vitis-idaea*):** Kowalska, Katarzyna. "Lingonberry (*Vaccinium vitis-idaea* L.) fruit as a source of bioactive compounds with health-promoting effects—a review." *International journal of molecular sciences* 22, 10 (12 May 2021): 5126. doi:10.3390/ijms22105126.

Ryyti, Riitta, et al. "Beneficial effects of lingonberry (*Vaccinium vitis-idaea* L.) supplementation on metabolic and inflammatory adverse effects induced by high-fat diet in a mouse model of obesity." *PLOS one* 15, 5 (7 May 2020): e0232605. doi:10.1371/journal.pone.0232605.

346 **Maqui berry (*Aristotelia chilensis*):** Bribiesca-Cruz, Iván, et al. "Maqui berry (*Aristotelia chilensis*) extract improves memory and decreases oxidative stress in male rat brain exposed to ozone." *Nutritional neuroscience* 24, 6 (2021): 477–89. doi:10.1080/1028415X.2019.164543.

Genskowsky, Estefania, et al. "Determination of polyphenolic profile, antioxidant activity and antibacterial properties of maqui [*Aristotelia chilensis* (Molina) Stuntz] a Chilean blackberry." *Journal of the science of food and agriculture* 96, 12 (2016): 4235–42. doi:10.1002/jsfa.7628.

Rodríguez, Lyanne, et al. "A comprehensive literature review on cardioprotective effects of bioactive compounds present in fruits of *Aristotelia chilensis* Stuntz (maqui)." *Molecules* (Basel, Switzerland) 27, 19 (20 Sep. 2022): 6147. doi:10.3390/molecules27196147.

346 **TRIPHALA:** Ahmed, Suhail, et al. "Exploring scientific validation of triphala rasayana in Ayurveda as a source of rejuvenation for contemporary healthcare: an update." *Journal of ethnopharmacology* 273 (2021): 113829. doi:10.1016/j.jep.2021.113829.

Peterson, Christine Tara, et al. "Therapeutic uses of triphala in Ayurvedic medicine." *Journal of alternative and complementary medicine* (New York, NY) 23, 8 (2017): 607–14. doi:10.1089/acm.2017.0083.

Ibid. "Modulatory effects of triphala and manjistha dietary supplementation on human gut microbiota: a double-blind, randomized, placebo-controlled pilot study." *Journal of alternative and complementary medicine* (New York, NY) 26, 11 (2020): 1015-1024. doi:10.1089/acm.2020.0148.

Phetkate, Pratya, et al. "Significant increase in cytotoxic T lymphocytes and natural killer cells by triphala: a clinical phase I study." *Evidence-based complementary and alternative medicine* 2012 (2012): 239856. doi:10.1155/2012/239856.

347 **TULSI (*Ocimum sanctum*):** Cohen, Marc Maurice. "Tulsi—*Ocimum sanctum*: a herb for all reasons." *Journal of Ayurveda and integrative medicine* 5, 4 (2014): 251–59. doi:10.4103/0975-9476.146554.

Kamyab, Amir A'lam, et al. "Anti-inflammatory, gastrointestinal and hepatoprotective effects of *Ocimum sanctum* Linn: an ancient remedy with new application." *Inflammation & allergy drug targets* 12, 6 (2013): 378–84. doi:10.2174/187152811266613 1125110017.

Prakash, P., et al. "Therapeutic uses of *Ocimum sanctum* Linn (tulsi) with a note on eugenol and its pharmacological actions: a short review." *Indian journal of physiology and pharmacology* 49, 2 (2005): 125–31.

Suanarunsawat, Thamolwan, et al. "Lipid-lowering and antioxidative activities of aqueous extracts of *Ocimum sanctum* L. leaves in rats fed with a high-cholesterol diet." *Oxidative medicine and cellular longevity* 2011 (2011): 962025. doi:10.1155/2011/962025.

349 **TURMERIC (*Curcuma longa*):** Kocaadam, Betül, et al. "Curcumin, an active component of turmeric (*Curcuma longa*), and its effects on health." *Critical reviews in food science and nutrition* 57, 13 (2017): 2889–95. doi:10.1080/10408398.2015.1077195.

Vaughn, Alexandra R., et al. "Effects of turmeric (*Curcuma longa*) on skin health: a systematic review of the clinical evidence." *Phytotherapy research* 30, 8 (2016): 1243–64. doi:10.1002/ptr.5640.

Zeng, Liuting, et al. "The efficacy and safety of *Curcuma longa* extract and curcumin supplements on osteoarthritis: a systematic review and meta-analysis." *Bioscience reports* 41, 6 (2021): BSR20210817. doi:10.1042/BSR20210817.

349 **VALERIAN ROOT (*Valeriana officinalis*):** Shinjyo, Noriko, et al. "Valerian root in treating sleep problems and associated disorders—a systematic review and meta-analysis." *Journal of evidence-based integrative medicine* 25 (2020): 2515690X20967323. doi:10.1177/2515690X20967323.

349 **a tried-and-true remedy for treating insomnia:** Bent, Stephen, et al. "Valerian for sleep: a systematic review and meta-analysis." *American journal of medicine* 119, 12 (2006): 1005–12. doi:10.1016/j.amjmed.2006.02.026.

349 **valerenic acid and valerenol have been shown:** Benke, Dietmar, et al. "GABA A receptors as in vivo substrate for the anxiolytic action of valerenic acid, a major constituent of valerian root extracts." *Neuropharmacology* 56, 1 (2009): 174–81. doi:10.1016/j.neuropharm.2008.06.013.

349 **VANILLA (*Vanilla planifolia*):** Bezerra-Filho, Carlos S. M., et al. "Therapeutic potential of vanillin and its main metabolites to regulate the inflammatory response and oxidative stress." *Mini reviews in medicinal chemistry* 19, 20 (2019): 1681–93. doi:10.2174/1389557519666190312164355.

349 **a phenolic compound with powerful antioxidant:** Singletary, K. "Vanilla: potential health benefits." *Nutrition today* 55, 4 (Jul./Aug. 2020): 186–96. doi:10.1097/NT.0000000000000412.

Index

Italic page numbers indicate photos.

A

abhyanga massage, 215
acai berry, *71*, 146, *147*, 344
acid reflux remedies, 288
adaptogenic mushroom latte, *240*
adaptogens, 82, *83–85*, 85
    for adjusting to stress, 57
    amla berry, *302*, 302–303
    ashwagandha root, *304*, 304–305
    astragalus root, *305*, 305–306
    cordyceps, 314, *314*
    current renaissance of, 85
    ginseng root, 318, *318*
    goji berry, 319, *319*
    for immunity boost, 293
    introducing kids to, 297
    licorice root, *325*, 325–326
    maca root, *327*, 327–328
    medicinal mushrooms, 328, *329*, 330–331
    reishi, *335*, 335–336
    resources for, 352
    rhodiola, *336*, 336–337
    schisandra berry, 339, *339*
    shatavari root, 342, *342*
    tulsi, 347, *347*
adaptogens (Protocol step 5), 235–259
    FAQs for, 259
    getting started with, 238–239
    options for, 244–247
    plants and other ingredients for, 236, *236–237*
    recipes for, 249–255
    sample daily menus for, 241
    saturating your day in, 240
aging, 175
Agni-Kindling Honey, 114, 123
air element, 28, 29
alfalfa leaf, 146, *146*
allergy remedies, 289
allspice, 102, *103*
aloe vera, *74*, 75, 176, *177*, 182, 193, 302, *302*
ama, 44

amaros, 106
American ginseng root, *237*
amla berry, 82, 146, *147*, 236, *236*, 237, *302*, 302–303, *345*
antimicrobial effects, 63
antioxidants
    in cacao, 168
    in culinary herbs and spices, 63
    digestive-supporting, 40
    in green tea, 139
    in Indian diet, 65
    in nutritives, 70, 72
    in pepper, 8
aperitifs, 109, 110, 114, 115
apothecary. *See* home apothecary
arnica flower harvest, *9*
aromas, 60, 200
aromatic bitters, 101, *106*, 106–107, *107*
aromatic essential oils, 97
    buying and administering, 202
    digestive-supporting, 40, 101
    in herbs and spices, 61, 63, 94, 101
    as nervines, 78, 79, 197, *199*, 199–203, 212
    resources for, 353
    in Traditional Chinese Medicine, 78, 79
aromatic herb-infused water, 210
aromatic herbs, *14–15*, 61, 101
aromatic resins, 78, 79, 215, 353
aromatic spices, 101
aromatic woods, 78, 79, 353
artichoke leaf, *104*, 105, 303, *303*
asavas, 97
ashitaba, 146, *146*, 154, 304, *304*
Ashwagandha and Shatavari Coconut Replenisher, 245, 250
Ashwagandha Deep Rest Replenisher, 246, 253
ashwagandha root, 85, *236*, 237, *304*, 304–305
astragalus root, *236*, 237, *305*, 305–306
autonomic nervous system, 48
avipattikar, 115

Ayurveda, 11, 25
    abhyanga in, 215
    ama in, 44
    asavas in, 97
    in design of protocol, 27
    detoxification function in, 44
    on diet, 38
    digestive function in, 40
    digestive system in, 38
    flavor in, 68
    ghee in, 186
    ojas in, 55
    prana in, 32
    prajnaparadha in, 32
    resources for formulas, 352
    sama in, 112
    self-massage in, 215
    universal elements in, 28, 29

B

balance in body, 28–29. *See also* imbalance
    endocrine system, 55–56
    for individual constitutions, 91
    nervous system, 78
    restoring, 82
bancha, *141*, 142
basil, 102, *102*, *103*
basil leaf, 305, *305*
basil seed, 176, *177*, 182, 307, *308*
basil seed pudding, 183
bay leaf, 102, *103*
bedside table, *282–283*, 283
beginning Plant Medicine Protocol, 260–265
bellflowers, 146, *146*
beta brain waves, 48
bitter greens, *104*, 105, *105*, 116, 297. *See also* bitters
bitter liquors, 114–115. *See also* liquors
bitter melon, *104*, 105
bitters, 67, 104, *104–105*, 105. *See also* culinary herbs, spices, and bitters (Protocol step 1)
    aromatic, 101, *106*, 106–107, *107*
    artichoke leaf, 303, *303*

burdock root, *307*, 307–308
dandelion, 315, *315*
in detoxification, 44, 101, 110
digestive-supporting, 41, 101, 110
formulas and supplements of, 115
gentian root, *316*, 316–317
introducing kids to, 297
milk thistle, 331, *331*
resources for, 352–353
tinctures of, 97
triphala, 346, *346*
bitters bar, 109
black licorice candy, 77, *77*, 184
black pepper, 8, 9, *9*, 102, *102*, *103*
bloating remedies, 290–291
blood, 50, 170
Blue Poppy-Seed Sleep Elixir, 211, *222–223*, 224
body. *See also* essential body systems
in balance, 28–29
early warning signs from, 38
mind-body connection, 33
mind-body integration, 78
as scientific instrument, 35
unique constitution of, 33
wisdom of the, 32
brain, 46
brain waves, 48
buckwheat, 176, *176*
burdock root, *104*, 105, 146, *147*, *307*, 307–308
burning resins, 215

C

cacao, *104*, 105, *105*, 168–171, 353
Cacao Adaptogenic Energy Balls, *190–191*, 246, 255
Cacao-Reishi-Cordyceps Latte, 244, 249
Cacao Rose CBD Bliss Latte, 212, *213*, 221
California poppy, *198*, 199, 308, *308*
calmatives. *See* nervine calmatives
camu camu, 146, *147*
cannabidiol (CBD), *198*, 199, 211
cannabis, *198*, 199, 309, *309*
capsules, *96*, 97
cardamom, *10*, 102, *103*

Cardamom Hills of Kerala, 65
carob, 105, *105*
cause and effect principle, 32
CBD. *See* cannabidiol
ceremonial oils, 201
Chaga Chai Latte, 244, *248*, 249
chaga mushrooms, 237, *237*, *329*, 330
chai tea, 115
chamomile, *198*, 199, *309*, 309–310
Chamomile Latte, 221, *222*
chan seeds, 176, *176*
Chia-Aloe-Lime Rehydrator, 183, *192*, 193
chia seed, 176, *176*, 182, *310*, 310–311
chia seed pudding, 183
chicory root, *104*, 105, 146, *147*
children
home spaces for, 284, *284–285*
and medicinal plants, 296–297
chile, 102, *102*
chives, 102, *103*
chlorella, 311, *311*
chyawanprash, 246
cilantro, 102, *102*, 146, *147*
cinnamon, 63, 102, *102*, 313, *313*
Cinnamon Tea, 115, 128
citrus oils, 201
citrus peels, 67, 105, *105*, *312*, 313–314
cloves, 102, *103*
coca leaves, *42*
cod liver oil, 186
coffee, 105, *105*, 244
cold infusions, *95–96*, 96, 183
cold remedies, 290
colon, 43
condiments, 108, 110, 116
constipation remedies, 290–291
cordyceps, 82, 236, 237, *237*, 314, *314*, *329*
core energy, 55–57
coriander, 102, *103*
Coriander, Cumin, and Fennel Tea, 115, 128
cough remedies, 291
culinary herbs, spices, and bitters (Protocol step 1), 101–143
aromatic bitters, *106*, 106–107, *107*
FAQs for, 257
getting started with, 108

heat of spices, 112, *112*, *113*
options for, 114–117
plants and other ingredients for, 102, *102–105*, 105
plantventure for, 136–143
recipes for, 122–135
sample daily menus for, 111
saturating your day in, 110
spice blends, 118–119, *119*
sprinkles and toppers, 120, *120–121*
culinary herbs and spices, *62*, 63, *64–65*, 65, 102, *102–103*
basil leaf, 305, *305*
cinnamon, 313, *313*
citrus peels, *312*, 313–314
digestive-supporting, 40–41
garlic, *315*, 315–316
gingerroot, 317, *317*
for immunity boost, 293
introducing kids to, 297
rosemary, 338, *338*
turmeric, *347*, 347–348
vanilla, 349, *349*
cumin, 102, *103*
curries, 118, *119*

D

dandelion, 315, *315*
Dandelion, Chicory, and Carob Latte, 117, 127
dandelion greens, 105, *105*, 154
dandelion root, *104*, 105
Dandy Blend, *104*, 105
Darwin, Charles, 55
decoctions, 94, *95*, 96, 244
dehydration, 50, 52, 175, 180
Demulcent Hydration Balls, 183, 188, *190–191*
Demulcent Powder Blend, 182, 188
demulcents, *74*, 75, *76–77*
aloe vera, 302, *302*
basil seed, 307, *308*
chia seed, *310*, 310–311
cold infusions of, 96
digestive-supporting, 41
hibiscus, *321*, 321–322
for hydration, 52
for immunity boost, 293
introducing kids to, 297
Irish moss, 322, *322–323*
licorice root, *325*, 325–326
linden, *326*, 326–327

demulcents, *(continued)*
    marshmallow root, 328, *328*
    psyllium husk, *334*, 334–335
    resources for, 353
    shatavari root, *342*, *342*
    slippery elm, *343*, 343–344
demulcents (Protocol step 3),
    175–195
    FAQs for, 258
    getting started with, 178
    morning rituals for, 186–187
    options for, 182–184
    plants and other ingredients for,
      176, *176–177*
    recipes for, 188–195
    sample daily menus for, 181
    saturating your day in, 180
desk, *280–281*, 281
detoxification, 43–45
    bitters for, 67, 101, 110
    with demulcents, 75
    and essential oils, 200
    health impact of, 101
    nutritives in, 70
    water in, 50
detoxifying herbs, 67
    artichoke leaf, 303, *303*
    burdock root, *307*, 307–308
    citrus peels, *312*, 313–314
    milk thistle, 331, *331*
    triphala, 346, *346*
diet(s)
    in Ayurveda, 38
    Indian, 65
    plants in, 59
    traditional, 63
diffusing essential oils, 202, 204,
    204
digestifs, 109, 110, 114, 115, 117
digestion, 67, 101, 110
digestive system, 38, 40–41, 44,
    45, 53
dill, 102, *102*
dining room, 276, *276–277*
*Divine Farmer's Classic of Materia
    Medica* (Sheng), 35
draksha, 114
dukkah, 120, 135
dulse, 176, *176*, *340*, 341

E

earth element, 28, 29
elderberry, 146, *147*, 344, *345*

eleuthero, *236*, 237
elimination, 40, 41, 43, 67, 70
elixirs, *150*, 153, 162, *162*, 171,
    183, 208, 210, 211
emergency medicine, *22*, 23
emotions, 49
endocrine system, 44, 55–57
energy
    with adaptogens, 235
    bitters for, 67
    core, 55–57
    for digestion, 38
    and flavor, 68
    and hydration, 50, 53
entryway, *270–271*, 271
enzymes, 44
essential body systems, 37–57
    core energy, 55–57
    detoxification, 43–45
    digestive system, 38, 40–41
    hydration, 50, *51*, 52–53
    nervous system, 46, 48–49
essential oils. *See* aromatic
    essential oils

F

FAQs, 90, 257–259
    for adaptogens (step 5), 259
    for culinary herbs, spices, and
      bitters (step 1), 257
    for demulcents (step 3), 258
    for nervines (step 4), 258–259
    for nutritives (step 2), 257
Farm to Pharmacy, 11–12
Farmers' markets, 148, *148*
fennel, 102, *103*
fenugreek, 102, *102*
fermented foods, 116
Fernet-Branca, 106
fire element, 28, 29
flavors, 60, 68
floral oils, 197, 201
floral water, *30*
flowers, extracting, 94
flu remedies, 290
fragrant relaxants, 78, 79, 197, 198,
    198–199
    chamomile, *309*, 309–310
    digestive-supporting, 41
    Greek mountain tea, *320*,
      320–321
    honeybush, *322*, *322*
    introducing kids to, 297

    lavender, *323*, 323–324
    lemon balm, *324*, 324–325
    lemon verbena, 325, *325*
    linden, *326*, 326–327
    peppermint, 334, *334*
    rooibos, 322, *322*
    rosemary, 338, *338*
    spearmint, 334, *334*
    teas or infusions of, 204
    vanilla, 349, *349*
frankincense oil, 201
Franklin, Benjamin, 50
functional medicine professionals,
    22, 23

G

galangal, 102, *103*
GALT (gut-associated lymphoid
    tissue), 40
Gammel Dansk, 106
garlic, 63, 102, *103*, *315*,
    315–316
garnishes, 154
gastrointestinal (GI) tract, 38–40,
    44
    demulcents in, 75, 176
    microbes in, 63
    and vagus nerve, 46, 48
    water in, 52, 53
genmaicha, *140*, 142
gentian root, *104*, 105, *316*,
    316–317
GERD remedies, 288
ghee, 186
GI tract. *See* gastrointestinal tract
ginger, 63, 102, *103*, 317, *317*
ginger "pizza," 114
Ginger Shots, 114, 124, *125*
Ginger-Turmeric Shots, 124, *125*
ginseng, 56, 82, *236*, 237, *237*,
    242–243, 243, 246, 318, *318*
Ginseng-Ginger Lemon Tonic, 245,
    250
goji berry, *236*, 237, *237*, 319, *319*,
    345
Goji-Chrysanthemum-Pomegranate
    Eye-Brightening Elixir, 153,
    157, *157*
Goldthread, 9, 10–12, *92–93*, 93
gomasio, 120
gotu kola, 146, *147*, *319*, 319–320
Gotu Kola and Lime Clarity Elixir,
    153, 162, *162*

Greek mountain tea, 17, *198*, 199, *208–209*, 210, 218, *219*, *320*, 320–321
green pepper, 102, *103*
Green Power Powder Blend, 152, 158
green tea, *66*, 67, 105, *105*, 136–143, 353
greens, *104*, 105, *105*, 116, 154, 297
Gremolata, 116, 120, 130
guayusa, *104*, 105
gut, 40, 53
gut-associated lymphoid tissue (GALT), 40
gymnostema, *236*, 237
gyokuro, *141*, 143

H

hawthorn berry, *345*
he shou wu, *236*, 237
healing power of nature, 32
health
  decline in, 37
  digestion and detoxification impacting, 101
  functions sustaining, 70 (*See also individual functions*)
  and hydration, 50, 52
  pursuit of, 55
  as verb, 33
Health-Care Pyramid, *22*, 22–23
healthy living, elements of, 21
Heart Health Tea Blend, 153, 158
heart-rate variability (HRV), 48
heat, of spices, 112, *112*, *113*
helichrysum oil, 200
herbal liquors, 97
herbal powders, 96
herbs. *See also specific herbs*
  aromatic, *14–15*, 61, 101
  bitter, *104*, 105, *105* (*See also bitters*)
  culinary (*See* culinary herbs and spices)
  extractions from, 94
  pulse dosing with, 216–217
  resources for, 355
  storage of, 99
hibiscus, 146, *147*, 176, *321*, 321–322
hijiki, *340*
hingvastak, 115

Hippocrates, 32, 43
hojicha, *140*, 142
holy basil. *See* tulsi (holy basil)
home apothecary, 287–297
  acid reflux and GERD, 288
  allergies, 289
  boosting immunity, 293
  for children, 296–297
  colds and flus, 290
  constipation and bloating, 290–291
  coughs, 291
  muscle tension, 292
  plants for, 61
  sore throat, 292
Homemade Nutritive Tea Blend, 156
honey, 186, 246, 253
honeybush, 199, *199*, *322*, *322*
Honeybush Latte, 218, *222–223*
hops, 199, *199*
hormones, 44, 55, 67, 235
horseradish (wasabi), 63, 102, *102*
horsetail, 146, *146*
Horta Vrasta, 110, 133, 154
hot infusions, 94, *95–96*, 96
HRV (heart-rate variability), 48
hydration, 44, 50, *51*, 52–53, 75
hydrosols, 97

I

Il Marchese, 107
imbalance
  in core energy, 57
  in detoxification system, 44–45
  in digestion, 38, 41
  in hydration system, 50, 53
  in nervous system, 49
immune cells, 40, 50
immune system, 43, 45, 200, 293
immunity, 235, 293
Indian diet, 65
inflammation
  basis for, 40
  and demulcents, 176
  health issues from, 40
  and hydration, 53
  reduced by culinary herbs and spices, 63
  from toxins overload, 45
infusions, 94, *95–96*, 96
  adaptogenic, 145
  demulcents, 182, 183

fragrant relaxants, 204
  nervines, 210
Irish moss, 176, *177*, *322*, 322–323, *340*
Irish Moss–Cacao Nib Elixir, 183, *185*, 188
Irish Moss Gel, 183, 188

J

jams, *150*, 155, 246
Japanese green tea, *66*, 67, 136–143
Japanese matcha, 17–18, *18*
jasmine oil, 199, *199*
jatamansi oil, 200
Jerusalem artichoke, 176, *177*
jing, 55
joints, 45, 49, 50, 53
juicing, 153
jujube dates, 146, *147*

K

kabuse cha, *141*, 143
kava, 18, 199, *199*, 226, *227–231*, 229–231
Kava Koolada, 211, 224, *225*
kelp, 176
kidneys, 43
Kitchari, 117, 134, *134*
kitchen, 272, *272–273*
know thyself principle, 33
kombu, *340*, 341
Korean ginseng, *56*, 82, *237*, *242–243*, 243
kukicha, *140*, 142
Kuna people, 168, 170

L

lattes, herbal, 211
lavender, *47*, 80, *80–81*, 199, *199*, *323*, 323–324
Lavender Flower Latte, 221, *223*
lavender oil, 200
leaky gut syndrome, 40, 75
leaves, extracting, 94
lemon balm, 199, *199*, *324*, 324–325
lemon verbena, 199, *199*, 325, *325*
lemongrass, 102, *103*
licorice candy, 77, *77*, 184

licorice root, *76–77*, 77, 176, *177*, *325*, 325–326

linden, *48*, 78, 79, 176, *198, 326*, 326–327

lingonberry, 344, *345*, 346

lion's mane mushrooms, *236*, 237, *329*, 330

liquors, 67, 97, *106*, 106–107, *107*, 114–115

liver, 43–45, 70

living room, 278, *278–279*

longevity, 208

lozenges, demulcent, 184

lungs, 43

lymphatic system, 40, 43

M

maca chicha, 85

maca root, 85, 236, 237, *237*, *327*, 327–328

Maca-Vanilla-Coconut Tonifying Honey, 246, 253

mace, 102, *103*

maitake mushrooms, 236, 237, *237*, *329*, 330

Mango–Basil Seed Pudding, 183, 194, *195*

manuka honey, 176, *177*, 186–187, *187*

maqui berry, 346

marshmallow root, 176, *176*, 328, *328*

mastic resin, *104*, 105

matcha, 17–18, *18*, 66, 67, *138*, *141*, 353

Matcha Latte, *206*, 211, 220, *220*

medicinal mushrooms, 236, *236–237*, 237, 328, 329, 330–331. *See also specific mushrooms*

    chaga, *329*, 330

    cordyceps, 82, *329*

    for immunity boost, 293

    lion's mane, *329*, 330

    maitake, *329*, 330

    reishi, 82, *329*, 335, 335–336

    shiitake, *329*, 330

    turkey tail, *329*, 330

medicinal plants, 8–12, 59–85

    adaptogens, 82, *83–85*, 85

    bitters and detoxifying herbs, 67

    and children, 296–297

    culinary herbs and spices, *62*, 63, *64–65*, 65

    demulcents, *74*, 75, *76–77*

    digestive-supporting, 40–41

    in Health-Care Pyramid, 22, *22*, 23

    nervines, 78–80, *79–81*

    nutritives, 70, *71–73*, 72

    as only one aspect of wellness, 21

    phytochemicals in, 59

    in Plant Medicine Protocol, 16, 19, 21, 88

    potency spectrum for, 60–61

    power of, 17–19

menus. *See* sample daily menus

metabolism, 38, 43, 63

microalgae supplements and powders, 153

microbiome, 40, 45, 53, 63, 75

micronutrients, 44, 60, 70

milk thistle, *104*, 105, 331, *331*

Milk Thistle Detox-Enhancing Dukkah, 116, 135

mind-body connection, 33

mind-body integration, 78

Minimum Daily Doses, 88

    for adaptogens, 241

    for culinary herbs, spices, and bitters, 111

    for demulcents, 181

    for nervines, 207

    for nutritives, 151

mint, 199, *199*

Mint Chocolate Chip–Green Power Smoothie, 152, 159, *160–161*

mizuna, *104*, 105

moringa, 72, *72–73*, 146, *146–147*, 332, *332*

morning rituals, demulcents in, 186–187

mucous membranes, 75

Mukhwas, 116, 135

mullein flowers, *294–295*

muscle tension remedies, 292

muscles, 45, 49, 53

mushrooms. *See* medicinal mushrooms

mustard greens, 105, *105*

mustard seed, 102, *102*

N

natural medicine, 8–12

    defined, 27

    essential body systems, 37–57

    in Health-Care Pyramid, 22, *22*

    medicinal plant categories, 59–85

    principles of, 25, 27–33

    tenets of, 32–33

natural medicine professionals, *22*, 23

nature, 28–29, 32

nerves, 46

nervine calmatives, 78, 79, 197, 198, *198–199*

    California poppy, 308, *308*

    cannabis, 309, *309*

    passionflower, *333*, 333–334

    skullcap, 343, *343*

    valerian root, *348*, 348–349

nervines, 78–80, *79–81*

    groups of herbs within, 78, 79 (*See also specific groups*)

    resources for, 353–354

    tinctures of, 97

nervines (Protocol step 4), 197–231

    essential oils, 200–203

    FAQs for, 258–259

    getting started with, 204–205

    options for, 210–213

    plants and other ingredients for, 198, *198–199*

    plantventure for, 226–231

    pulse dosing for sleep, 216–217

    recipes for, 218–225

    rituals for, *214*, 214–215

    sample daily menus for, 207

    saturating your day in, 106

nervous system, 46, 48–49, 78

nettles, 146, *147*, *332*, 332–333

Nettles Soup, 154, *166*, 167

neurotransmitters, 46, 78, 136, 200

nopal cactus, 176

nori, 146, *147*, 154, *340*, 341

nutmeg, 102, *102*, 199, *199*

Nutmeg-Saffron Deep Sleep Elixir, 211, *223*, 224

nutrition, detoxification and, 44

Nutritive Green Power Balls, 153, 163, *190–191*

nutritives, 70, *71–73*, 72

    amla berry, *302*, 302–303

    ashitaba, 304, *304*

    burdock root, *307*, 307–308

    chlorella, 311, *311*

    dandelion, 315, *315*

    goji berry, 319, *319*

    gotu kola, *319*, 319–320

    hibiscus, *321*, 321–322

for immunity boost, 293
introducing kids to, 297
moringa, 332, *332*
nettles, 332, 332–333
plant profiles, 311, *311*
resources for, 354
rose hips, 337, *337*
super berries, 344, *345*, 346
nutritives (Protocol step 2),
145–171
FAQs for, 257
getting started with, 148–149
options for, 152–155
plants and other ingredients for,
146, *146–147*
plantventure for, 168–171
recipes for, 156–167
sample daily menus for, 151
saturating your day in, 150
Nyponsoppa, 72, 155, 165, *165*

O

oat tops, 146, *146*
oats, 176
oatstraw, 146, *146*
oils, 40, 55. *See also* aromatic
essential oils
ojas, 55
okra, 176
olive leaf, 105, *105*
olive oil, 176, *176*, 186
"On the Go" collection, 264,
264–265
adaptogens, 239, *239*
culinary herbs, spices, and
bitters, 109, *109*
demulcents, 179, *179*
nervines, 205, *205*
nutritives, 149, *149*
options, 90
for adaptogens (step 5), 244–247
for culinary herbs, spices, and
bitters (step 1), 114–117
for demulcents (step 3), 182–184
for nervines (step 4), 210–213
for nutritives (step 2), 152–155
oregano, 63, 102, *103*

P

palm inhalations, 78, 202, 215, *215*
pandan leaf, 102, *103*
paprika, 102, *103*

Paracelsus, 107
parasympathetic nervous system,
46, 48
parsley, 102, *103*, 146, *146*
Parsley Chimichurri, 154, 164
passionflower, *198*, 199, *333*,
333–334
Pasteur, Louis, 293
Peanut Butter–Maca–Goji Berry
Smoothie, 245, 250
peppermint, 334, *334*
peppermint elixir, 210
performance and recovery,
151–155
phytochemicals, 59, 63, 65, 68
pickled foods, 116
piperine, 8
Plant Medicine Protocol, 19–20,
87–265
adaptogens (step 5), 235–255
beginning your, 260–265
culinary herbs, spices, and bitters
(step 1), 101–143
demulcents (step 3), 175–195
FAQs for, 257–259
goal of, 19
nervines (step 4), 197–231
nutritives (step 2), 145–171
personalization of, 92
preparations for, 94–97
steps in, 20, 88–90 (*See also
individual steps*)
tools for, *98*, 99
universal benefits of, 92
using whole, unprocessed plants
in, 89
plant-powered day, sample of, 262
plant-powered home, 267, 269–297
bedside table, *282–283*, 283
children's spaces, *284*, 284–285
desk, *280–281*, 281
dining room, 276, *276–277*
entryway, *270–271*, 271
home apothecary, 287–297
kitchen, 272, *272–273*
living room, 278, *278–279*
refrigerator, 274, *274–275*
plant-powered protocol, 16, 19–21.
See also Plant Medicine
Protocol
plant profiles, 301–349
aloe vera, 302, *302*
amla berry, *302*, 302–303
artichoke leaf, 303, *303*

ashitaba, 304, *304*
ashwagandha root, *304*,
304–305
astragalus root, 305, 305–306
basil leaf, 305, *305*
basil seed, 307, *308*
burdock root, *307*, 307–308
California poppy, 308, *308*
cannabis, 309, *309*
chamomile, 309, 309–310
chia seed, *310*, 310–311
chlorella, 311, *311*
cinnamon, 313, *313*
citrus peels, *312*, 313–314
cordyceps, 314, *314*
dandelion, 315, *315*
garlic, 315, 315–316
gentian root, 316, 316–317
gingerroot, 317, *317*
ginseng root, 318, *318*
goji berry, 319, *319*
gotu kola, *319*, 319–320
Greek mountain tea, *320*,
320–321
hibiscus, *321*, 321–322
honeybush, 322, *322*
Irish moss, 322, 322–323
lavender, 323, 323–324
lemon balm, 324, 324–325
lemon verbena, 325, *325*
licorice root, 325, 325–326
linden, *326*, 326–327
maca root, 327, 327–328
marshmallow root, 328, *328*
medicinal mushrooms, 328, *329*,
330–331
milk thistle, 331, *331*
moringa, 332, *332*
nettles, 332, 332–333
passionflower, *333*, 333–334
peppermint, 334, *334*
psyllium husk, 334, 334–335
reishi, *335*, 335–336
rhodiola, *336*, 336–337
rooibos, 322, *322*
rose hip, 337, *337*
rosemary, 338, *338*
schisandra berry, 339, *339*
sea vegetables, 339, *340*,
341–342
shatavari root, 342, *342*
skullcap, 343, *343*
slippery elm, *343*, 343–344
spearmint, 334, *334*

plant profiles, *(continued)*
    spirulina, 311, *311*
    super berries, 344, *345*, 346
    triphala, 346, *346*
    tulsi, 347, *347*
    turmeric, *347*, 347–348
    valerian root, *348*, 348–349
    vanilla, 349, *349*
plantain leaf, 176, *177*, 183
plants
    medicinal, 61 (*See also* medicinal
      plants)
    phytochemicals in, 59
    potency spectrum for, 60–61
    sunlight transformed by, 63
plants and other Protocol
    ingredients, 90
    for adaptogens (step 5), 236,
      236–237
    for culinary herbs, spices, and
      bitters (step 1), 102, *102–105*,
      105
    for demulcents (step 3), 176,
      176–177
    for nervines (step 4), 198,
      198–199
    for nutritives (step 2), 146,
      146–147
plantventures, 20, *92–93*
    cacao, 168–171
    at Goldthread, *92–93*, 93
    Japanese green tea, 136–143
    kava, 226, *227–231*, 229–231
poppy seeds, 199, *199*
potency spectrum, 60–61
powder blends
    amounts and storage of, 159
    demulcents, 182, 188
    nutritives, 152, 158
powdered extracts, 96–97
    adaptogenic, 238, *239*
    nutritives, 152
    resources for, 355
powders, 96–97, 99
    adaptogenic, 238, *239*, 244
    microalgae, 153
    resources for, 355
prana, 32
prajnaparadha, 32
Prebiotic Fiber Blend, 183, 194
preparations for Plant Medicine
    Protocol, 94–97
prevent and optimize principle,
    33

principles of natural medicine, 25,
    27–33
    body in balance, 28–29
    tenets of natural medicine,
      32–33
psyllium husk, 176, *177*, *334*,
    334–335
pulse dosing for sleep, 216–217
"purification tonics," 67

Q
qi, 32, 49, 206

R
Ramazzotti, 106
Ramazzotti, Ausano, 106
red clover, 146, *147*
red pepper, 102, *103*
red pepper flakes, 102, *103*
refrigerator, 274, *274–275*
reishi mushrooms, 82, 236, 237,
    237, 329, *335*, 335–336
relaxants, 78–80. *See also* fragrant
    relaxants
resins
    aromatic, 78, 79, 215, 353
    burning, 215
    mastic, *104*, 105
respiratory oils, 201
rhodiola, *236*, 236–237, *336*,
    336–337
rituals
    demulcents in, 186–187
    for demulcents (step 3), 186–187
    for nervines (step 4), 214–215
rooibos, 199, *199*, 322, *322*
roots, bitter, *104*, 105, *105*. *See also*
    bitters
"roots tonic" wines, 97
rose hips, 146, *147*, 155, 337, *337*,
    345
rose hips soup, 155, 165, *165*
Rose Hips Super Berry Antioxidant
    Jam, *150*, 155, 163
rose oil, 200, *201*
rose petals, *198*, 199
rosemary, 102, *103*, 338, *338*

S
saffron, 102, *103*, 199, *199*
sage, 102, *103*

sama, 112
samgyetang, 243
sample daily menus, 90
    for adaptogens (step 5), 241
    for culinary herbs, spices, and
      bitters (step 1), 111
    for demulcents (step 3), 181
    for nervines (step 4), 207
    for nutritives (step 2), 151
    for plant-powered day, 262
Samst, Klaus, 107
saturating your day, 87–90
    in adaptogens (step 5), 240
    in culinary herbs, spices, and
      bitters (step 1), 110
    in demulcents (step 3), 180
    in nervines (step 4), 106
    in nutritives (step 2), 150
schisandra berry, 82, *83*, 85, 236,
    237, *237*, 339, *339*, *345*
Schisandra Berry–Rose Energizing
    Lemonade, 245, *252*, 253
Sea Vegetable Sprinkles, 164
sea vegetables, 146, *147*, 154, 339,
    340, 341–342
    dulse, 176, *176*, *340*, 341
    Irish moss, 176, *177*, *322*,
      322–323, *340*
    kombu, *340*, 341
    nori, 146, *147*, 154, *340*, 341
sencha, *140*, 142
senses, 35, 200
shatavari root, 176, *177*, 237, *237*,
    342, 342
shen, 78, 79
Shen Nong, *34*, 35
shiitake mushrooms, 236, 237, *237*,
    329, 330
Shiso, Shiitake, and Burdock
    Kinpira, 117, *132*, 133
shiso leaf, 146, *147*
skin, 43, 45, 50
skullcap, *198*, 199, 343, *343*
sleep
    ashwagandha for, 82
    and detoxification, 44
    nervines for, 205, *205*, 206,
      210–212
    and nervous system imbalance,
      49
    pulse dosing for, 216–217
    rehydrating after, 75
slippery elm, 176, *177*, *343*,
    343–344

smoothies, *150*, 159
  adaptogens in, 238, 245, 250, 251
  setup for, 148, *148*
sore throat remedies, 292
sourgrass, *104*, 105
space element, 28, 29
Sparkling Rosemary Limeade, 115, 126, *126*
spearmint, 334, *334*
spice blends, 109, 116, 118–120, *119–121*
spice rack, 108
spices, 108. *See also specific spices*
  aromatic, 61, 101
  culinary (*See* culinary herbs and spices)
  heat of, 112, *112–113*
  in Indian diet, 65
  origination of, 63
  storage of, 99
spinal cord, 46
spirulina, 311, *311*
Spring Cleaning Tonic, 117, 128
Spring Salad with Wild Greens, 116, 130, *131*
sprinkles, 110, 120, *120–121*, 154, 164
star anise, 102, *103*
storage, 99, 178
Strawberry Shatavari Smoothie, 245, 251, *251*
stress
  adapting to, 82
  adaptogens in reducing, 235
  and core energy, 55, 57
  and dehydration, 50
  and heart-rate variability, 48
  nervines for reducing, 206, 210–212
  and nervous system imbalance, 49
  as "silent killer," 57
  from social isolation, 229
Strong Infusion, 152, 156
sugar, 91
sunlight, stored, 63
super berries, 146, *147*, 344, *345*, 346
  acai berry, 344
  amla berry, *302*, 302–303, *345*
  elderberry, 344, *345*
  goji berry, 319, *319*, *345*
  hawthorn berry, *345*

lingonberry, 344, *345*, 346
  maqui berry, 346
  rose hips, 337, *337*, *345*
  schisandra berry, 339, *339*, *345*
Super Berry Power Powder Blend, 152, 158
Super Berry Power Smoothie, 152, 159, *160–161*
Super Seed Topper, 164
Super Sonic Tonic, 263, *263*, 266, *266*
superfoods, nutritives as, 70, 145
supplements, 70, 89
  adaptogens, 247
  bitters, 115
  demulcents, 184
  for digestion, 109
  microalgae, 153
  resources for, 354–355
sweeteners, 91, *91*
sympathetic nervous system, 46, 50, 206

T
tablets, *96*, 97, 184
tarragon, 102, *102*
tatsoi, *104*, 105
TCM. *See* Traditional Chinese Medicine
tea station, 204
teas, 94. *See also specific types*
  bitters in, 67
  of demulcents, 183
  for digestion and detoxification, 115, 117
  of fragrant relaxants, 204
  of nervines, 210
  of nutritives, 153, 156, 158
  storage of, 99
tencha, *140*
tension
  muscle, 49, 292
  and nervous system imbalance, 49
thoughts, nervous system and, 49
thyme, 63, 102, *102*
tinctures, 97, 216–217, 354–355
tonics, 67, *150*, 263, 354
tools, for Plant Medicine Protocol, 98, 99
toppers, 110, 116, 120, *120–121*, 154, 164

toxins, 40, 43–45. *See also* detoxification
traditional caffeinated plants, 117
Traditional Chinese Medicine (TCM), 11, 25
  abundant energy in, 55
  aromatic essential oils in, 78, 79
  "dampness" in, 44–45
  in design of protocol, 27
  detoxification in, 43–45
  flavors in, 68
  hydration function in, 50
  immune system in, 293
  jing in, 55
  nervous system function in, 49
  qi in, 32, 49, 206
  resources for formulas, 355
  shen in, 78, 79
  Shen Nong in, *34*, 35
  yin-yang in, 50
traditional cultures, 17–18
traditional diets, 63
trikatu, 115
triphala, 346, *346*
triphala powder, *104*, 105
triphala tablets, 117
tropical spices, 17
tulsi (holy basil), 82, 199, *199*, 236, 347, *347*
Tulsi Rose Chai, 127
tulsi tea, 246
turkey tail mushrooms, 236, 237, *237*, *329*, 330
turmeric, 63, 102, *103*, *347*, 347–348
Turmeric Balls, 114, 123, *190–191*
Turmeric Golden Milk Latte, 115, 127
Turmeric-Orange-Lime Shots, 124, *125*
turmeric shots, 114

U
Underberg, 107
Underberg, Hubert, 107
universal elements, 28, 29

V
vagus nerve, 46, 48
valerian root, 199, *199*, *348*, 348–349
vanilla, 102, *102*, 349, *349*

Vietnamese Artichoke Elixir, 115,
129, *129*
vitamins, 70
Voltaire, 27

W

wakame, *340*
wasabi (horseradish), 63, 102, *102*
wastes
detoxification of, 43
in digestive system, 40
and hydration, 50
water
aromatic herb-infused, 210
demulcent, 182
floral, *30*
hydration, 50, *51*, 52–53
hydration-enhanced, 182
pure source of, 178
water element, 28, 29
water preparations, 94, *95–96*, 96
watercress, *104*, 105
weeds, eating, 154
Wei Qi Soup, 247, *254*, 255
Western medicine, 10, 22, *22*, 23
wild bitter greens, 116
wines, 67, 97
wisdom of the body, 32
woods, aromatic, 78, 79, 353
World Health Organization, 27

X

Xocoatl, 168, 171, *171*

Y

yams, 176
yerba maté, 105, *105*
yin-yang, 50
ylang-ylang oil, 199, *199*
yuzu kosho, 120

Z

za'atar, 120

Photography Credits

All images are by Kelsey Fugere except for the following:

Courtesy of the author: pages 4–5; 9; 10; 14–15; 23; 24–25; 26–27; 30–31; 36–37; 39; 42; 47; 48; 51; 52; 54; 56; 62; 66; 72–73; 79; 80–81; 83; 92–93; 95, left and top right; 107; 137; 138; 139; 148, right; 157; 169; 170; 172–173; 187; 208–209; 214; 227; 228; 229; 230; 232–233; 234–235; 268–269; 286–287; 294–295; 296; 302–311; 313–328; 331–339; 342–343; 346–349; 350–351; and 372

Elin Azganun: pages 300–301

GettyImages/The Image Bank/Danny Lehman: pages 64–65

iStock/borchee: page 217

iStock/Brasil2: pages 84–85

iStock/Daniel Balakov: page 201

iStock/Edalin: page 240

iStock/Future Artist: page 74

iStock/Kanawa_Studio: pages 100–101

iStock/Milaspage: pages 196–197

iStock/solidcolours: page 215

iStock/wagnerokasaki: page 71

Joesboy: pages 34–35

Shutterstock/lzf: pages 58–59

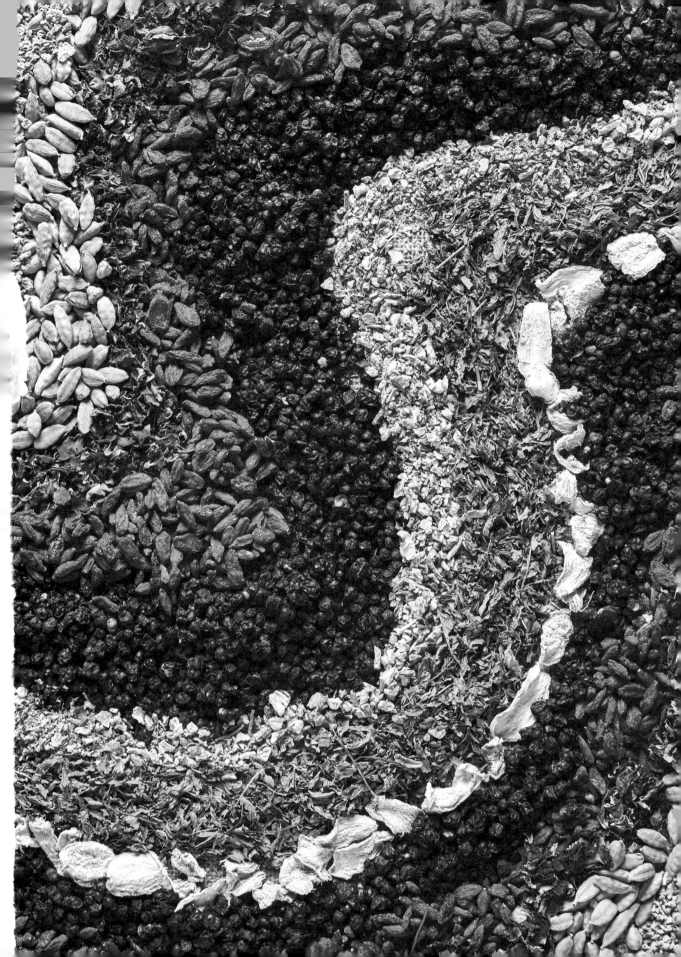

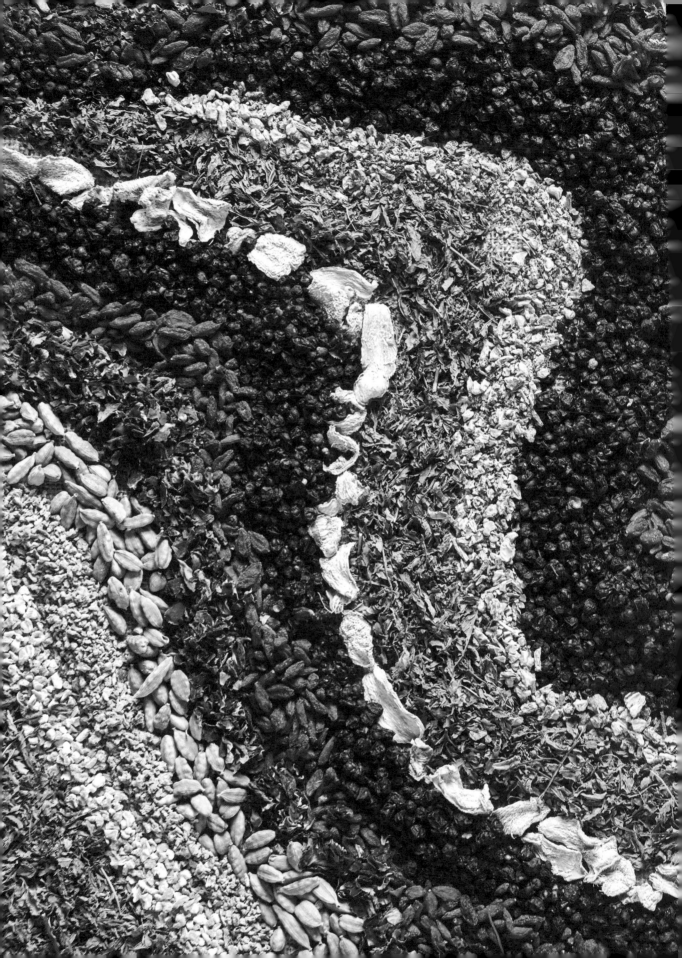